T0229886

Metabolic Syndrome and Cardiovascular Disease

Metabolic Syndrome and Cardiovascular Disease

Epidemiology, Assessment, and Management

Edited by

Andrew J. Krentz, MD, FRCP
Consultant in Diabetes & Endocrinology
Southampton University Hospitals
Honorary Senior Clinical Lecturer
University of Southampton
Southampton, U.K.

Nathan D. Wong, PhD, MPH, FACC, FAHA
Professor and Director, Heart Disease Prevention Program
Division of Cardiology, Department of Medicine, School of Medicine
University of California, Irvine
Irvine, California, U.S.A.
Adjunct Professor of Epidemiology
School of Public Health, University of California, Los Angeles
Los Angeles, California, U.S.A.

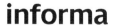

informa
healthcare

New York London

Informa Healthcare USA, Inc.
52 Vanderbilt Avenue
New York, NY 10017

© 2007 by Informa Healthcare USA, Inc.
Informa Healthcare is an Informa business

No claim to original U.S. Government works

10 9 8 7 6 5 4 3 2 1

International Standard Book Number-10: 1-4200-6676-5 (Paperback)
International Standard Book Number-13: 978-1-4200-6676-0 (Paperback)

This book contains information obtained from authentic and highly regarded sources. Reprinted material is quoted with permission, and sources are indicated. A wide variety of references are listed. Reasonable efforts have been made to publish reliable data and information, but the author and the publisher cannot assume responsibility for the validity of all materials or for the consequences of their use.

No part of this book may be reprinted, reproduced, transmitted, or utilized in any form by any electronic, mechanical, or other means, now known or hereafter invented, including photocopying, microfilming, and recording, or in any information storage or retrieval system, without written permission from the publishers.

For permission to photocopy or use material electronically from this work, please access www.copyright. com (http://www.copyright.com/) or contact the Copyright Clearance Center, Inc. (CCC) 222 Rosewood Drive, Danvers, MA 01923, 978-750-8400. CCC is a not-for-profit organization that provides licenses and registration for a variety of users. For organizations that have been granted a photocopy license by the CCC, a separate system of payment has been arranged.

Trademark Notice: Product or corporate names may be trademarks or registered trademarks, and are used only for identification and explanation without intent to infringe.

Visit the Informa Web site at
www.informa.com

and the Informa Healthcare Web site at
www.informahealthcare.com

To all our colleagues in research and healthcare
who have done so much in understanding the causes and
treatments of metabolic syndrome and cardiovascular disease
and to the millions of volunteers who participated in the studies
mentioned in this book. Without all your generosity and efforts,
this book could not exist.

Andrew J. Krentz
Nathan D. Wong

Preface

The term "metabolic syndrome" denotes a clustering of traditional and emerging risk factors for atherothrombotic cardiovascular disease. Moreover, individuals who satisfy the current diagnostic criteria that define the syndrome are also at substantially increased risk of developing Type 2 diabetes—itself a coronary heart disease risk equivalent. Central obesity and insulin resistance are core features of the syndrome, which has come to be recognized as a major global threat to vascular health in the 21st century. The time is optimal for a textbook dedicated to this important issue.

The metabolic syndrome has adverse implications for many aspects of vascular function ranging from endothelial function, the microvascular tree, medium-sized arteries, and large conduit vessels. Furthermore, gathering evidence suggests that interactions between small and large vessel disease may be more important than perhaps has previously been appreciated.

There are fears that the successes in reducing cardiovascular mortality in recent decades may soon be reversed. Fueled by the explosion of obesity, the syndrome is characterized by the clustering of classic and emerging risk factors for cardiovascular disease. No longer is it appropriate to regard obesity, glucose intolerance and diabetes, hypertension, and dyslipidemia as separate entities to be treated in individual clinical settings (e.g. the diabetes clinic, hypertension clinic, etc.). If one of the components of the metabolic syndrome is discovered, then steps should be taken to determine whether others are also present, and for implementing comprehensive approaches aimed toward treating the constellation of metabolic risk factors. This can be accomplished by simple clinical and biochemical tests and a multidisciplinary team approach implementing lifestyle and pharmacologic treatment.

This new paradigm presents challenges for clinicians involved in the assessment and management of individuals with metabolic syndrome. This rapidly moving area is being driven by advances in clinical and basic science. The latter are informing strategies for risk stratification and optimization of nonpharmacologic and drug-based treatment.

v

Our objective in bringing this book into print has been to present a state-of-the-art account of the salient issues for a clinically-oriented readership. In this endeavor, we are pleased to have been joined by an international team of experts, each recognized in his or her field. Various chapters cover epidemiology, diagnosis, risk assessment, vascular biology, lifestyle measure, management of hyperglycemia, dyslipidemia, and hypertension, and strategies for maximizing compliance to treatment recommendations. We hope that the book will not only be of academic interest but will provide helpful practical guidance to primary care physicians, diabetologists, cardiologists, dietitians, and other healthcare professionals involved in the prevention and treatment of vascular disease.

A better understanding of the mechanisms that cause cardiovascular risk factors to cluster together to the long-term detriment of so many individuals should facilitate more effective measures for prevention and treatment. Scientists working in epidemiology, basic science, drug discovery, and clinical trials each have roles to play in unraveling what is proving to be a major public health crisis.

It has been a pleasure working with colleagues from around the world and with the staff of Informa Healthcare. We welcome feedback from readers in the expectation that the text will require updating in the future, given the rapidly increasing scientific knowledge and developments in the field.

Andrew J. Krentz
Nathan D. Wong

Acknowledgments

We give special thanks to our contributors, many renowned in their respective areas of specialization, for their devotion, without which this text would not be possible. We also thank our colleagues for their inspiration and our students among whom will emerge tomorrow's leaders in the field. This text would not have been possible without the considerable efforts of Vanessa Sanchez and Joseph Stubenrauch of Informa Healthcare and Laura Damask, Alicia Mott, Joanne Jay, and Paula Garber of the Egerton Group in producing this text. Finally, we wish to thank our families and acknowledge the sacrifices they have made to make this text possible.

Contents

Contributors

K. George M. Alberti   Department of Endocrinology and Metabolism, Imperial College, London, U.K.

Ezra A. Amsterdam   Department of Medicine, Division of Cardiology, University of California, Davis, California, U.S.A.

Christopher D. Byrne   Endocrinology and Metabolism Unit, Southampton General Hospital, University of Southampton, Southampton, U.K.

Robin P. Choudhury   Department of Cardiovascular Medicine, University of Oxford, John Radcliffe Hospital, Oxford, U.K.

Prakash C. Deedwania   Cardiology Division, University of California San Francisco School of Medicine and Fresno Central San Joaquin Valley Medical Education Program, Fresno and Stanford University, Palo Alto, California, U.S.A.

Regina Dodis   Department of Medicine, University of Rochester School of Medicine, Rochester, New York, U.S.A.

Vivian Fonseca   Department of Medicine, Diabetes Program, Tulane University Health Sciences Center, New Orleans, Louisiana, U.S.A.

Stanley S. Franklin   Heart Disease Prevention Program, Department of Medicine, University of California, Irvine, California, U.S.A.

John E. Gerich   Department of Medicine, University of Rochester School of Medicine, Rochester, New York, U.S.A.

Gang Hu   Department of Epidemiology and Health Promotion, National Public Health Institute, and Department of Public Health, University of Helsinki, Helsinki, Finland

Ali Jawa   King Edward Medical University, Lahore, Pakistan

C. Tissa Kappagoda   Department of Medicine, Division of Cardiology, University of California, Davis, California, U.S.A.

Andrew J. Krentz   Southampton University Hospitals, University of Southampton, Southampton, U.K.

Hanna-Maaria Lakka   Department of Public Health and Clinical Nutrition, University of Kuopio, Kuopio, Finland

Timo A. Lakka   Department of Physiology, Institute of Biomedicine, University of Kuopio, and Kuopio Research Institute of Exercise Medicine, Kuopio, Finland

Justin M. S. Lee   Department of Cardiovascular Medicine, University of Oxford, John Radcliffe Hospital, Oxford, U.K.

Jaakko Tuomilehto   Department of Epidemiology and Health Promotion, National Public Health Institute, and Department of Public Health, University of Helsinki, Helsinki, Finland and South Ostrobothnia Central Hospital, Seinäjoki, Finland

Natalia B. Volkova   Department of Internal Medicine, University of California San Francisco, Fresno, California, U.S.A.

Sara Wild   Public Health Sciences, University of Edinburgh, Edinburgh, U.K.

Nathan D. Wong   Heart Disease Prevention Program, Department of Medicine, Division of Cardiology, School of Medicine, University of California–Irvine, Irvine, California, U.S.A.

Paul Z. Zimmet   Department of Medicine, International Diabetes Institute, Victoria, Australia

Introduction

Metabolic Syndrome and Cardiovascular Disease is a comprehensive text addressing the cardiovascular risk factors and consequences associated with this important condition, a concept that has evolved over much of the past century, but which has received renewed and heightened attention over the past decade. It has been known for several decades that risk factors for atherosclerotic cardiovascular disease often cluster together. This knowledge is the basis for multifactorial algorithms to predict risk for cardiovascular disease. The Framingham Heart Study produced the first risk-prediction algorithms, but more recently, similar risk engines have been created from other databases of prospective studies. These risk-prediction tools have included all of the established atherosclerotic cardiovascular disease risk factors and provide the basis for estimates of global risk. Only recently have efforts been made to identify particular patterns of risk factors that have a common origin. The metabolic syndrome is one such pattern that has generated much interest in recent years.

Two lines of evidence have merged to produce the metabolic syndrome concept. These different origins have not been fully integrated and account for much of the debate that surrounds the syndrome. The first of these has been the recognition that obesity is strongly associated with multiple risk factors and undoubtedly contributes significantly to them. These include hypertension, hypercholesterolemia, hypertriglyceridemia, low levels of high-density lipoproteins, and hyperglycemia. In spite of much research on these metabolic complications of obesity, researchers in this field never consolidated all of them into a syndrome. But certainly it was recognized that prevention and treatment of obesity is the foundation of management of these risk factors.

During this same period, researchers in the diabetes field identified a metabolic state called insulin resistance. It was characterized by resistance to the actions of insulin and hyperinsulinemia. Insulin resistance was first recognized as a major contributing factor to Type 2 diabetes. However, in 1998, Dr. Gerald Reaven presented the hypothesis that insulin resistance also can be a cause of risk factors of metabolic origin. Among these risk factors he first identified were hypertension, low high-density lipoproteins levels, and hypertriglyceridemia. Although Dr. Reaven called the clustering of risk factors with insulin resistance and hyperinsulinemia tighten by the name syndrome X, others shortly thereafter changed the name to insulin resistance syndrome. Several different names have been used as alternatives for the metabolic syndrome. Besides metabolic syndrome X, and insulin resistance syndrome, there are the dysmetabolic syndrome, metabolic syndrome X, the deadly quartet, CHAOS, and the cardiometabolic syndrome. Often the name chosen is meant to highlight one or another feature of the syndrome. Recently some investigators have raised the question of whether a clustering of metabolic risk factors should be called a "syndrome" at all. This is a semantic issue, but most researchers believe that the term "syndrome" is appropriate for a clustering of risk factors of metabolic origin. For another decade, the metabolic syndrome/insulin resistance syndrome remained a topic of research interest, but did not become an entity for clinical identification. But in 1998, the World Health Organization Working Group on Definition of Diabetes attempted to formulate criteria for the diagnosis of the metabolic syndrome. These criteria were based on the assumption that insulin resistance is the major cause of the syndrome. Subsequently, other organizations have made an effort to reformulate diagnostic criteria both to add simplicity and to include the key features of the syndrome. Over the next eight years, diagnostic criteria have been suggested by the European Group for Study of Insulin Resistance, the United States National Cholesterol Education Program Adult Treatment Panel III, the American Association of Clinical Endocrinology, the International Diabetes Federation, and the American Heart Association/National Heart, Lung, and Blood Institute. The World Health Organization definition was influential in concept but lacking in clinical utilization. The simplicity of the Adult Treatment Panel III definition, however, was attractive to many researchers and clinicians and has sparked great interest. Subsequently, the International Diabetes Federation and American Heart Association/National Heart, Lung, and Blood Institute made minor modifications to the Adult Treatment Panel III criteria. The two are very similar, and use the same risk factors and cut points for diagnosis. This similarity provides enough harmonization to make the two essentially interchangeable for diagnosis.

The metabolic syndrome has been strongly associated with risk for atherosclerotic cardiovascular disease. When Gerald Reaven introduced syndrome X, it identified a clustering of factors related to insulin resistance and predicting risk for atherosclerotic cardiovascular disease. Currently accepted metabolic risk factors for atherosclerotic cardiovascular disease are

- Atherogenic dyslipidemia
- Vascular dysfunction
- Dysglycemia
- A prothrombotic state
- A proinflammatory state

Atherogenic dyslipidemia consists of

■ Elevated apolipoprotein B including elevated levels of triglyceride and small low-density lipoprotein particles
■ Reduced levels of high-density lipoproteins

There is general agreement that most apolipoprotein B-containing lipoproteins are atherogenic, whether contained in the low-density lipoprotein or very low-density lipoprotein fractions. The relationship between low levels of high-density lipoprotein and atherogenesis is less well understood. Several causative mechanisms have been proposed, e.g., reduced reverse cholesterol transport, loss of protection against low-density lipoprotein oxidation within the arterial wall, and reduction of anti-inflammatory properties. The extent to which a low high-density lipoprotein level contributes to atherogenesis must await controlled clinical trials with high-density lipoprotein-raising drugs. Such trials are currently underway.

Vascular dysfunction is manifest by elevations in blood pressure and by endothelial dysfunction. The former is known to be atherogenic, whereas the latter may be. The role of endothelial dysfunction in the development of atherosclerosis is still under investigation. Finally, some investigators believe that vascular dysfunction may play a direct role in the development of insulin resistance and other metabolic risk factors.

Dysglycemia can take several forms: high–normal plasma glucose, impaired glucose tolerance, impaired fasting glucose, and clinical hyperglycemia (Type 2 diabetes). A variety of mechanisms have been proposed whereby elevations in plasma glucose can directly promote atherogenesis. In addition, higher glucose levels cause microvascular disease. There is growing evidence that microvascular disease may secondarily cause macrovascular disease. Some investigators question whether the metabolic syndrome and Type 2 diabetes can coexist. According to these investigators, Type 2 diabetes subsumes the metabolic syndrome. Without question, most patients with Type 2 diabetes exhibit current diagnostic criteria for the metabolic syndrome. It must be pointed out, however, that current criterion for the diagnosis of Type 2 diabetes is based entirely on plasma glucose cut points. Further, an alternate view is that Type 2 diabetes is essentially a severe form of the metabolic syndrome. This view is justified by those to point out that it is characterized by multiple metabolic risk factors. Clearly the two conditions have many common pathogenic features.

A prothrombotic state is characterized mainly by elevations of plasminogen activator inhibitor-1. Nevertheless, several other coagulation abnormalities have been reported in patients with the metabolic syndrome. Some of these include

■ Platelet dysfunction
■ Elevated fibrinogen
■ Elevated von Willebrand factor
■ Elevated factor VII
■ Elevated tissue plasminogen activator antigen

- Elevated factor V Leiden
- Elevated protein C
- Elevated antithrombin II

Abnormalities in coagulation and thrombolysis have been implicated both in atherogenesis itself and in propagation of thrombi following disruption of atherosclerotic plaques.

The proinflammatory state associated with the metabolic syndrome appears to have several features. First, circulating levels of inflammatory cytokines are raised. These high levels appear to be derived largely from adipose-tissue beds. Second, in muscle and liver, an excessive influx of fatty acids can elicit the formation of intracellular inflammatory pathways that can induce insulin resistance. Third, the metabolic syndrome is accompanied by increases in acute phase proteins, such as C-reactive protein. Several reports suggest that these proteins may have proatherogenic properties. And finally, there is a cellular inflammatory response in the arterial way secondary to interaction with the known metabolic risk factors; this inflammatory response may be heightened by increases in circulating inflammatory cytokines.

As indicated above, each of the components of the metabolic syndrome has been implicated in atherogenesis. Because of their colinearity within the syndrome, it has been difficult to dissect the relative contributions of each to atherosclerotic cardiovascular disease events. For this reason, the metabolic syndrome can be considered to be a multiplex cardiovascular risk factor. The metabolic syndrome belongs in the category of causative risk factors similar to individual risk factors of cigarette smoking, hypercholesterolemia, and hypertension. The introduction of a multiplex risk factor is something new to the cardiovascular field, and not surprisingly, the understanding of the place of the metabolic syndrome in cardiovascular risk has been slow in development.

The question has arisen whether the risk for metabolic syndrome as a whole is greater than the sum of the risk factors of its individual components. This is a complex question, but can be addressed in several ways. First, epidemiological studies suggest that multiple risk factors are synergistic in raising risk and not just additive. This synergism has long been called multiplicative risk . Second, several of the risk components, e.g., elevated apolipoprotein B, a prothrombotic state, and a proinflammatory state, are not usually measured in clinical practice. Consequently, their contribution to risk is not identified with the typical clinical measures. Third, some of the measured risk factors, such as low high-density lipoprotein cholesterol, may be predictive but not necessarily causative; thus, the individual risk factors that are used for prediction may be only markers for the true causative factors accompanying the syndrome. And fourth, the metabolic syndrome is a progressive disorder, that is, it worsens over time. Consequently, risk measured at any one time underestimates the long-term risk accompanying the syndrome.

Considerable confusion has arisen regarding the relation of the component metabolic risk factors to the risk surrogates (categorical risk markers) for these factors that are the basis for clinical diagnosis. In both updated Adult Treatment Panel III and International Diabetes Federation formulations of the risk the following surrogates are included:

- Serum triglycerides <150 mg/dL (<1.7 mmol/L)
- High-density lipoprotein cholesterol < 40 mg/dL (<1.0 mmol/L) in men, and <50 mg/dL (<1.3 mmol/L) in women
- Blood pressure <130 mmHg systolic, and <85 mmHg diastolic
- Fasting glucose <100 mg/dL (<5.6 mmol/L)
- Increased waist circumference (population-dependent thresholds)

The following waist circumference thresholds are recommended:

- Non-Asian <94 cm in men (<102 cm in U.S. men); <80 cm in women (<88 cm in U.S. women)
- Asian <90 cm in men; <80 cm in women

The higher waist circumference in U.S. men and women relates in large part to practicality because of the high prevalence of obesity. However, recent studies have shown that in the United States, a similar prevalence of metabolic syndrome exists by International Diabetes Federation and updated Adult Treatment Panel III criteria.

International Diabetes Federation requires that elevated waist circumference be present for a diagnosis of the metabolic syndrome. Adult Treatment Panel III does not require this when other risk surrogates are present. According to both criteria, when three or more (3+) risk markers are present, a diagnosis of the metabolic syndrome can be made. It has been shown that most persons with 3+ metabolic markers are affected with all of the metabolic risk factors that constitute the metabolic syndrome.

Although the metabolic syndrome is multifactorial in origin, the pathogenesis can be simplified into two general categories of causation. The first category can be called metabolic susceptibility. For the syndrome to develop there must be an underlying propensity. Reaven and other workers have suggested that this susceptibility be called insulin resistance. Without question, most people who exhibit the metabolic syndrome also manifest insulin resistance. Even so, the metabolic connection between insulin resistance and the multiple components of the syndrome have not been elucidated. One view holds that insulin resistance, or concomitant hyperinsulinemia, is a direct cause of all of the components of the syndrome. Certainly, insulin resistance contributes directly to the dysglycemia of prediabetes and Type 2 diabetes. On the other hand, the mechanistic link between insulin resistance and other components—atherogenic dyslipidemia, vascular dysfunction, and prothrombotic and proinflammatory states—remains to be clarified. The possibility exists that other causes that are responsible for these abnormalities also produce insulin resistance. If so, insulin resistance may be a marker for the presence of these underlying causes without itself being a direct causative factor. Thus, more research is needed to understand the mechanistic basis of metabolic susceptibility for the metabolic syndrome.

Several factors appear to contribute to metabolic susceptibility. Among these are physical inactivity, advancing age, adipose-tissue disorders, certain drugs, and ethnic, racial, and family propensity. At a more mechanistic level, susceptibility has been related to deficiencies and maldistribution of adipose tissue, loss of muscle mass, genetic defects in insulin-signaling pathways, and other genetic variations. All of these changes are associated with insulin resistance, but whether the latter is a cause or a marker of the several components of the metabolic syndrome is yet to be determined. Certainly, the possibility must be considered that these susceptibilities act on development of metabolic syndrome components in ways that are independent of insulin resistance.

The second large category of causation for syndrome is an excess in body fat. This typically is a manifestation of energy overload. It results in either overweight or obesity. Epidemiological studies show that increases in obesity in a population are accompanied by increases in the prevalence of the metabolic syndrome. Thus, obesity can be viewed as the driving force behind the metabolic syndrome. This is true even for individuals who are metabolically susceptible. Still, obesity is particularly likely to precipitate the syndrome in persons who are susceptible based on other factors. The mechanisms whereby obesity worsens the syndrome is a subject of intense research interest. Recent discoveries show that an excess in body fat is accompanied by abnormalities in release of many factors from adipose tissue. Among these are increased outputs of nonesterified fatty acids, resistin, angiotensinogen, and others. All of these have been implicated in systemic metabolic abnormalities related to the metabolic syndrome. In addition, adiponectin, a putative protective adipokine, is reduced with obesity. Consequently, obesity and its accompanying abnormalities may be a direct cause of several of the metabolic syndrome constituents. The actions of these several adipokines represent an area of great importance in research on the development of the metabolic syndrome.

One of the features of the metabolic syndrome is a tendency to accumulate fat in tissues outside of adipose tissue. This is called ectopic fat. Two prime locations are muscle and liver. In muscle, ectopic fat accumulation is accompanied by insulin resistance. The pathways whereby excess fatty acids in muscle cause insulin resistance are becoming better understood. In liver, ectopic fat accumulation, called fatty liver, is accompanied by insulin resistance and increased outputs of glucose and very low-density lipoprotein triglyceride. The pathways underlying these changes are only partially understood. The reasons for ectopic fat accumulation have not been fully elucidated. One possibility is that patients with the metabolic syndrome may be relatively deficient in adipose-tissue storage capacity. Most of the body fat is normally stored in subcutaneous adipose tissue. If fat storage capacity is limited, caloric overload may result in accumulation of fat elsewhere, hence excess ectopic fat. An example of this phenomenon occurs in patients with lipodystrophy—which is characterized by a loss of body fat, particularly subcutaneous fat. Patients with lipodystrophy typically have large accumulations of ectopic fat and many metabolic complications. One of the features of ectopic fat accumulation is the presence of excess intraperitoneal (visceral) fat. Thus, visceral obesity can be viewed as a marker of a relative deficiency of subcutaneous fat stores.

The above model of the pathogenesis of the metabolic syndrome provides a rational approach to its management. Highest priority goes to prevention and/or treatment of obesity. Second is modification of metabolic susceptibility. And third is to treat residual risk-factor components of the syndrome. A few comments can be made about each.

To reduce the burden of metabolic syndrome in society, obesity prevention deserves a high priority for public health. This is true for all nations of the world. Changing lifestyles can largely account for the rising prevalence of the syndrome throughout the world. For much of the world, life is becoming more sedentary and food is increasingly available. Both lead to energy overload and obesity. Society is ill prepared to reverse this trend. But both governments and society at large must recognize the consequences of allowing obesity to develop unchecked. Greater national commitments to modifying the structure of daily life habits will be required to reverse this unfortunate trend.

For individuals who have developed obesity, management requires intervention by the healthcare community. Priority in clinical management should go to persons in whom obesity has elicited the metabolic syndrome. A major challenge to the healthcare system is to develop more efficient lifestyle interventions. This may require creation of clinical management structures that do not currently exist in most medical settings. In overweight/obese subjects with the metabolic syndrome, the primary goal is to reduce body weight by 10% in the first year. If this can be achieved, a secondary goal is to reduce weight to the desirable range, e.g., a body mass index less than 25 kg/m^2. To achieve these goals, a combination of caloric restriction, behavior modification, and increased physical activity will be required.

The second aim in management of the metabolic syndrome is to reduce metabolic susceptibility. The most practical means for achieving this aim is to enhance physical activity. Regular exercise will lower insulin resistance, improve cardiovascular risk factors overall, and reduce risk for cardiovascular events through multiple mechanisms. Further any secondary causes of metabolic susceptibility should be appropriately treated. Drug treatment of metabolic susceptibility is problematic. However, insulin sensitizers are promising. Included in this list are metformin and thiazolidinediones. The pharmaceutical industry is engaged in intensive research to develop new agents for reducing susceptibility to the metabolic syndrome; but at present, this field of research is in its infancy.

The third therapeutic approach is to favorably modify each of the risk-factor components of the syndrome with drug therapies. It is appropriate to use absolute risk estimates to guide choice and intensity of drug therapy. Several risk-assessment tools are available for estimating absolute risk. Among these are Framingham and PROCAM risk scoring. Others are under development.

Eventually, population-based risk scoring will be available so that absolute risk can be estimated from equations that factor in the baseline risk of the population. Some investigators have attempted to estimate absolute risk from the components of the metabolic syndrome alone. This is a mistake. The components of the syndrome do not incorporate all of the contributions to global cardiovascular risk.

Recently, the American Diabetes Association has introduced a multiple-component risk algorithm called Archimedes. This algorithm estimates what is called cardiometabolic risk . This term can be taken to refer to all cardiovascular diseases of atherosclerotic origin plus all other diseases of metabolic origin. Among the metabolic diseases are prediabetes, diabetes, fatty liver, cholesterol gallstones, polycystic ovarian syndrome, and obstructive sleep apnea. The current Archimedes algorithm includes multiple risk factors but at present only predicts absolute risk for cardiovascular disease and diabetes. Presumably as it is developed it will extend to predict other metabolic diseases. This ambitious program currently is a work in progress, and it will have to be validated with a variety of databases.

First-line therapy for atherogenic dyslipidemia is to reduce apolipoprotein B levels. Statin drugs are the most effective apolipoprotein B-lowering drugs. Other drugs that lower apolipoprotein B levels in patients with elevated triglycerides are ezetimibe, fibric acids, and nicotinic acid. The latter two also raise high-density lipoprotein-cholesterol levels, which may provide additional risk reduction. Currently, other drugs are under development that raise high-density lipoprotein concentrations. Whether these drugs produce incremental risk reduction awaits on-going clinical trials.

The primary target of vascular dysfunction is an elevated blood pressure. Many investigators favor use of drugs that dampen the renin-angiotensin system in patients with the metabolic syndrome. This is particularly the case for those patients who have Type 2 diabetes. Calcium-channel blockers are effective blood-pressure lowering agents, and generally are devoid of metabolic side effects. Beta-blockers and diuretics both can worsen insulin resistance, but may be required to achieve blood pressure goals in some patients.

The major unresolved question about glucose elevations in the prediabetes range is whether glucose-lowering drugs are indicated to prevent progressive hyperglycemia. Without doubt clinical hyperglycemia is a risk factor for both macrovascular and microvascular diseases. But is it enough just to treat hyperglycemia when it reaches the level of Type 2 diabetes? Ongoing clinical trials are discussing this question.

At present, there are no specific therapies for a prothromobotic state other than antiplatelet drugs, notably, aspirin. If patients with the metabolic syndrome have reached a level of risk high enough, the benefits of aspirin therapy outweigh the potential side effects—particularly bleeding complications. Further, there is currently no specific treatment for a proinflammatory state other than a reduction through lifestyle changes.

In summary, the metabolic syndrome as a multiplex cardiovascular risk factor is growing in importance as the world's population becomes increasingly sedentary and overweight. First and foremost, this is a public health problem. But the medical community has an important role to play in the management of the metabolic syndrome as a risk factor, just as they do for single risk factors such as smoking, hypertension, and hypercholesterolemia. *Metabolic Syndrome and Cardiovascular Disease* will help provide healthcare providers, researchers, and educators with the tools necessary to help combat this important problem on a global scale.

Scott M. Grundy, MD, PhD
Professor of Internal Medicine
Distinguished Chair in Human Nutrition
Director, Center for Human Nutrition
University of Texas, Southwestern Medical Center
Dallas, Texas, U.S.A.

1

Metabolic Syndrome: Nomenclature, Definition, and Diagnosis

K. George M. Alberti

Department of Endocrinology and Metabolism, Imperial College, London, U.K.

Paul Z. Zimmet

Department of Medicine, International Diabetes Institute, Victoria, Australia

SUMMARY

- Metabolic syndrome can be defined as a cluster of interrelated risk factors that are associated with an increased risk of diabetes and cardiovascular disease (CVD).
- Confusion has reigned because of a variety of diagnostic criteria for the metabolic syndrome proposed by different organizations, although these criteria largely identify similar groups of individuals.
- Recent definitions by the International Diabetes Federation (IDF) and the American Heart Association/National Heart, Lung and Blood Institute (AHA/NHLBI) have clarified matters in providing greater refinement and agreement on criteria for diagnosing the metabolic syndrome.
- There is agreement that the main measurable components of the metabolic syndrome are central obesity, impaired fasting blood glucose, elevated blood pressure, elevated triglycerides, and high-density lipoprotein-cholesterol (HDL-C).
- The metabolic syndrome provides a practical, clinical, easy-to-use diagnostic set for early detection of those at risk worldwide and in primary-care settings.
- Long-term prospective studies are needed to refine and improve the criteria and increase their utility in identifying persons at future risk of diabetes and CVD.

INTRODUCTION

Worldwide, CVD continues to be the major cause of mortality and morbidity, with its incidence increasing alarmingly in the developing world. Diabetes is rising in tandem due to increasing obesity and decreasing physical activity and fuelling the increase in CVD. Anything which can lead to better knowledge of the causes, earlier detection, and possible prevention of these twin epidemics is to be welcomed, hence the widespread interest in the metabolic syndrome over recent years. There has, however, been considerable confusion over its nomenclature, diagnostic criteria, and clinical usefulness. There has also been confusion between whether it is a disease, a pathophysiological construct, or a diagnostic tool—or all three—and indeed doubts have been expressed as to whether it exists at all (1,2). At its simplest, it is a cluster of interrelated risk factors for CVD and diabetes, which coincide more often than by chance alone. We would stress that the metabolic syndrome is an evolving concept, which does indeed have a clinical role and has stimulated much interest in the pathological basis of the cluster.

HISTORY

This clustering of cardiometabolic risk factors was first pointed out by Kylin more than eight decades ago when he described the association between hypertension, hyperglycemia, and gout (3). This was closely followed by a highly perceptive paper by the Spanish endocrinologist Maranon who specifically stated that hypertension was a prediabetic condition as was obesity and perhaps also gout (4). He suggested that diet was essential to prevent and treat those abnormalities! The next significant contribution was that of Vague who in a series of painstaking studies showed that upper body or android obesity was associated with the metabolic abnormalities found in hypertension and hyperglycemia (5). This paved the way for Bjorntorp who later demonstrated abnormalities of the hypothalamo–pituitary–adrenal axis in people with android/central obesity (6). The last of the historical studies was that of Avogaro et al. who described the association of obesity, hyperinsulinemia, hypertriglyceridemia, and hypertension (7) but failed to pursue this.

THE INSULIN RESISTANCE ERA

Modern interest in the clustering of cardiovascular and diabetes risk factors started with the epochal paper of Reaven in 1988 (8). He described Syndrome X as a clustering of hyperinsulinemia, hyperglycemia, hypertension, raised very–low-density lipoprotein-triglycerides, and low levels of HDL-C with the suggestion that insulin resistance was the underlying etiological factor. Importantly he also suggested that changes in nonesterified fatty acids played a pivotal role in the interaction between hyperinsulinemia, glucose intolerance, and insulin resistance. He showed that insulin resistance correlated with each of the other factors and suggested that people with this cluster were at an increased risk of CVD. This in fact followed many years of speculation as to whether hyperinsulinemia

Table 1 Abnormalities Associated with Insulin Resistance

Raised blood pressure
Dysglycemia
Hyperuricemia
Dyslipidemia
  Increased VLDL-triglycerides
  Low HDL-cholesterol
  Increased small dense LDL particles
Endothelial dysfunction
  Increased levels of adhesion molecules
  Decreased endothelial-dependent vasodilatation
Hypercoaguability
  Increased PAI-1
  Increased fibrinogen
Abnormal inflammatory markers
  Increased hs-CRP

Abbreviations: Hs-CRP, high sensitivity C-reactive protein; VLDL, very–low-density lipoprotein; LDL, low-density lipoprotein; HDL, high-density lipoprotein; PAI, plasminogen activator inhibitor. *Source*: From Ref. 8.

could cause atherogenic abnormalities. Epidemiological studies had shown associations between hyperinsulinemia and subsequent CVD (9) and some in vitro studies were highly suggestive (10). Following Reaven's seminal paper, many other abnormalities were shown to be associated with insulin resistance and the syndrome was renamed "the insulin resistance syndrome" (Table 1). Further studies also showed the predictive power of both insulin resistance and raised serum insulin levels with regard to CVD (11,12). It is worth stressing that Reaven was putting forward a pathophysiological construct rather than a clinical or diagnostic tool and much confusion has occurred due to the lack of appreciation of the difference. It should be emphasized that obesity was not included as a core component of the original syndrome X.

THE METABOLIC SYNDROME

An explosion of studies followed Reaven's original description. A variety of other factors were shown to be associated with the core components of syndrome X, many of which were also associated with insulin resistance, as shown in Table 1. The most important of these was obesity, which became recognized as being associated with all other factors in the cardiovascular risk cluster. A range of new names have been applied to the cluster including metabolic syndrome, metabolic syndrome X, cardiovascular metabolic syndrome, chronic cardiovascular risk factor clustering syndrome, plurimetabolic syndrome, dysmetabolic syndrome, cardiometabolic syndrome and "deadly quartet" as well as insulin resistance syndrome (13). In general, metabolic syndrome became the accepted term and tended to be favored over insulin resistance syndrome as it carried fewer connotation of etiology. There were however no agreed major components or cutoff points for those components with most authors using their own arbitrary cutoff points. This led a World Health Organization (WHO) consultation group to attempt to produce a working definition (14,15).

CRITERIA AND DEFINITIONS OF THE METABOLIC SYNDROME

The World Health Organization Definition

The premise for the WHO effort in defining the metabolic syndrome was the lack of any international definition. They carefully stated that their new definition did not imply causality and should be viewed as a starting point—a working definition to allow comparisons and further work and to be improved upon when more information was available (14,15). In particular, they felt that data were needed to support the relative importance of each component. Table 2 shows the WHO criteria. The original blood pressure criterion in the provisional publication (14) of 160/90 mmHg was lowered to 140/90 mmHg in the final publication (15). The members of the group were largely diabetes specialists and it is not surprising that they felt that glucose intolerance, impaired glucose tolerance (IGT) or diabetes, and/or insulin resistance were essential components of the syndrome together with two or more out of raised arterial pressure, raised triglycerides, and/or low levels of HDL-C, central obesity or body mass index (BMI) $\geq$ 30 kg/m^2, and microalbuminuria. Most of these were based on Reaven's suggestions for syndrome X with the notable addition of obesity and microalbuminuria, the latter having already been shown to be an important CVD risk factor, particularly in patients with Type 2 diabetes (16,17), as well as being associated with insulin resistance (18). Other possible components of the syndrome such as hyperuricemia, coagulation disorders, and raised circulating levels of plasminogen activator inhibitor-1 were mentioned but not deemed necessary for recognition of the syndrome.

Table 2   World Health Organization Criteria for the Metabolic Syndrome

---

Essential component:
   Impaired glucose regulation or diabetes and/or insulin resistance (under hyperinsulinemic conditions, glucose uptake below lowest quartile for background population)

Plus two of the following:
   Raised arterial pressure ($\geq$ 140/90 mmHg)
   Raised plasma triglycerides ($\geq$ 1.7 mmol/L; 150 mg/dL) and/or low HDL-cholesterol (<0.9 mmol/L; 35 mg/dL in men: <1.0 mmol/L, 39 mg/dL in women)
   Central obesity (males: waist-to-hip ratio >0.90; females: waist-to-hip ratio > 0.85) and/or BMI > 30 kg/m^2
   Microalbuminuria (urinary albumin excretion rate $\geq$ 20 g/min or albumin:creatinine ratio $\geq$ 30 mg/g)

Abbreviations: HDL, high-density lipoprotein; BMI, body mass index.

It was recognized at the time that insulin resistance was not easy to measure and that there were no standardized criteria for determining whether insulin resistance was present in a given individual. Pragmatically, however, anyone with dysglycemia or diabetes was likely to be insulin resistant. One important point was that the relative importance of central rather than total obesity was noted although it was assumed that once the BMI was greater than 30 kg/m^2, the person was likely to be centrally obese as well. It is also worth noting that IGT as well as impaired fasting glucose (IFG) and diabetes was included as a qualifying dysglycemic condition—indeed it was felt that IGT was a much better cardiovascular risk indicator than IFG (19).

The European Group for the Study of Insulin Resistance Definition

The European Group for the Study of Insulin Resistance (EGIR) produced their own definition shortly after the publication of the WHO report (Table 3). They initially objected to the use of the term "metabolic" in that they argued that it included nonmetabolic items and suggested reverting to the term "insulin resistance syndrome" (21). It is

Table 3 European Group for the Study of Insulin Resistance and National Cholesterol Education Program Adult Treatment Panel III (Original and Revised) Criteria for the Metabolic Syndrome

European Group for the Study of Insulin Resistance

Insulin resistance (defined as hyperinsulinemia, top 25% of fasting insulin values among the nondiabetic population) plus two or more of:
  Central obesity: waist circumference ≥ 94 cm in males and ≥ 80 cm in females
  Dyslipidemia: triglycerides > 2.0 mmol/L (190 mg/dL) or high-density lipoprotein-cholesterol < 1.0 mmol/L (40 mg/dL)
  Hypertension: blood pressure ≥ 140/90 mmHg and/or medication
  Fasting plasma glucose ≥ 6.1 mmol/L (110 mg/dL)

National Cholesterol Education Program Adult Treatment Panel III Criteria for the Metabolic Syndrome

Three or more of the following:
  Central obesity: waist circumference > 102 cm in males or > 88 cm in females
  Hypertriglyceridemia: triglycerides ≥ 150 mg/dL (1.7 mmol/L) [a]or on medication for elevated triglycerides
  Low HDL-cholesterol: <40 mg/dL (1.04 mmol/L) in males or <50 mg/dL (1.29 mmol/L) in females [a]or on medication for low HDL-cholesterol
  Hypertension: blood pressure ≥ 130/85 mg [a]or on medication for hypertension
  Fasting plasma glucose ≥ 110 mg/dL (6.1 mmol/L) [[a]≥ 100 mg/dL (5.5 mmol/L) or on medication for hyperglycemia]

Note: Prothrombotic and proinflammatory states (not essential for diagnosis).
Abbreviation: HDL, high-density lipoprotein.
[a]Represent changes made in the revised criteria.
Source: From Ref. 20.

worth noting that they were a study group performing epidemiologic studies on insulin resistance so their stance was hardly surprising. They also suggested that fasting insulin be used as a surrogate for insulin resistance as this was easier to usein epidemiologic studies than a standard clamp and anyway correlated well with more formal insulin resistance measurements (22). It was slightly surprising that they did not use the most common method for measurement of insulin sensitivity in the basal state—the Homeostatic Model Assessment (HMA) technique. They also excluded all diabetic people from their definition as it was not possible to measure insulin resistance—whereas WHO included people with a diagnosis of diabetes—on the grounds that virtually all such people would be insulin resistant. Dysglycemia was represented purely by a raised fasting glucose level but below the diabetic threshold, i.e., 6.1 to 6.9 mmol/L (110–125 mg/dL) again on the grounds that an oral glucose tolerance test was not practical for their epidemiological studies, following the American Diabetes Association (ADA) recommendations. They excluded microalbuminuria and also used different cutoff points for lipids following the Second Joint Task Force of European and other Societies on Coronary Prevention. Importantly they suggested using waist girth as a measure of central obesity and also a better index of visceral adipose tissue than waist-to-hip ratio (23), choosing the values suggested by Lean et al. as indicating an appropriate risk level (24). The full report appeared in 2002 and they finished with the perceptive comment that the usefulness of identifying and treating the syndrome (whatever its name) and the definition needed long-term studies and delineation of the pathophysiology and etiology of the syndrome (25).

National Cholesterol Education Program-Adult Treatment Panel III Criteria

Shortly after the initial response of EGIR, the Adult Treatment Panel III (ATP III) of the National Cholesterol Education Program (NCEP) in the United States published a comprehensive report on treatment of high cholesterol in adults (26). Within this report they recognized the existence of the metabolic syndrome as a major contributor to cardiovascular risk. They included abdominal obesity, atherogenic dyslipidemia [low HDL-C, raised triglycerides, and small low-density lipoprotein (LDL) particles], raised blood pressure, insulin resistance (with or without glucose intolerance), and prothrombotic and proinflammatory states. A strong emphasis of the definition was to recognize people at high risk of CVD in addition to the conventional risk factors of low-density lipoprotein-cholesterol (LDL-C), smoking, and family history. They produced a pragmatic, practical set of criteria to aid the detection of individuals at risk (Table 3). Very simply, people had to meet three of the five criteria, which were similar to those of the WHO group but also showed some significant differences. Central adiposity was represented by waist girth as with EGIR, but the levels chosen equate to a BMI of 30+ kg/m^2 whereas the EGIR values equated to a BMI of 25, which in turn picked out more people than the original WHO waist-to-hip ratio. Some of the rationale for the ATP III choice was that their value focused on a higher risk group of individuals, and given the high prevalence of overweight/obesity in the United States, the lower cutoff point would have identified too many people. Another important point was that HDL-C and raised triglycerides could count separately whereas in the WHO criteria it was either/or. Blood pressure was also slightly lower for the ATP III definition (130/85 mmHg or higher) than for the other two definitions and like EGIR they restricted glucose to the fasting state, for practical reasons, but did include known diabetes. Insulin resistance was not included due to difficulties in measurement in routine practice (27).

American College of Endocrinology Criteria

Shortly after publication of ATP III, the American College of Endocrinology (ACE) published a modified version of ATP III. It preferred the name insulin resistance syndrome—looking on insulin resistance as the prime component although for practical reasons, measurement of insulin resistance was not included. Lipid and blood pressure cut points were the same as for ATP III. Postprandial glucose was included, as with WHO, as well as fasting blood glucose. Obesity was excluded on the somewhat spurious grounds that abdominal obesity contributes to insulin resistance rather than being a risk factor itself, but was included as a factor that increased the likelihood of the syndrome being present. Thus only four criteria were listed and no set number of abnormalities had to be present. The more criteria that an individual had the more likely they were to be insulin resistant, and by inference, the greater the risk of CVD (and diabetes). Much emphasis was placed on history and clinical judgment. Because of these reasons, this definition is less helpful in making a definite diagnosis or in prevalence studies.

International Diabetes Federation Criteria

Following publication of the ATP III criteria, a plethora of publications appeared on the prevalence of the metabolic syndrome in different parts of the world; some used ATP III criteria, others used the WHO recommendations, and many used both. In general, not dissimilar total prevalence figures appeared in the comparative studies although concordance rates were relatively poor (13,28). Thus in Australia, the prevalence of the metabolic syndrome in a nondiabetic adult population was 20.7% using the WHO definition compared with 15.8% with EGIR and 18.2% using ATP III; half were positive with all three definitions and two-thirds were positive with both WHO and ATP II (28,29). Similar results were obtained with the Diabetes Epidemiology Collaborative Analysis of Diagnostic Criteria in Europe study in Europe (DECODE) (30).

It was apparent that some form of consensus was required. Some of the differences between the three major sets of criteria were undoubtedly due to the nature of the different groups producing them. The WHO group were diabetologists and EGIR (and ACE) focussed on insulin resistance primarily, whilst ATP III came from lipidologists and cardiologists looking for a tool to help identify people at high risk of CVD, above and beyond LDL-C, smoking, and family history. The IDF Task Force on epidemiology therefore convened a group representing the three main factions to see whether an agreed set of criteria could be produced, which would then form the basis of long-term studies so that in the future the criteria could be refined and modified. It was felt that there was a strong need for one simple definition/diagnostic tool for clinical practice, which could be used relatively easily in any part of the world by any physician to identify patients at high risk of diabetes and/or CVD. The group also deemed it necessary to focus not just on the statistical clustering of the putative components of the syndrome but also to look at predictive power for CVD and—to a lesser extent—diabetes.

An initial part of the discussion focused on whether the syndrome was indeed a syndrome in its own right. A syndrome is defined as a complex of symptoms and signs or biochemical findings for which the precise cause is unknown and where the components coexist more than would be expected by chance alone (31). This is indeed the case as we showed in Mauritius and others have shown repeatedly. One problem is whether components are causally related to each other or are caused by other aspects of the syndrome. In pragmatic terms this does not matter, although it is important if one is to advance understanding of the pathogenesis of the syndrome. Several studies have attempted to look at this in more detail using modelling approaches and cluster analysis. The earlier ones showed from two to four clusters with principal component analysis (32–34), although using confirmatory factor analysis one recent study has suggested that there is a single underlying factor (35).

Overall there was agreement that abdominal obesity, insulin resistance, atherogenic dyslipidemia, elevated blood pressure, elevated plasma glucose, proinflammatory states, and prothrombotic states were part of the syndrome—in line with the suggestions of ATP III. For practical worldwide use, it was obvious that not all of these could be included in the diagnostic set. It was agreed that central obesity, raised triglycerides (or specific treatment thereof), reduced HDL-C (or specific treatment), raised blood pressure (or previous treatment), and raised fasting glucose or previously treated Type 2 diabetes should be the core components (29). These are shown in detail in Table 4.

There was discussion as to whether HDL-C and triglycerides were genuinely separate components. In the WHO view, they counted as a single abnormality whereas ATP III had them as separate components, but it was felt that the latter should be used for consistency. It was agreed for practical reasons that it was not possible to measure insulin resistance as there was no simple measurement available or indeed international standardization of methods. It was deemed highly likely that those with central adiposity and two or more other abnormalities would indeed be insulin resistant. The biggest changes regarded central adiposity. First it was felt that the ATP III criteria were too high and would miss many people with moderate visceral adiposity but who still had an increased likelihood of developing CVD or diabetes. The EGIR values were therefore adopted. Second it was felt inappropriate to use a single value for everyone regardless of ethnic group. WHO

Table 4 International Diabetes Federation Criteria for the Metabolic Syndrome

Essential component:
Central obesity: waist circumference ≥ 94 cm Europid males; ≥ 90 cm South Asian, Chinese and Japanese males; ≥ 80 cm females[a]

Plus two of the following:
Raised triglycerides:
≥ 1.7 mmol/L (150 mg/dL) or specific treatment
Reduced HDL-cholesterol
<1.03 mmol/L (40 mg/dL) in males
<1.29 mmol/L (50 mg/dL) in females or specific treatment
Raised blood pressure
Systolic ≥ 130 mm Hg or
Diastolic ≥ 85 mm Hg or specific treatment
Raised fasting plasma glucose
≥ 5.6 mmol/L (100 mg/dL) or previously diagnosed diabetess

Abbreviation: HDL, high-density lipoprotein.
[a]If body mass index is more than 30 kg/m^2, waist circumference measurement is not required. For ethnic South and Central Americans use South Asian recommendations, for sub-Saharan Africans, Eastern Mediterranean, and Middle East use Europid recommendations until further data available.
Source: From Ref. 29.

had already issued revised BMI criteria and definitions of obesity for people of Asian origin (36,37) recognizing that South Asians for example will have more central adipose tissue for the same BMI as Europids, particularly males. Levels, which predict other features of the metabolic syndrome in different ethnic groups, were therefore sought. In Singapore, Tan et al. showed that 89 cm for males and 79 cm for females were the best values using receiver operating characteristic analyses (38) whilst 85 cm in males and 80 cm in females were found in a Chinese study (39). Values of 90 cm and 80 cm in males and females, respectively, were therefore selected. In Japanese, 85 cm in males and 90 cm for females were suggested based on correlation studies with visceral adipose tissue (40) but subsequent studies have not supported this (41) and IDF now recommends using the same figures as in other Asian populations (42).

A major change from other criteria was to make increased waist girth a sine qua non. It was felt that in the presence of two other components this would equate to significant risk. It had the major added advantage that it enabled waist measurement to be used as an initial screening tool, which in many parts of the world and in primary care would greatly simplify detection of people at risk and save considerable cost. There was concern that this might miss significant numbers of people genuinely at risk, but by using the lower waist girth cut points this risk has been considerably diminished.

The same lipid and blood pressure values were chosen as for ATP III (which follow international recommendations) but the lower glucose value of 5.6 mmol/L (100 mg/dL) was chosen as this was the more recent recommendation of ADA.

Several studies have now been published comparing IDF and ATP III criteria (43–45). In general, higher prevalence values have been shown with the new IDF suggestions. The differences were not as great as might be expected by the obligatory need for increased waist girth by IDF—partly because of the higher cut point for ATP III. The fear that people would be missed with the new IDF criteria who would be picked up by ATP III has been realized to only a small extent—again because of the lower IDF waist size requirement. Thus only 5% to 15% of those detected by ATP III were not picked up by IDF (unpublished observations). Overall in the United States, the unadjusted prevalence of the metabolic syndrome using ATP III was 33.7% in males and 35.4% in females compared with 39.7% and 38.1%, respectively, using IDF (43). However the overlap was not great and only longitudinal studies will be able to indicate which of these criteria are the most sensitive and specific screening tool.

American Heart Association/National Heart, Lung and Blood Institute Criteria

Most recently, the NCEP-ATP III definition has undergone a revision in the AHA/NHLBI scientific statement on the diagnosis and management of the metabolic syndrome (20). Many of these bring ATP III in line with the new IDF recommendations. Given the recent ADA revision of the lower cut point of IFG to 5.6 mmol/L (100 mg/dL), this lower cut point has now been adopted in the revised definition. In addition, the elevated triglyceride criterion now includes those taking medication for hypertriglyceridemia (even if their triglycerides are now normal), and the HDL-C criterion also includes those on medication for low HDL-C (Table 3). Similarly the blood pressure recommendations have been clarified. The new statement also comments on possible ethnic differences and that lower waist values may be adopted in certain ethnic groups. These revisions undoubtedly will increase the prevalence of metabolic syndrome.

ETIOLOGY OF THE METABOLIC SYNDROME

Although a detailed discussion about etiology is beyond the scope of this chapter, some comment is needed here as it has an impact on both nomenclature and criteria for the syndrome. As stated above, modern views of the syndrome derive from Reaven's syndrome X where he hypothesized an etiologic role for insulin resistance. This has been argued over now for nearly two decades and one school believes firmly that it is the basis of the syndrome. It is certainly closely related to several of the components, and several metabolic pathways have been proposed linking insulin resistance to the other factors (46,47). An alternative hypothesis is that visceral adiposity is the predominant etiologic factor. Certainly visceral adipose tissue is metabolically extremely active and releases fatty acids and a range of adipokines. The increased fatty acids could contribute to the insulin resistance as could the adipokines with several having direct effects in promoting atherogenesis. More recently, it has been suggested that low-grade inflammation underlies or exacerbates the syndrome. Whether visceral adiposity actually caused insulin resistance continues to be debated (48,49). It is likely that both visceral adiposity and insulin resistance play major roles, with genetic factors also involved. Thus it is likely that South Asians are genetically more predisposed to insulin resistance than those of European origin. Certainly considerable heterogeneity is likely between individuals. These possibilities are discussed in greater detail in the AHA/NHLBI scientific statement (20). Further detailed studies are needed as suggested by IDF (29).

PROBLEMS WITH THE DEFINITION AND CRITERIA

Several stringent criticisms have been levelled at both the nomenclature and the whole concept of the metabolic syndrome (1,2,50). The most thoughtful of these came in a joint statement from the ADA and the European Association for the Study of Diabetes (1). They criticised the use of the term syndrome—which was unjustified as discussed above. Any clustering of factors, which occurs by more than chance alone, qualifies for the term. They also commented on the confusion between different criteria—ignoring the IDF definition, which attempted to pull together the different criteria being used, further strengthened by the recent update of the ATP III definition. The spurious argument was also raised that the etiology of the syndrome is unknown and confused. This is why it is termed a syndrome and not a disease, although there are now clear pointers to etiology. It is also worth commenting that in a rapidly evolving field, criteria will change as more knowledge is acquired. There were criticisms as to whether the metabolic syndrome was a useful indicator of CVD or diabetes risk—or added anything to the individual components. Even if the risk is purely additive, it will be helpful in identifying people at increased risk—and there are compelling data suggesting that the risk is indeed more than the sum of the parts (51,52). There is also the benefit in detecting people with marginal elevations of several of the risk factors when they might not be treated for a single borderline abnormality.

It has also been suggested that the metabolic syndrome is a poorer indicator of cardiovascular or diabetes risk than using the Framingham score for CVD or "prediabetes" or fasting glucose for diabetes respectively. This conveys a misunderstanding of the role of the metabolic syndrome. It has never been suggested that it is an indicator of absolute risk, but rather relative risk. Clearly it does not cover *all* CVD risk factors but purely the cluster of interrelated metabolic factors. Thus unlike the Framingham risk score, total cholesterol, smoking, and family history are not included. It could be that taking simply the metabolic syndrome, LDL-C, and smoking in a simple risk score would be useful for overall risk. The metabolic syndrome appears to convey a 50% to threefold increase in risk for CVD and a much greater risk for diabetes (53,54).

The biggest argument concerns clinical utility of the syndrome. It is argued by the specialist diabetologists that more is to be gained by measuring all risk factors when one sees a patient with diabetes or others at risk. The IDF and

AHA/NHLBI would argue that focusing on the metabolic syndrome ensures that at all levels of healthcare, attention is drawn clearly to CVD risk and risk of diabetes. In particular, the IDF criteria with the basic screening tool of waist measurement allow for a relatively simple stepwise approach with particular attention to *early* detection of those at risk so that intervention can start when it is most likely to be beneficial.

Nonetheless there are still problems with the metabolic syndrome. In order to be of practical value it must be simple. Equal weight is given to all components and cut points used for continuous variables. Risk engines, which can take such factors into account, are attractive but of limited utility for worldwide use. Attempts have been made to develop a slightly more sophisticated model with use of a score chart, which looks helpful but will require testing (55). On the other hand, if the intention is primarily to draw attention to those at risk so that appropriate lifestyle advice can be given or drug therapy instituted, then a relatively crude indicator will suffice. Finally there is still uncertainty as to whether the correct variables are being measured. Prospective studies are needed to test out new variables such as markers of inflammation, endothelial dysfunction, and hypercoaguability. Further work on the undoubtedly complex etiology of the syndrome may also indicate new markers—and treatments. Time alone will tell whether the syndrome is a true pathophysiologic construct or just a helpful guide to clinicians and patients.

CONCLUSIONS

Over the past 10 years, there has been burgeoning interest in the clustering of a particular group of risk factors for diabetes and CVD. Various names have been applied to this cluster, the most common of which are metabolic syndrome and insulin resistance syndrome. The former is preferred as it carries fewer etiologic implications and is more directly applicable to CVD risk. Various definitions have been tried with some confusion resulting. More recently, the IDF and AHA/NHBLI have produced criteria, which are very close. Many epidemiologic studies have been performed showing that the syndrome is becoming increasingly common worldwide. The field continues to evolve rapidly and undoubtedly criteria will change as new knowledge is gained. The syndrome is particularly useful in a practical clinical sense in drawing attention to those at increased risk of CVD and diabetes and allowing early intervention. Over the next decade, new criteria based on long-term prospective studies will appear and will allow more precise prediction of risk, particularly allowing for ethnic variation.

REFERENCES

1. Kahn R, Buse J, Ferrannini E, et al. The metabolic syndrome: time for a critical reappraisal: joint statement of the American Diabetes Association and the European Association for the Study of Diabetes. Diabetes Care 2005; 28:2289–2304.
2. Reaven GM. The metabolic syndrome: is this diagnosis necessary? Am J Clin Nutr 2006; 83:1237–1247

3. Kylin E. Studien ueber das Hypertonie-Hyperglyka "mie-Hyperurika" miessyndrom. Zentralblatt fuer Innere Medizin 1923; 44:105–127

4. Maranon G. "Pradiabetische Zustande". Abhandlungen aus den grenzgebiete der Inneren Secretion. Wisenschafthliche Verlags Buchhandlung Rudolf Novak & C. Budapest Leipzig 1927:12–42.

5. Vague J. Sexual differentiation, a factor affecting the forms of obesity. Presse Med 1947; 30:339–340.

6. Bjorntorp P. "Portal" adipose tissue as a generator of risk factors for cardiovascular disease and diabetes. Arteriosclerosis 1990; 10:493–496.

7. Avogaro P, Crepaldi G, Enzi G, Tiengo A. Associazione de iperlipidemia, diabete mellito e obesita di medio grado. Acta Diabetol Lat 1967; 4:36–41.

8. Reaven GM. Role of insulin resistance in human disease. Diabetes 1988; 37:1595–1607.

9. Pyorala K. Relationship of glucose tolerance and plasma insulin to the incidence of coronary heart disease: results from two population studies in Finland. Diabetes Care 1979; 2:131–141.

10. Stout RW, Vallance-Owen J. Insulin and atheroma. Lancet 1969; i:1078–1080.

11. Despres J-P, Lamarche B, Mauriege P, et al. Hyperinsulinemia as an independent risk factor for ischemic heart disease. New Engl J Med 1996; 334:952–957.

12. Yip J, Facchini FS, Reaven GM. Resistance to insulin-mediated glucose disposal as a predictor of cardiovascular disease. J Clin Endocrinol Metab 1998; 83:2773–2776.

13. Ford ES. Prevalence of the metabolic syndrome in US populations. In: Grundy SM, ed. Metabolic Syndrome. Endocrin Metab Clin North Am 2004; 33:333–350.

14. Alberti KG, Zimmet PZ. Definition, diagnosis and classification of diabetes mellitus and its complications. Part 1:diagnosis and classification of diabetes mellitus. Provisional report of a WHO Consultation. Diabet Med 1998; 15:539–553.

15. World Health Organization. Definition, diagnosis and classification of diabetes mellitus and its complications. Part 1: diagnosis and classification of diabetes mellitus. WHO/NCD/NCS/99.2. Geneva: Department of Noncommunicable Disease Surveillance, 1999.

16. Schmitz A, Vaeth M. Microalbuminuria: a major risk factor in non-insulin-dependent diabetes. A 10-year follow-up study of 503 patients. Diabet Med 1988; 5:126–134.

17. Kuuisto J, Mykkanen L, Pyorala K, Laakso M. Hyperinsulinemic microalbuminuria. A new risk indicator for coronary heart disease. Circulation 1995; 91:831–837.

18. Mykkanen L, Zaccaro DJ, Wagenknecht LE, Robbins DC, Gabriel M, Haffner SM. Microalbuminuria is associated with insulin resistance in nondiabetic subjects: the Insulin Atherosclerosis Study. Diabetes 1998; 47:793–800.

19. The Decode Study Group. Glucose tolerance and cardiovascular mortality: comparison of fasting and 2-hr diagnostic criteria. Arch Intern Med 2001; 161:397–404.

20. Grundy SM, Cleeman JI, Daniels SR, et al. Diagnosis and management of the metabolic syndrome. An American Heart Association/National Heart, Lung and Blood Institute Scientific Statement. Circulation 2005; 112:2735–2752.

21. Balkau B, Charles MA. Comment on the provisional report from the WHO consultation: European Group for the Study of Insulin Resistance (EGIR). Diabet Med 1999; 16:442–443.

22. Laakso M. How good a marker is insulin level for insulin resistance? Am J Epidemiol 1993; 137:959–965.

23. Pouliot M, Despres J, Melieux S, et al. Waist circumference and abdominal sagittal diameter: best simple anthropometric measures of abdominal visceral adipose tissue accumulation and related cardiovascular risk in men and women. Am J Cardiol 1994; 73:460–468.

24. Lean MEJ, Han TS, Seidell JC. Impairment of health and quality of life in people with large waist circumference. Lancet 1998; 351:863–866.

25. Balkau B, Charles MA, Drivsholm T, et al. European Group for the Study of Insulin Resistance (EGIR): frequency of the WHO metabolic syndrome in European cohorts, and an alternative definition of an insulin resistance syndrome. Diabetes Metab 2002; 28:364–376.

26. Expert Panel on Detection, Evaluation, and Treatment of High Blood Cholesterol in Adults. Executive Summary of the third report of the National Cholesterol Education Program (NCEP) Expert Panel on Detection, Evaluation, and Treatment of High Blood Cholesterol in Adults (ATP III). JAMA 2001; 285:2486–2492.

27. Malik S, Wong ND, Franklin SS, et al. Impact of the metabolic syndrome on mortality from coronary heart disease, cardiovascular disease, and all causes in United States Adults. Circulation 2004; 110:1239–1244.

28. Cameron AJ, Shaw JE, Zimmet P. The metabolic syndrome: prevalence in worldwide populations. Metabolic Syndrome. Endocrinol Metab Clin 2004; 33:351–376.

29. Alberti KGMM, Zimmet P, Shaw J. Metabolic syndrome-a new world-wide definition. A consensus statement from the International Diabetes Federation. Diabet Med 2006; 23:469–480.

30. Hu G, Qiao Q, Tuomilehto J, et al. Prevalence of the metabolic syndrome and its relation to all–cause and cardiovascular mortality in nondiabetic European men and women. Arch Intern Med 2004; 164:1066–1076.

31. Last JM, ed. A Dictionary of Epidemiology. 3rd ed. New York: Oxford University Press, 1995:180.

32. Hodge AM, Boyko EJ, de Courten M, et al. Leptin and other components of the metabolic syndrome in Mauritius: a factor analysis. Int J Obes Relat Metab Disord 2001; 25:126–131.

33. Meigs JB, D'Agostino RB, Wilson PFW, Cupples LA, Nathan DM, Singer DE. Risk variable clustering in the insulin resistance syndrome. Diabetes 1997; 46:1594–1600.

34. Novak S, Stapleton LM, Litaker JR, Lawson KA. A confirmatory factor analysis evaluation of the coronary heart disease risk factors of metabolic syndrome with emphasis on the insulin resistance factor. Diabetes Obes Metab 2003; 5:388—396.

35. Pladevall M, Singal B, Williams LK, et al. A single factor underlies the metabolic syndrome. A confirmatory factor analysis. Diabetes Care 2006; 29:113–122.

36. World Health Organisation, Western Pacific Region. The Asia-Pacific Perspective. Redefining Obesity and its Treatment. WHO/IASO/IOTF, 2000.

37. WHO Expert Consultation. Appropriate body-mass index for Asian populations and its implications for policy and intervention strategies. Lancet 2004; 363:157–163.

38. Tan CE, Ma S, Wai D, Chew SK, Tai ES. Can we apply the National Cholesterol Education Program Adult Treatment Panel definition of the metabolic syndrome to Asians. Diabetes Care 2004; 27:1182–1186.

39. Lin WY, Lee LT, Chen CY, et al. Optimal cut-off values for obesity: using simple anthropometric indices to predict cardiovascular disease risk factors in Taiwan. Int J Obes Relat Metab Disord 2002; 26:1232–1238.

40. Japanese Society for the Study of Obesity. The Examination Committee of Criteria for "Obesity Disease" in Japan. Circulation J 2002; 66:987–992.
41. Hara K, Yokoyama T, Matsushita Y, Tanaka H, Horikoshi M, Kadowaki T, Yoshike N. A proposal for the cutoff point of waist circumference for the diagnosis of metabolic syndrome in the Japanese population. Diabetes Care 2006; 29:1123–1124.
42. Alberti KGMM, Zimmet P, Shaw J for the IDF Epidemiology Task Force Consensus Group. The metabolic syndrome-a new worldwide definition. Lancet 2005; 366:1059–1062.
43. Ford ES. Prevalence of the metabolic syndrome defined by the International Diabetes Federation among adults in the U.S. Diabetes Care 2005; 28:2745–2749.
44. Lorenzo C, Villena A, Serrano-Rios M, et al. Diabetes Care 2006; 29:685–691.
45. Deepa M, Farooq S, Datta M, Deepa R, Mohan V. Prevalence of metabolic syndrome using WHO, ATP III and IDF definitions in Asian Indians: the Chennai urban rural epidemiology study. Diab Metab Res Rev 2006:22. In press.
46. Reaven G. The metabolic syndrome or the insulin resistance syndrome? Different names, different concepts, and different goals. Endocrinol Metab Clin North Am 2004; 33:283–303.
47. Eckel RH, Grundy SM, Zimmet PZ. The metabolic syndrome. Lancet 2005; 365:1415–1428.
48. Lebovitz HE, Banerji MA. Point: visceral adiposity is causally related to insulin resistance. Diabetes Care 2005; 28:2322–2325.
49. Miles JM, Jensen MD. Counterpoint: visceral adiposity is not causally related to insulin resistance. Diabetes Care 2005; 28:2326–2328.
50. Kahn R. The metabolic syndrome (emperor) wears no clothes. Diabetes Care 2006; 29:1693–1696.
51. Grundy SM. Metabolic syndrome: connecting and reconciling cardiovascular and diabetes worlds. J Am Coll Cardiol 2006; 47:1093–1100.
52. Yusuf S, Hawken S, Ounpuu S, et al. Obesity and the risk of myocardial infarction in 27,000 participants from 52 countries: a case-control study. Lancet 2005; 366:1640–1649.
53. Wilson PWF, D'Agostino RB, Parise H, Sullivan L, Meigs JB. Metabolic syndrome as a precursor of cardiovascular disease and Type 2 diabetes mellitus. Circulation 2005; 112:3066–3072.
54. Ford ES. Risks for all-cause mortality, cardiovascular disease, and diabetes associated with the metabolic syndrome. Diabetes Care 2005; 28:1769–1778.
55. Hillier TA, Rousseau A, Lange C, et al. Practical way to assess metabolic syndrome using a continuous score obtained from principal components analysis. Diabetologia 2006; 49:1528–1535.

2

Epidemiology and Cardiovascular Disease Risk Assessment in the Metabolic Syndrome

Nathan D. Wong

Heart Disease Prevention Program, Department of Medicine, Division of Cardiology, School of Medicine, University of California–Irvine, Irvine, California, U.S.A.

SUMMARY

■ The metabolic syndrome is present in nearly 40% of U.S. adults; its prevalence varies substantially according to the definition used as well as population and ethnic group studied. In the United States, Hispanics have the highest prevalence among major ethnic groups.

■ The metabolic syndrome, even in the absence of diabetes, is associated with an increased risk of cardiovascular disease, stroke, and total mortality, and is related to an increased risk for the development of diabetes.

■ Initial evaluation of coronary artery disease risk in metabolic syndrome subjects without diabetes involves global risk estimation using Framingham or other algorithms for risk prediction.

■ Screening for novel risk factors such as C-reactive protein, as well as subclinical atherosclerosis (from carotid ultrasound, computed tomography, or ankle-brachial index), can refine the estimation of cardiovascular disease risk.

■ The American Heart Association and U.S. National Heart, Lung, and Blood Institute have recently released revised guidelines for the diagnosis and clinical management of the metabolic syndrome, which include treatment goals based in part on global risk assessment and evidence of subclinical atherosclerosis.

INTRODUCTION

The metabolic syndrome is a clustering of risk factors known to promote or increase the risk of development of cardiovascular disease (CVD). Recent estimates show that approximately one-third of the adult population of developed countries are characterized by metabolic syndrome, by different definitions. The metabolic syndrome, even in the absence of diabetes, is associated with an increased risk of CVD and total mortality, and is related to an increased risk of the development of diabetes. Those with diabetes are considered a cardiovascular risk equivalent and warrant aggressive management of underlying risk factors to optimize prevention of CVD. Initial evaluation of coronary artery disease risk involves global risk estimation using Framingham or other algorithms for risk prediction. The UKPDS risk engine is suitable for use in subjects with preexisting diabetes. Further, consideration of screening for novel risk factors such as C-reactive protein, as well as subclinical atherosclerosis (from carotid ultrasound, computed tomography, or ankle-brachial index), can further refine the estimation of future CVD risk. The presence of subclinical atherosclerosis or elevated levels of C-reactive protein can potentially modify recommended treatment goals for lipid and other cardiovascular risk factors.

PREVALENCE AND EPIDEMIOLOGY

The metabolic syndrome is a constellation of interrelated risk factors of metabolic origin that appears to directly promote the development of atherosclerotic CVD. The contributing risk factors most widely recognized include atherogenic dyslipidemia, elevated blood pressure, and elevated plasma glucose. Recent data on adults in the U.S. during 1999 to 2002 show a prevalence (age-adjusted) of the metabolic syndrome of 34.4% among men and 34.5% among women, using the National Cholesterol Education Program (NCEP) definition; and with higher estimates of 40.7% and 37.1%, respectively, using the International Diabetes

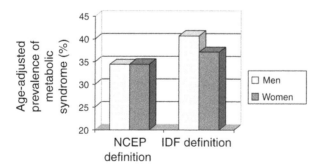

Figure 1 Prevalence of metabolic syndrome by NCEP and IDF definitions, U.S. Adults, National Health and Nutrition Examination Survey 1999–2002. *Abbreviations*: NCEP, National Cholesterol Education Program; IDF, International Diabetes Federation. *Source*: Adapted from Ref. 1.

Federation (IDF) definition (Fig. 1) (1). Earlier data among U.S. adults examined during 1988 to 1994 show a substantially lower prevalence of approximately 25% (2). Moreover, in comparing increases in prevalence from 1988–1994 to 1999–2000 among U.S. adults, Ford et al. (3) noted increases in prevalence to be most dramatic among women (increase of 23.5% during this time period) and attributable primarily to increases in high blood pressure, waist circumference, and hypertriglyceridemia.

Wide variations in the prevalence of the metabolic syndrome are observed across ethnic groups within the United States and among other parts of the world, and depend on the definition used. In a large U.K. population–based study, South Asians had the highest prevalence of the metabolic syndrome (29% in men and 32% in women using the NCEP definition) and European women the lowest (14%) (4); and in a large study involving 11 European cohorts, prevalence using a modified World Health Organization (WHO) definition was slightly higher in men (15.7%) than in women (14.2%) (5). Among nearly 10,000 adults in Greece, age-adjusted prevalences of metabolic syndrome were shown to be 24.5% using the NCEP ATP III definition versus 43.4% using the IDF definition (6). Lower prevalence rates were recently noted using the ATP III definition among 2100 Italian adults: 18% in women and 15% in men (7).

Ethnicity-specific data among U.S. adults from the most recent National Health and Nutrition Examination Survey (NHANES) 2001–2002 surveys show the highest prevalence among Mexican Americans, but prevalence among African Americans, in particular males, is lower than in whites (Fig. 2) (1). In the Mexico City Diabetes Study, some of the highest prevalences are noted; the most recent prevalence estimates from 1997 to 1999 show 39.9% of men and 59.9% of women to have the metabolic syndrome, representing little change from 1990 to 1992 among men (38.9%), but a decrease in women (65.4%). Increases in prevalence were attributed to elevated waist circumference, elevated fasting glucose, and

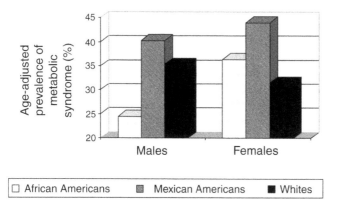

Figure 2 Prevalence of metabolic syndrome by ethnicity and gender, U.S. Adults, National Health and Nutrition Examination Survey 1999–2002. *Source*: Adapted from Ref. 1.

low levels of high-density lipoprotein cholesterol (HDL-C) (8). These data, however, contrast with a nationwide study in Mexico involving 2158 men and women aged 20 to 69 years, where the age-adjusted prevalence of the metabolic syndrome was noted to be 13.6% using WHO criteria and 26.6% using the NCEP ATP III definition (and 9.2% and 21.4%, respectively, among those without diabetes) (9). Among Asian populations, lower prevalences are generally noted. Among Hong Kong Chinese, metabolic syndrome prevalence was noted to be 9.6% using the NCEP definition and 13.4% using the WHO definition (10). Higher prevalences were more recently noted among Hong Kong Chinese in another study: 16.7% using the NCEP definition, but 21.2% if incorporating lower waist circumference criteria recommended for Asians by the WHO (≥80 cm for men and (90 cm for women) (11). Among 1230 Korean adults aged 30 to 79 years, the prevalence of the metabolic syndrome according to modified WHO criteria was 21.8% in men and 19.4% in women; however, this increased to 34.2% in men and 38.7% in women using the modified NCEP definition (12). Among Japanese and Mongolian adults, using ATP III criteria, metabolic syndrome prevalences were only 6% and 12%, respectively; however, these estimates did not factor in lower WHO-recommended waist circumference cut points for Asians (13).

Data are limited regarding the prevalence of the metabolic syndrome and diabetes in children and adolescents. Most of the data available have come from the United States and no such reports are available in the European Caucasian population, although the problem appears to be of a lesser magnitude there. An urgent need to establish internationally acceptable criteria for defining and screening for the metabolic syndrome in children and adolescents has been called for (14). The most recently published data among U.S. adolescents aged 12 to 19 years from the NHANES 1999–2000 shows a prevalence of the metabolic syndrome of 6.4%, using the NCEP, modified for age, compared to 4.2% in NHANES III (1988–1992). A greater prevalence was noted in male compared to female adolescents (9.1% vs. 3.7%), and 32% of overweight (based on BMI ≥ 95th percentile for age and sex) adolescents had the metabolic syndrome (15). In a school-based cross-sectional study of 1513 black, white, and Hispanic teens, the overall prevalence of NCEP-defined metabolic syndrome was 4.2% and WHO-defined metabolic syndrome 8.4%; among obese teens, this increased to 19.5% and 38.9%, respectively. Moreover, nonwhite teens were more likely to have the metabolic syndrome defined by WHO criteria (16).

A summary of studies reporting on the prevalence of the metabolic syndrome appears in Table 1.

CARDIOVASCULAR RISK IN PERSONS WITH THE METABOLIC SYNDROME

Prediction of Cardiovascular Events and Mortality

Persons with diabetes are considered to be a coronary artery disease (CAD) risk equivalent according to the NCEP (18). In the absence of prior myocardial infarction

(MI), they have a similar risk of future cardiovascular mortality as persons with a prior MI without diabetes. The presence of both diabetes and prior MI is associated with an even higher risk of cardiovascular mortality (19). Those who have the metabolic syndrome but do not have diabetes can be shown to have a wide spectrum of risk. Applying Framingham global risk algorithms to the U.S. population with the metabolic syndrome but without diabetes identifies 45% of men and 42% of women to be at intermediate risk (10–20%) of CAD and another 20% of men and 2% of women at high risk (>20%) of CAD in the next 10 years (20). While the vast majority (>75%) of these persons have increased waist circumference, blood pressure, and triglycerides, and depressed HDL-C levels, 58% of men and 63% of women with the metabolic syndrome also have levels of low-density lipoprotein cholesterol (LDL-C) of 130 mg/dL (3.4 mmol/L) or higher (Fig. 3) (20). We have additionally shown (by statistically controlling lipids and blood pressure using Framingham risk algorithms) (20) that approximately 80% of CAD events could potentially be prevented by control of blood pressure, LDL-C, and HDL-C to optimal levels in persons with the metabolic syndrome without diabetes (Fig. 4).

Moreover, it has been recently shown that the combination of diabetes and the metabolic syndrome is associated with a much higher prevalence of CAD and even those with the metabolic syndrome in the absence of diabetes have a higher prevalence of CAD than those with diabetes who do not have the metabolic syndrome (Fig. 5) (21). Conversely, among those with preexisting atherosclerotic

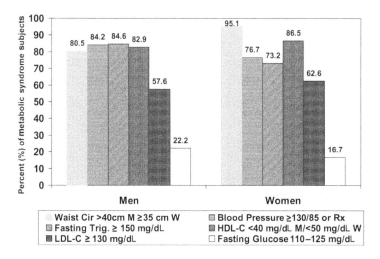

Figure 3 Prevalence of metabolic syndrome risk factors among U.S. adults with metabolic syndrome (but without diabetes), National Health and Nutrition Examination Survey 1988–1994. *Abbreviations*: HDL-C, high-density lipoprotein cholesterol; LDL-C, low-density lipoprotein cholesterol. *Source*: Adapted from Ref. 20.

Table 1 Prevalence of Metabolic Syndrome in Various Populations

References	Population	Prevalence of metabolic syndrome
1	3601 U.S. adult men and women (NHANES 1999–2002)	Age-adjusted prevalences: NCEP definition: 34.4% (men), 34.5% (women); IDF definition: 40.7% (men), 37.1% (women); NCEP definition: Whites: 35.4%(men), 31.5% (women), African Americans: 24.5% (men), 36.4% (women), Mexican Americans: 40.3% (men), 44.0% (women)
4	U.K. multiethnic adult men and women aged 40–69 yr (n = 2346 European Caucasians,1711 South Asians, and 803 African-Carribeans)	South Asians: WHO definition: 46% men, 31% women, NCEP definition: 29% men,32% women; European Caucasians: WHO definition: 19% men,9% women, NCEP definition: 18% men[A J19], 14% women
5	11 European cohorts, n = 6156 men and 5356 women aged 30–89 yr	WHO definition: 15.7% (men), 14.2% (women)
6	Greek adults, n = 9669	NCEP definition: 24.5%, IDF definition: 43.4%
7	Italian adults aged 19 yr and older (n = 2100)	NCEP definition: 18% (women), 15% (men)
8	Mexico City Diabetes Study (n = 2282 adults, 1990–1992; n = 1764, 1993–1995; n = 1754, 1997–1999)	NCEP definition: 38.9% (1990–1992), 43.4% (1993–1995), and 39.9% (1997–1999) in men and 65.4%, 65.7%, and 59.9% in women, respectively
9	Mexican adults aged 20 = 69 (nationwide population-based study, n = 2158)	WHO definition: 13.6%, NCEP definition: 26.6% (9.2% and 21.4%, respectively, in those without diabetes)
10	Hong Kong Chinese adults (n = 1513)	Modified NCEP definition (with Asian WHO waist cut points (80 cm for men and (90 cm for women: 9.6%, WHO definition: 13.4%
11	Hong Kong Chinese adults	NCEP criteria: 16.7%; Modified NCEP criteria (with Asian WHO waist cut points (80 cm for men and (90 cm for women): 21.2%

12	Korean adults aged 30–79 yr (n = 1230)	Modified WHO criteria: 21.8% men, 19.4% women; Modified NCEP criteria: 34.2% (men), 38.7% (women)
13	Japanese and Mongolian adults	NCEP criteria: 6% Japanese, 12% Mongolians
15	Adolescents aged 12–19 yr (n = 991)	Modified NCEP criteria: 4.2% (1988–1992), 6.4% (1999–2000); males 9.1%, females 3.7%
16	Adolescents (n = 1513) (school-based cross-sectional study)	NCEP definition: 4.2%, WHO definition 8.4%
17	Patients with cardiovascular morbidities	NCEP definition: overall 46%, peripheral arterial disease patients 58%, CAD patients 41%, cerebrovascular disease patients 43%, abdominal aortic aneurysm patients 47%

Abbreviations: CAD, coronary artery disease; IDF, International Diabetes Federation; NCEP, National Cholesterol Education Program; NHANES, National Health and Nutrition Examination Survey.

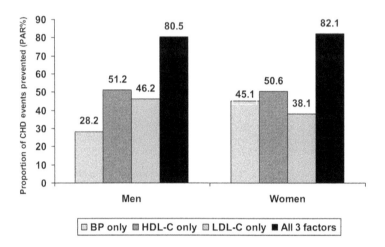

Figure 4 Proportion of CAD events potentially preventable from optimal control of BP (to <120 mmHg/<80 mmHg), LDL-C (to <100 mg/dL) and HDL-C (to >60 mg/dL) in men and women. *Abbreviations*: BP, blood pressure; LDL-C, low-density lipoprotein cholesterol; HDL-C, high-density lipoprotein cholesterol; CAD, coronary artery disease. *Source*: Adapted from Ref. 20.

vascular disease, the metabolic syndrome is highly prevalent. Among a cross-sectional survey of 1117 patients with CAD, cardiovascular disease, peripheral vascular disease, or abdominal aortic aneurysm, the overall prevalence of the metabolic syndrome was noted to be 46%: it was 58% in those with peripheral vascular disease, 41% in those with CAD, 43% in those with CVD, and 47% in those with abdominal aortic aneurysm. Moreover, age did not impact on these prevalences (17).

In a recently published meta-analysis of risks for all-cause mortality, CVD, and diabetes, Ford (22) noted that among studies that used the exact NCEP definition of the metabolic syndrome, relative risks [and 95% confidence intervals (CI)] associated with the metabolic syndrome were 1.27 (0.90–1.78) for all-cause mortality, 1.65 (1.38–1.99) for CVD, and 2.99 (1.96–4.57) for diabetes. For the WHO definition, corresponding estimates were 1.37 (1.09–1.74), 1.93 (1.39–2.67), and 2.60 (1.55–4.38), respectively. The authors concluded population-attributable fractions of the metabolic syndrome to be 6% to 7% for all-cause mortality, 12% to 17% for CVD, and 30% to 52% for diabetes.

We recently demonstrated in the U.S. population of men and women a twofold greater risk of mortality from CAD and CVD in persons with the metabolic syndrome; even those with the metabolic syndrome but without diabetes and those with only one or two metabolic syndrome risk factors were at an increased risk of death from CAD and CVD. Increased risks associated with the metabolic syndrome held similarly for men as they did for women. Moreover,

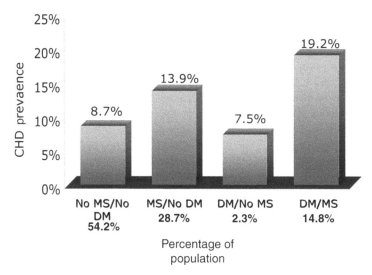

Figure 5 Prevalence of coronary artery disease by presence/absence of metabolic syndrome and diabetes, U.S. Adults, National Health and Nutrition Examination Survey 1988–1994. *Source*: Adapted from Ref. 21.

those with diabetes had a similar risk of future mortality as those with preexisting CVD. Those with both diabetes and preexisting CVD had the highest risk (Fig. 6) (23).

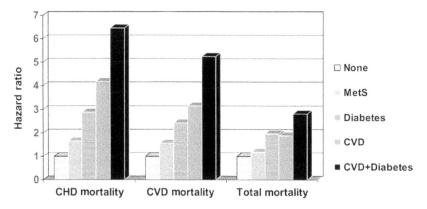

Figure 6 CVD and total mortality in U.S. men and women ages 30 to 74: age, gender, and risk-factor adjusted Cox regression, National Health and Nutrition Examination Survey II follow-up ($n = 6255$). In comparison to those with neither metabolic syndrome, diabetes, nor CVD, Metabolic syndrome: $p < 0.05$ for CAD mortality and $p < 0.01$ for CVD mortality; diabetes, CVD, and CVD plus diabetes: $p < 0.001$ for CAD, CVD, and total mortality. *Abbreviations*: CVD, cardiovascular disease; CAD, coronary artery disease. *Source*: Adapted from Ref. 23.

In the large meta-analysis of 11 prospective European cohort studies (5) involving 6156 men and 5356 women without diabetes aged 30 to 89 years and followed for a median of 8.8 years, the hazard ratios (HRs) for all-cause and cardiovascular mortality were 1.44 (95% CI = 1.17–1.84) and 2.26 (1.61–3.17), respectively, in men and 1.38 (1.02–1.87) and 2.78 (1.57–4.94), respectively, in women. These observations are consistent with other reports documenting the prognostic importance of the metabolic syndrome among 6447 men in the West of Scotland study where it predicted both incident diabetes (HR = 3.50, 95% CI = 2.51–4.90) and CAD events (HR = 1.30, 95% CI = 1.00–1.67) (24), and among 1209 Finish men followed for 11.4 years, increased CVD mortality (2.6 to 4.2–fold increased risk depending on definition used) and total mortality (1.9 to 3.3–fold increased risk depending on definition used) (25).

Other U.S. population–based studies have also demonstrated a relation of the metabolic syndrome to cardiovascular event risk. In the Framingham Offspring Study, Rutter et al. (26) showed an age, sex, and CRP-adjusted HR for the metabolic syndrome of 1.8 (95% CI = 1.4–2.5) for predicting incident CVD events over seven years. Moreover, among 12,089 black and white middle-aged individuals in the Atherosclerosis Risk in Communities (ARIC) study, where the metabolic syndrome was found to be prevalent in 23% of those without diabetes or prevalent CVD at baseline, over an average 11 years of follow-up, those with versus without the metabolic syndrome were 1.5 to 2 times more likely to develop CAD in risk factor–adjusted analyses. However, the metabolic syndrome did not improve risk prediction beyond that achieved by the Framingham risk score (27). In 2175 elderly subjects in the Cardiovascular Health Study, the metabolic syndrome defined by the ATP III but not WHO criteria was associated with a significant 38% increased risk (HR = 1.38, 95% CI = 1.06–1.79) of coronary or cerebrovascular events (28). In the San Antonio Heart Study (29), among 2815 subjects aged 24 to 64 years, the NCEP metabolic syndrome definition predicted all-cause mortality (multivariable HR = 1.47, 95% CI = 1.13–1.92), but not the WHO metabolic syndrome definition; among those without diabetes or prior CVD, the NCEP metabolic syndrome definition predicted only cardiovascular mortality (HR = 2.01, 95% CI = 1.13–3.57); there was evidence also for stronger relations of the metabolic syndrome with cardiovascular mortality in women compared to men. Also, among a large, primarily healthy cohort of 19,223 men who underwent a clinical examination and fitness examination, adjusted relative risks for all-cause and cardiovascular mortality were 1.29 (1.05–1.57) and 1.89 (1.36–2.60), respectively among those with versus without metabolic syndrome (30). Additional adjustment for cardiorespiratory fitness, however, resulted in associations being no longer significant. Finally, among the largest and most recently reported population-based studies, among 10,950 men in the Multiple Risk Factor Intervention Trial (MRFIT) (31), modified NCEP–defined metabolic syndrome was associated with increased HRs over a median of 18.4 years of follow-up for total mortality [1.21 (1.13–1.29)], CVD mortality [1.49 (1.35–1.64)], and CAD mortality [1.52 (1.34–1.70)], with elevated blood glucose and low HDL-C being the factors most predictive of CVD mortality among men with the metabolic syndrome.

A summary of studies reporting on cardiovascular events and mortality associated with the metabolic syndrome appears in Table 2.

Prediction of Stroke

The risk of stroke associated with the metabolic syndrome among subjects with preexisting CAD has recently been reported. Among 14,284 subjects with CAD, of which 26% had the metabolic syndrome, those with the metabolic syndrome but without diabetes had a 1.49-fold greater odds for ischemic stroke or transient ischemic attacks (95% CI = 1.20–1.84), whereas those with diabetes had a 2.29-fold increased odds (95% CI = 1.88–2.78); risks were higher in women than in men (32). Case–control studies have also recently reported on the association of the metabolic syndrome with stroke. In a Japanese study, among 197 stroke survivors and 356 matched controls, the metabolic syndrome was associated with a significant 3.1-fold greater odds of stroke (33). Another case–control study in Greece involving 163 stroke survivors aged 70 years and above and 166 controls, in risk factor–adjusted analyses, the metabolic syndrome was associated with a 2.6-fold greater odds of stroke (34).

Metabolic Syndrome Risks Among Subjects with Known Cardiovascular Disease

Among subjects with established CVD, the metabolic syndrome is also associated with future cardiovascular event risk. Among subjects with acute coronary syndromes within the Myocardial Ischemia Reduction with Aggressive Cholesterol Lowering (MIRACL) trial, 38% of patients met the criteria for the metabolic syndrome; those with the metabolic syndrome had a HR of 1.49 (95% CI = 1.24–1.79) for the primary endpoint of death, nonfatal MI, cardiac arrest, or recurrent unstable myocardial ischemia (35). Within the GISSI-Prevenzione Trial among 11,232 patients with a prior MI, those with the metabolic syndrome had a 29% greater risk of death and 23% greater risk of major cardiovascular events; these risks were amplified in diabetic patients (68% and 47%, respectively) (36). Finally, of interest are data from the Scandinavian Simvastatin Survival Study (4S), which showed, among 3933 nondiabetic subjects with known CAD, that those with the metabolic syndrome have at least as great a reduction (if not greater) in the risk of total mortality (relative risk 0.54), coronary mortality (relative risk 0.39), or major CAD events (relative risk 0.59) as those without the metabolic syndrome (0.72, 0.62, and 0.71, respectively) (37).

GLOBAL RISK ASSESSMENT IN THE METABOLIC SYNDROME AND DIABETES

Given these observations, intensified efforts to screen and adequately treat persons with the metabolic syndrome are needed. The NCEP (18) has provided a

Table 2 Studies Examining Relation of Metabolic Syndrome to Cardiovascular Events and Mortality

References	Population	Findings
22	Meta-analysis of prospective studies from 1998 to 2004, variable length of follow-up	NCEP definition: RR[a] = 1.27 (0.90–1.78) for all-cause mortality, 1.65 (1.38–1.99) for CVD, and 2.99 (1.96–4.57) for diabetes; WHO definition: 1.37 (1.09–1.74) for all-cause mortality, 1.93 (1.39–2.67) for CVD, 2.60 (1.55–4.38) for CAD
23	6255 subjects aged 30–75 yr (representing 64 million U.S. adults), NHANES II follow-up study, 13.3 yr follow-up	NCEP metabolic syndrome definition: multivariable HRs: 2.02 (1.42–2.89) CAD mortality, 1.82 (1.40–2.37) for CVD mortality, 1.40 (1.19–1.66) for total mortality
5	11 prospective European cohort studies (n = 6156 men and 5356 women), variable length of follow-up	Modified WHO definition: multivariable HRs: men: 1.44 (1.17–1.84) all-cause mortality, 2.26 (1.61–3.17) cardiovascular mortality; women: 1.38 (1.02–1.87) all-cause mortality, 2.78 (1.57–4.94) cardiovascular mortality
24	6447 men, West of Scotland Coronary Prevention Study, 4.9 yr follow-up	NCEP definition: HR = 1.76 (1.44–2.15) for CAD events and 3.50 (2.51–4.90) for diabetes; multivariable HR for CAD events 1.30 (1.00–1.67)
25	1209 Finnish men (Kuopio Ischemic Heart Disease Risk Factor Study), 11.4 yr follow-up	NCEP definition: multivariable HR = 2.9 (1.2–7.2) to 4.2 (1.6–10.8) for CAD mortality; WHO definition: multivariable HR = 2.9 (1.2–6.8) to 3.3 (1.4–7.7) for CAD mortality, 2.6 (1.4–5.1) to 3.0 (1.5–5.7) for CVD mortality, and 1.9 (1.2–3.0) to 2.1 (1.3–3.3) for all-cause mortality
26	3037 men and women, Framingham Offspring Study, 7 yr follow-up	Age, sex, and CRP-adjusted HR for metabolic syndrome: 1.8 (1.4–2.5)
27	12,089 Black and White adults (Atherosclerosis Risk in Communities study), 11 yr follow-up	NCEP definition: relative risks for CAD 1.5 (men) and 2 (women)

28	2175 elderly adults free of CVD at baseline (Cardiovascular Health Study), 4.1 yr follow-up	NCEP criteria: HR for coronary or cerebrovascular events 1.38 (1.06–1.79). No relation of metabolic syndrome to events with WHO criteria
29	2815 men and women aged 24–64 yr, San Antonio Heart Study, 12.7 yr follow-up	All-cause mortality multivariable HR = 1.47 (1.13–1.92) for NCEP definition and 1.27 (0.97–1.66) for WHO definition. CVD mortality: NCEP definition: 4.65 (2.35–9.21) for women and 1.82 (1.14–2.91) for men; WHO definition: 2.83 (1.55–5.17) for women and 1.15 (0.72–1.86) for men
30	19,223 men aged 20 to 83 yr, variable follow-up time	RR for all-cause mortality 1.29 (1.05–1.57) and for CVD mortality 1.89 (1.36–2.60)
31	10,950 men, Multiple Risk Factor Intervention Trial, median 18.4 yr of follow-up	Modified NCEP definition: adjusted HRs for: total mortality 1.21 (1.13–1.29), CVD mortality 1.49 (1.35–1.64), and CAD mortality 1.51 (1.34–1.70)

[a]95% confidence intervals in parenthesis.

Abbreviations: CAD, coronary artery disease; CRP, C-reactive protein; CVD, cardiovascular disease; HR, hazard ratio; NCEP, National Cholesterol Education Program; NHANES, National Health and Nutrition Examination Survey; RR, relative risk.

clinically useful definition of the metabolic syndrome, which has been widely disseminated through the medical community and has been recently updated (38). Recently, investigators have shown this definition to be robust, predicting CVD events in a manner similar to that of the WHO definition, which differs from the NCEP definition in that it requires glucose intolerance or hyperinsulinemia as one of the required criteria (29). Moreover, the IDF has recently proposed a definition requiring abdominal obesity by waist circumference thresholds (including lower cut points for Asians and European whites) plus two other criteria (same as NCEP criteria) (39).

In persons with the metabolic syndrome who do not have diabetes, initial evaluation of risk can utilize determination of Framingham risk scores (Fig. 7) (18), given the significant heterogeneity in estimated risk of persons with the metabolic syndrome. Older persons or those who are smokers or have increased total or LDL-C levels, even if only minimal elevations of defined metabolic syndrome risk factors are present, may be at an intermediate or higher risk of CAD. Also, one critical caveat in the use of Framingham risk or other global risk algorithms is that they often do not include critical metabolic syndrome risk factors such as fasting glucose or elevated triglycerides, which while possibly not providing additive predictive value in a *general* population, could be critically important in stratifying risk in those with the metabolic syndrome. Therefore, in situations where a calculated global risk score results in a borderline figure (e.g., 18–19%, 10-year risk), the presence of significant metabolic risk factors not included in the global-risk algorithm may warrant the individual being stratified to a higher risk stratum (e.g., >20% or CAD–risk equivalent status in this case). A recent scientific statement on the clinical management of the metabolic syndrome released by the American Heart Association and National Heart, Lung, and Blood Institute (NHLBI) (36) noted, however, that the Framingham algorithms do capture most of the risks for CVD in persons with the metabolic syndrome and that adding obesity, triglycerides, and fasting glucose does not appear to increase the power of prediction.

For those with diabetes, the United Kingdom Prospective Diabetes Study (UKPDS) in 2001 developed a risk engine based on data from 4540 male and female patients with diabetes for predicting the risk of new CAD events. Unlike previously published equations, this model was diabetes-specific and incorporated glycemia, systolic blood pressure, and lipid levels in addition to age, sex, ethnic group, smoking status, and time since diagnosis of diabetes (40). Recent reports have examined the performance of this risk engine in relation to the Joint British Societies (JBS) risk calculator (41) and the earlier version of the Framingham risk equations that incorporated diabetes status (42). Among 700 Type 2 diabetes patients, the UKPDS risk calculator identified a higher mean 10-year CAD risk (21.5%) than the JBS risk calculator (18.3%) (39). The more recent report compared the ability of UKPDS to the Framingham risk equation to predict events that actually occurred among 428 subjects with newly diagnosed Type 2 diabetes followed for a median of 4.2 years. The Framingham risk equations significantly underestimated the overall number of cardiovascular events by 33% and coronary

Estimate of 10-Year Risk for **Men**
(Framingham Point Scores)

Age, y	Points
20-34	-9
35-39	-4
40-44	0
45-49	3
50-54	6
55-59	8
60-64	10
65-69	11
70-74	12
75-79	13

Total Cholesterol, mg/dL	Points				
	Age 20-39 y	Age 40-49 y	Age 50-59 y	Age 60-69 y	Age 70-79 y
<160	0	0	0	0	0
160-199	4	3	2	1	0
200-239	7	5	3	1	0
240-279	9	6	4	2	1
≥280	11	8	5	3	1

	Points				
	Age 20-39 y	Age 40-49 y	Age 50-59 y	Age 60-69 y	Age 70-79 y
Nonsmoker	0	0	0	0	0
Smoker	8	5	3	1	1

HDL, mg/dL	Points
≥60	-1
50-59	0
40-49	1
<40	2

Systolic BP, mm Hg	If Untreated	If Treated
<120	0	0
120-129	0	1
130-139	1	2
140-159	1	2
≥160	2	3

Point Total	10-Year Risk, %
<0	<1
0	1
1	1
2	1
3	1
4	1
5	2
6	2
7	3
8	4
9	5
10	6
11	8
12	10
13	12
14	16
15	20
16	25
≥17	≥30

Estimate of 10-Year Risk for **Women**
(Framingham Point Scores)

Age, y	Points
20-34	-7
35-39	-3
40-44	0
45-49	3
50-54	6
55-59	8
60-64	10
65-69	12
70-74	14
75-79	16

Total Cholesterol, mg/dL	Points				
	Age 20-39 y	Age 40-49 y	Age 50-59 y	Age 60-69 y	Age 70-79 y
<160	0	0	0	0	0
160-199	4	3	2	1	1
200-239	8	6	4	2	1
240-279	11	8	5	3	2
≥280	13	10	7	4	2

	Points				
	Age 20-39 y	Age 40-49 y	Age 50-59 y	Age 60-69 y	Age 70-79 y
Nonsmoker	0	0	0	0	0
Smoker	9	7	4	2	1

HDL, mg/dL	Points
≥60	-1
50-59	0
40-49	1
<40	2

Systolic BP, mm Hg	If Untreated	If Treated
<120	0	0
120-129	1	3
130-139	2	4
140-159	3	5
≥160	4	6

Point Total	10-Year Risk, %
<9	<1
9	1
10	1
11	1
12	1
13	2
14	2
15	3
16	4
17	5
18	6
19	8
20	11
21	14
22	17
23	22
24	27
≥25	≥30

Figure 7 Estimation of 10-year risk of coronary artery disease. *Source*: From Ref. 18.

events by 32%, compared with a lower and nonsignificant underestimation of CAD events of 13% by the UKPDS risk engine, although both performed similarly in terms of discrimination and calibration for a 15% 10-year CAD risk threshold (42).

ASSESSMENT OF NOVEL RISK FACTORS FOR ENHANCING RISK EVALUATION

There is interest as to whether the addition of newer risk factors such as C-reactive protein (CRP), fibrinogen, and small dense LDL will further add to predicting risk in persons with the metabolic syndrome. In the Nurses' Health Study, Ridker et al. showed that among those with the metabolic syndrome, age-adjusted incidence rates of future CVD events were 3.4 and 5.9 per 1000 person-years for those with CRP levels of ≤3 and >3 mg/L, with additive effects of higher CRP levels also seen for those with four to five metabolic syndrome risk factors (43). Framingham investigators recently reported that CRP levels provide additive value over the metabolic syndrome in predicting CVD events (26). In addition, we have recently published in the NHANES 1999–2000 sample that those with increased CRP levels and the metabolic syndrome have a similar odds of CVD as those with diabetes who have low CRP levels, and those with diabetes and high CRP levels to be at the highest odds of CVD (Fig. 8) (44). A similar report we have published also shows an enhanced likelihood of peripheral arterial disease in U.S. adults with the metabolic syndrome and diabetes who have elevated CRP levels (45). Moreover, it has been recommended that CRP be considered a criterion for that metabolic syndrome and incorporated into the coronary risk score (46), and its measurement in such individuals may be appropriate given the American Heart Association/Centers for Disease Control guidelines for measurement of CRP among persons at intermediate global risk of CVD (47). The role of other novel risk markers such as fibrinogen,

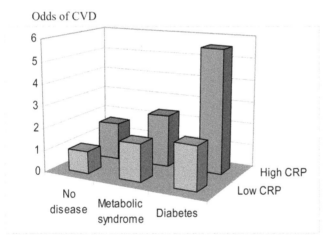

Figure 8   Odds of CVD in those with metabolic syndrome (without diabetes) or Diabetes Mellitus (DM), stratified by CRP levels (low, <1 mg/L; intermediate, 1–3 mg/L; and high, >3 mg/L) from National Health and Nutrition Examination Survey 1999–2000 data. Compared to those with neither Metabolic syndrome nor DM and low CRP, odds for CVD = 1.99 ($p < 0.05$) for those with no disease and high CRP, 2.67 ($p < 0.05$) for those with Metabolic syndrome and intermediate CRP, 3.33 ($p < 0.0001$) for those with Metabolic syndrome and high CRP, 3.21 ($p < 0.05$) if DM and low CRP, 6.01 ($p < 0.001$) for DM and intermediate CRP, and 7.73 ($p < 0.001$) for those with DM and high CRP. *Abbreviations*: DM, diabetes; CRP, C-reactive protein; CVD, cardiovascular disease. *Source*: Adapted from Ref. 44.

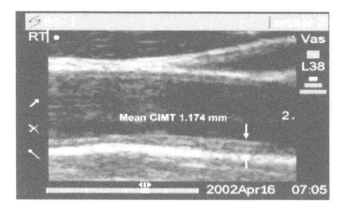

Figure 9 Example of carotid B-mode ultrasound showing increased carotid intimal medial thickness.

interleukin-1 (IL-1), IL-6, and adiponectin levels in providing additive risk stratification in persons with the metabolic syndrome needs to be established.

SCREENING FOR SUBCLINICAL ATHEROSCLEROSIS

The presence of subclinical atherosclerosis such as carotid ultrasound intimal medial thickness (IMT) (Fig. 9) (48), ankle-brachial index (49,50), or coronary artery calcium (CAC) (Fig. 10) (51–55) may also identify individuals with a

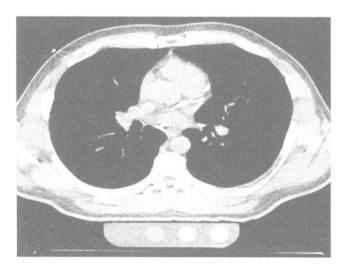

Figure 10 Example of computed tomography scan showing significant coronary artery calcium (score >400).

higher cardiovascular risk based on their demonstrated independent prognostic value. This may have important implications for persons with the metabolic syndrome, given the uncertainty of risk assessment on the basis of global risk assessment alone. Given recent recommendations to target atherosclerosis screening for those at intermediate global risk of CAD (defined as 6–20% risk in 10 years) (56), whereby those found to have clinically significant atherosclerosis could have their risk level "stratified upwards," e.g., reclassifying an intermediate risk individual as high risk, such screening may have implications for refining risk assessment in many persons with the metabolic syndrome. Although such screening in persons with diabetes could also offer improved risk stratification, since diabetes is considered a CAD risk equivalent and aggressive treatment guidelines already exist for those with diabetes, such evaluation is not normally recommended for those with diabetes (56).

We have demonstrated previously (57) the presence of the metabolic syndrome to be independently associated with an increased likelihood of CAC (compared to those without the metabolic syndrome), and those with diabetes to have the highest likelihood of CAC. Moreover, the prevalence of calcium among women with the metabolic syndrome was as high as in those with diabetes. Metabolic syndrome without diabetes was independently associated with an increased likelihood of CAC. Similarly, the NHLBI Family Heart Study has shown the metabolic syndrome to be independently associated with an increased likelihood of CAC and abdominal aortic calcification in both men and women after adjustment for other risk factors (58). Noteworthy is that approximately 40% of persons with the metabolic syndrome (but without diabetes) would be identified by global risk assessment showing >20% 10-year risk of CAD and/or would have CAC levels at or above the 75th percentile for age and gender (57), a level that has been indicated by the NCEP (18) to warrant more aggressive intervention [e.g., treating to a goal LDL-C of <100 mg/dL (2.6 mmol/L) instead of <130 mg/dL (3.4 mmol/L) as would be the case for most intermediate risk patients]. This suggests that potentially 40% of such individuals with the metabolic syndrome (but without diabetes) may be candidates for more aggressive risk factor management (e.g., as a CAD risk equivalent). Moreover, others have shown the metabolic syndrome to be associated with the prevalence and quantity of CAC, even after adjustment for 10-year Framingham CAD risk (59), further suggesting the potential utility of subclinical disease screening over global risk assessment. We have also shown that among persons with metabolic abnormalities (the metabolic syndrome or diabetes), there is an increased likelihood of myocardial ischemia from nuclear SPECT testing (60) at intermediate levels of CAC (e.g., 100–399) that is similar to those without such abnormalities who have higher levels of CAC (e.g., 400 or more).

Others have also examined the relation of the metabolic syndrome to other measures of subclinical atherosclerosis. In a random sample of 1153 French adults aged 35 to 65 years, the presence of metabolic syndrome was independently associated with the number of carotid and femoral plaques, carotid IMT, and pulse wave velocity, with odds ratios ranging from 1.80 to 2.15 using the NCEP definition and 1.48 to 1.97 when using the WHO definition (61). A recently published investigation from the aforementioned ARIC study showed a stepwise gradient in left ventricular mass by increasing number of metabolic syndrome disorders (none, any one, any two, and all three of the following: hypertension, dyslipidemia, and glucose intolerance) in both men and women (62). Also in a separate investigation of 14,502 black and white subjects in the ARIC study, comparing those with versus without metabolic syndrome, both prevalence of CAD (7.4% vs. 3.6%) as well as average carotid IMT (747 vs. 704 mm) were significantly greater in those with versus without metabolic syndrome (63). Finally, even among nondiabetic young subjects from the Bogalusa Heart Study ($n = 507$), composite carotid IMT increased significantly with the number of metabolic syndrome components present, and metabolic syndrome predicted composite carotid IMT (75th percentile by receiver operator curve characteristic (ROC) curves (64).

CONCLUSIONS

The metabolic syndrome is associated with an increased risk of future diabetes, CVD, and total mortality. While persons with diabetes are regarded as having CAD risk equivalence warranting aggressive clinical management, a wide spectrum of global risk is present in persons with metabolic syndrome (but without diabetes), necessitating careful assessment of cardiovascular risk. While initial global risk assessment utilizing Framingham or other risk algorithms is appropriate, consideration of novel risk markers and screening for subclinical atherosclerosis may improve risk stratification and identify those at greatest risk for future CVD events and mortality.

Both primary care and subspecialty physicians should regularly assess for the presence of multiple risk factors as well as metabolic syndrome at regular intervals in each patient, given the presence of metabolic syndrome in such a high proportion of middle-aged and older adults. Identification of metabolic syndrome will also get physicians accustomed to simultaneous treatment of multiple risk factors (particularly abdominal obesity, dyslipidemia, and elevated blood pressure), instead of the traditional model of treatment of risk factors in isolation. Most importantly, intensified efforts at lifestyle therapies including effective dietary and physical activity counseling done by trained individuals who can provide the necessary guidance and follow-up are needed and crucial if a significant impact is to be made on metabolic syndrome and its future complications.

REFERENCES

1. Ford ES. Prevalence of the metabolic syndrome defined by the International Diabetes Federation among adults in the U.S. Diabetes Care 2005; 28:2745–2749.
2. Ford ES et al. Prevalence of the metabolic syndrome in U.S. adults. JAMA 2002; 287:356–359.
3. Ford ES, Giles WHO, Mokdad AH. Increasing prevalence of the metabolic syndrome among U.S. adults. Diabetes Care 2004; 27:2444–2449.

4. Tillin T, Forhouhi N, Johnston DG, et al. Metabolic syndrome and coronary heart disease in South Asians, African-Caribbeans and white Europeans: a UK population-based cross-sectional study. Dibetologia 2005; 48:649–656.
5. Hu G, Qiao Q, Tuomilehto J, et al. Prevalence of the metabolic syndrome and its relation to all-cause and cardiovascular mortality in nondiabetic European men and women. Arch Intern Med 2004; 164:1066–1076.
6. Athyros VG, Ganotakis ES, Elisaf M, Mikhailidis DP. The prevalence of the metabolic syndrome using the National Cholesterol Education Program and International Diabetes Federation definitions. Curr Med Res Opin 2005; 21:1157–1159.
7. Miccoli R, Bianchi C, Odoguardi L, et al. Prevalence of the metabolic syndrome among Italian adults according to the ATP III definition. Nutr Metab Cardiovasc Dis 2005; 15:250–254.
8. Lorenzo C, Williams K, Gonzalez-Villalpando C, Haffner SM. The prevalence of the metabolic syndrome did not increase in Mexico City between 1990-1992 and 1997-1999 despite more central obesity. Diabetes Care 2005; 28:2480–2485.
9. Aguilar-Salinas CA, Rojas R, Gomez-Perez FJ, et al. High prevalence of metabolic syndrome in Mexico. Arch Med Res 2004; 35:76–81.
10. Ko GT, Cockram CS, Chow CC, et al. High prevalence of metabolic syndrome in Hong Kong Chinese-comparison of three diagnostic criteria. Diab Res Clin Pract 2005; 69:160–168.
11. Thomas GN, Ho SY, Janus ED, Lam KS, Hedley AJ, Lam TH. The US National Cholesterol Education Program Adult Treatment Panel III (NCEP ATP III) prevalence of the metabolic syndrome in a Chinese population. Diab Res Clin Pract 2005; 67:251–257.
12. Choi SH, Ahn CW, Cha BS, et al. The prevalence of the metabolic syndrome in Korean adults. Yonsei Med J 2005; 46:198–205.
13. Enkhmaa ZB, Shiwaku K, Anuurad E. Prevalence of the metabolic syndrome using the third report of the National Cholesterol Education Program Expert Panel on Detection, Evaluation, and Treatment of High Blood Cholesterol in Adults (ATP III) and the modified ATP III definitions for Japanese and Mongolians. Clin Chim Acta 2005; 352:105–113.
14. Molnar D. The prevalence of the metabolic syndrome and Type 2 diabetes mellitus in children and adolescents. Int J Obes Relat Metab Disord 2004; 28(suppl 3): S70–S74.
15. Duncan GE, Li SM, Zhou XH. Prevalence and trends of a metabolic syndrome phenotype among U.S. adolescents. Diabetes Care 2004; 27:2438–2443.
16. Goodman E, Daniels SR, Morrison JA, Huang B, Dolan LM. Contrasting prevalence of and demographic disparities in the World Health Organization and National Cholesterol Education Program Adult Treatment Panel III definitions of metabolic syndrome among adolescents. J Pediatr 2004; 145:445–451.
17. Gorter PM, Olijhoek JK, van der Graaf Y, Algra A, Rabelink TJ, Visseren FL; SMART Study Group. Prevalence of the metabolic syndrome in patients with coronary heart disease, cerebrovascular disease, peripheral arterial disease, or abdominal aortic aneurysm. Atherosclerosis 2004; 173:363–369.
18. Expert Panel on Detection, Evaluation, and Treatment of High Blood Cholesterol in Adults. Third report of the National Cholesterol Education Program (NCEP) Expert Panel on the Detection, Evaluation, and Treatment of High Blood Cholesterol in Adults (Adult Treatment Panel III): final report. Circulation 2002; 106:3143–3421.

19. Haffner SM, Lehto S, Ronnemaa T, Pyorala K, Laakso M. Mortality from coronary heart disease in subjects with Type 2 diabetes and in nondiabetic subjects with and without prior myocardial infarction. N Engl J Med 1998; 339:229–234.
20. Wong ND, Pio JR, Franklin SS, et al. Preventing coronary events by optimal control of blood pressure and lipids in patients with the metabolic syndrome. Am J Cardio 2003; 91:1421–1426.
21. Alexander CM, Landsman PB, Teutsch SM, Haffner SM. NCEP-defined metabolic syndrome, diabetes, and prevalence of coronary heart disease among NHANES III participants age 50 years and older. Diabetes 2003; 52:1210–1214.
22. Ford ES. Risks for all-cause mortality, cardiovascular disease, and diabetes associated with the metabolic syndrome: a summary of the evidence. Diabetes Care 2005; 28:1769–1778.
23. Malik S, Wong ND, Franklin SS, et al. Impact of the metabolic syndrome on mortality from coronary heart disease, cardiovascular disease, and all causes in United States adults. Circulation 2004; 110:1239–1244.
24. Sattar N, Gaw A, Scherbakova O, et al. Metabolic syndrome with and without C-reactive protein as a predictor of coronary heart disease and diabetes in the West of Scotland Coronary Prevention Study. Circulation 2003; 108:414–419.
25. Lakka HM, Laaksonen DE, Lakka TA, et al. The metabolic syndrome and total and cardiovascular mortality in middle-aged men. JAMA 2002; 288:2709–2716.
26. Rutter MK, Meigs JB, Sullivan LM, et al. C-reactive protein, the metabolic syndrome, and prediction of cardiovascular events in the Framingham Offspring Study. Circulation 2004; 110:380–385.
27. McNeill AM, Rosamond WD, Girman CJ, et al. The metabolic syndrome and 11-year incident cardiovascular disease in the atherosclerosis risk in communities study. Diabetes Care 2005; 28:385–390.
28. Scuteri A, Najjar SS, Morrell CH, Lakatta EG. The metabolic syndrome in older individuals: prevalence and prediction of cardiovascular events: the Cardiovascular Health Study. Diabetes Care 2005; 28:82–87.
29. Hunt KJ, Resendez RG, Williams K, Haffner SM, Stern MP. San Antonio Heart Study. National Cholesterol Education Program versus World Health Organization metabolic syndrome in relation to all-cause and cardiovascular mortality in the San Antonio Heart Study. Circulation 2004; 110:1251–1257.
30. Katzmarzyk PT, Church TS, Blair SN. Cardiorespiratory fitness attenuates the effects of the metabolic syndrome on all-cause and cardiovascular disease mortality. Arch Intern Med 2004; 164:1092–1097.
31. Eberly LE, Prineas R, Cohen JD, et al. Metabolic syndrome: risk factor distribution and 18-year mortality in the muiltiple risk factor intervention trial. Diabetes Care 2006; 29:123–130.
32. Koren-Morag N, Goldbourt U, Tanne D. Relation between the metabolic syndrome and ischemic stroke or transient ischemic attack: a prospective cohort study in patients with atherosclerotic cardiovascular disease. Stroke 2005; 36:1366–1371.
33. Kawamoto R, Tomita H, Oka Y, Kodama A. Metabolic syndrome as a predictor of ischemic stroke in elderly persons. Intern Med 2005; 44:922–927.
34. Milionis JH, Rizos E, Goudevenos J, Seferiadis K, Mikhailidis DP, Elisaf MS. Components of the metabolic syndrome and risk for first-ever acute ischemic nonembolic stroke in elderly subjects. Stroke 2005; 36:1372–1376.

35. Schwartz GG, Olsson AG, Szarek M, Sasiela WJ. Relation of characteristics of meta-bolic syndrome to short-term prognosis and effects of intensive statin therapy after acute coronary syndrome: an analysis of the Myocardial Ischemia Reduction with Aggressive Cholesterol Lowering (MIRACL) trial. Diabetes Care 2005;28:2508–2513.
36. Levantesi G, Macchia A, Marfisi R, et al. Metabolic syndrome and risk of cardiovas-cular events after myocardial infarction. J Am Coll Cardiol 2005; 46:277–283.
37. Pyorala K, Ballantyne CM, Gumbiner B, et al. Reduction of cardiovascular events by simvastatin in nondiabetic coronary heart disease patients with and without the meta-bolic syndrome: subgroup analysis of the Scandinavian Simvastatin Survival Study (4S). Diabetes Care 2004; 27:1735–1740.
38. Grundy SM, Cleeman JI, Daniels SR, et al. Diagnosis and management of the meta-bolic syndrome: an American Heart Association/National Heart Lung and Blood Institute Scientific Statement. Circulation 2005; 112.
39. International Diabetes Federation. Worldwide definition of the metabolic syndrome. Available at: http://www.idf.org/webdata/docs/IDF Meta-syndrome definition.pdf. Accessed August 24, 2005.
40. Stevens RJ, Kothari V, Adler AI, Stratton IM, Holman RR; on behalf of the United Kingdom Prospective Diabetes Study (UKPDS) Group. The UKPDS risk engine: a model for the risk of coronary heart disease in Type II diabetes (UKPDS 56). Clin Sci 2001; 101:671–679.
41. Song SH, Brown PM. Coronary heart disease risk assessment in diabetes mellitus: comparison of UKPDS risk engine with Framingham risk assessment function and its clinical implications. Diabet Med 2004; 21:238–245.
42. Guzder RN, Gatling W, Mullee MA, Mehta RL, Byrne CD. Prognostic value of the Framingham cardiovascular risk equation and the UKPDS risk engine for coronary heart disease in newly diagnosed Type 2 diabetes: results from a United Kingdom study. Diabet Med 2005; 22:554–562.
43. Ridker PM, Buring JE, Cook NR, Rifai N. C-reactive protein, the metabolic syndrome, and risk of incident cardiovascular events: an 8-year follow-up of 14,719 initially healthy American women. Circulation 2003; 107:391–397.
44. Malik S, Wong ND, Franklin SS, Pio J, Fairchild C, Chen R. Cardiovascular disease in U.S. persons with metabolic syndrome, diabetes, and elevated C-reactive protein. Diabetes Care 2005; 28:690–693.
45. Vu JD, Vu JB, Pio JR, et al. Impact of C-reactive protein on the likelihood of peripheral arterial disease in United States adults with the metabolic syndrome, diabetes mellitus and pre-existing cardiovascular disease. Am J Cardiol 2005; 96:655–658.
46. Ridker PM, Wilson PW, Grundy SM. Should C-reactive protein be added to meta-bolic syndrome and to assessment of global cardiovascular risk? [review]. Circulation 2004;109:2818–2825.
47. Pearson TA, Mensah GA, Alexander RW, et al. Markers of inflammation and cardio-vascular disease: application to clinical and public health practice: a statement for healthcare professionals from the Centers for Disease Control and Prevention and the American Heart Association. Circulation 2003; 107:499–511.
48. O'Leary DH, Polak JF, Kronmal RA, et al for the Cardiovascular Health Study Collaborative Research Group: carotid-artery intima and media thickness as a risk factor for myocardial infarction and stroke in older adults. Cardiovascular Health Study Collaborative Research Group. N Engl J Med 1999; 340:14–22.

49. Criqui MH, Langer RD, Fronek A, et al: Mortality over a period of 10 years in patients with peripheral arterial disease. N Engl J Med 1992; 326:381–386.
50. Criqui MH, Langer RD, Fronek A, Feigelson HS. Coronary disease and stroke in patients with large vessel peripheral arterial disease. Drugs 1991; 42(suppl 5):16–21.
51. Wong ND, Hsu JC, Detrano RC, Diamond G, Eisenberg H, Gardin JM. Coronary artery calcium evaluation by electron beam computed tomography: relation to new cardiovascular events. Am J Cardiol 2000; 86:495–498.
52. Arad Y, Spadaro LA, Goodman K, Newstein D, Guerci AD. Prediction of coronary events with electron beam computed tomography. J Am Coll Cardiol 2000; 36:1253–1260.
53. Kondos GT, Hoff JA, Sevrukov A, et al. Electron-beam tomography coronary artery calcium and cardiac events: a 37-month follow-up of 5,635 initially asymptomatic low to intermediate-risk adults. Circulation 2003; 107:2571–2576.
54. Shaw LJ, Raggi P, Schisterman E, Berman DS, Callister TQ. Prognostic value of cardiac risk factors and coronary artery calcium for all-cause mortality. Radiology 2003; 228:826–833.
55. O'Malley PG, Taylor AJ, Jackson JL, Doherty TM, Detrano RC. Prognostic value of coronary electron-beam computed tomography for coronary heart disease events in asyptomatic populations. Am J Cardiol 2000; 85:945–948.
56. Wilson PWF, Smith SC, Blumenthal RS, Burke GL, Wong ND. Task Force #4–How do we select patients for atherosclerosis imaging? In: 34th Bethesda Conference: can atherosclerosis imaging techniques improve the detection of patients at risk for ischemic heart disease. J Am Coll Cardiol 2003; 41:1898–1906.
57. Wong ND, Sciammarella MG, Polk D, et al. The metabolic syndrome, diabetes, and subclinical atherosclerosis assessed by coronary calcium. J Am Coll Cardiol 2003; 41:1547–1553.
58. Ellison RC, Zhang Y, Wagenknect LE, et al. Relation of the metabolic syndrome to calcified atherosclerotic plaque in the coronary arteries and aorta. Am J Cardiol 2005; 95:1180–1186.
59. Kullo IJ, Cassidy AE, Peyser PA, et al. Association between metabolic syndrome and subclinical coronary atherosclerosis in asymptomatic adults. Am J Cardiol 2004; 94:1554–1558.
60. Wong ND, Rozanski AR, Gransar H, et al. Metabolic syndrome increases the likelihood of inducible myocardial ischemia among patients with subclinical atherosclerosis. Diabetes Care 2005; 28:1445–1450.
61. Ahluwalia N, Drouet L, Ruidavets JB, et al. Metabolic syndrome is associated with markers of subclinical atherosclerosis in a French population-based sample. Atherosclerosis 2005; 26. In press.
62. Burchfiel CM, Skelton TN, Andrew ME. Metabolic syndrome and echocardiographic left ventricular mass in blacks: the Atherosclerosis Risk in Communities (ARIC) Study. Atherosclerosis 2006; 186:345–353.
63. McNeill AM, Rosamond WD, Girman CJ, et al. Prevalence of coronary heart disease and carotid arterial thickening in patients with the metabolic syndrome (The ARIC Study). Am J Cardiol 2004; 94:1249–1254.
64. Tzou WS, Douglas PS, Srinivasan SR. Increased subclinical atherosclerosis in young adults with metabolic syndrome: the Bogalusa Heart Study. J Am Coll Cardiol 2005; 46:457–463.

3

Metabolic Syndrome and Type 2 Diabetes Mellitus

Ali Jawa

King Edward Medical University, Lahore, Pakistan

Vivian Fonseca

Department of Medicine, Diabetes Program, Tulane University Health Sciences Center, New Orleans, Louisiana, U.S.A.

SUMMARY

■ The insulin resistance syndrome, also known as the metabolic syndrome, is a "cluster" of cardiovascular risk factors frequently, but not always, associated with obesity.

■ Several professional organizations including WHO, NCEP ATP III, and most recently IDF have defined the metabolic syndrome based on a combination of several clinical and biological parameters.

■ Several epidemiologic studies have shown that endogenous hyperinsulinemia is an independent risk factor for cardiovascular disease (CVD). Correction of insulin resistance is clearly important in the management of Type 2 diabetes mellitus and may decrease the risk for CVD.

■ Large-vessel atherosclerosis can precede the development of diabetes, suggesting that rather than atherosclerosis being a complication of diabetes, both conditions have common genetic and environmental antecedents; i.e., they spring from a "common soil."

■ Prevention and treatment of the metabolic syndrome and Type 2 diabetes mellitus include lifestyle modifications such as weight loss, diet, and physical exercise.

- Pharmacological agents such as metformin, thiazolidinediones, acarbose, and orlistat have also been shown to be effective in selected high-risk subjects.
- In combination with lifestyle modification wherever possible, these therapies offer hope for effective prevention of Type 2 diabetes mellitus and its consequences in high-risk patients.

INTRODUCTION

For most of the 20th century, cardiovascular disease (CVD) was identified as the major cause of morbidity and mortality in the developed world. During this period, there was considerable effort to understand the underlying biology of the disease and to identify the contributing risk factors. As risk factors were identified, it became apparent that more than one major factor was often present in the same individual. Toward the end of the century, the clustering of cardiovascular risk factors was first described, most notably the simultaneous presence of obesity, Type 2 diabetes mellitus, hyperlipidemia, and hypertension (1–3). Although insulin resistance (i.e., impaired insulin-stimulated glucose uptake) as a feature of Type 2 diabetes mellitus had been first described many years earlier (4), hyperinsulinemia (5,6), hyperlipidemia (7–9), obesity (10–13), and hypertension (10,11,14) were also found to be key features of Type 2 diabetes mellitus. In addition, a cluster of heart disease risk factors seemed clearly related to Type 2 diabetes mellitus (15). This risk-factor clustering, and its association with insulin resistance, led investigators to propose the existence of a unique pathophysiological condition called the "metabolic" (1–3) or "insulin resistance" (12) syndrome. This concept was unified and extended with the landmark publication of Reaven's 1988 Banting Medal award lecture (16).

Reaven postulated that insulin resistance and its compensatory hyperinsulinemia predisposed patients to hypertension, hyperlipidemia, and diabetes mellitus and thus was the underlying cause of much CVD. Although obesity was not included in Reaven's primary list of disorders caused by insulin resistance, he acknowledged that it, too, was correlated with insulin resistance or hyperinsulinemia, and that the obvious "treatment" for what he termed "syndrome X" was weight maintenance (or weight loss) and physical activity. Reaven's seminal paper was followed by many studies documenting the clustering of cardiovascular risk factors and their relationship to insulin resistance (17–25).

Over the last decade there has been a rapid increase in the prevalence of obesity. Comorbidities of obesity include Type 2 diabetes mellitus, hypertension, and lipid abnormalities, all of which contribute to CVD and are associated with endothelial dysfunction (26). These abnormalities frequently cluster in individuals and the term "metabolic syndrome" is now used to define this cluster. The syndrome is frequently (but not invariably) associated with insulin resistance and CVD.

The purpose of this chapter is to highlight what is known about the relationship between the metabolic syndrome and Type 2 diabetes mellitus and to discuss the pathophysiological links between these conditions that may have implications for prevention and treatment.

METABOLIC SYNDROME

The insulin resistance syndrome, also known as the metabolic syndrome (the term "metabolic syndrome" has now taken hold in the medical literature), is a "cluster" of cardiovascular risk factors frequently, but not always, associated with obesity. Reaven first drew attention to the association of insulin resistance with obesity, Type 2 diabetes, high-plasma triglycerides, and low plasma levels of high-density lipoprotein (HDL) cholesterol (16). Since its original description, there has been much experimental, clinical, and epidemiological data to support the association of this syndrome with CVD (27). Factor analyses including only risk factor variables proposed to be central components of the insulin resistance syndrome predicted the risk of coronary artery disease (CAD) and stroke independently of other risk factors (28).

Additionally, other cardiovascular risk factors have been frequently included in the description of the syndrome. These include inflammation, abnormal fibrinolysis, and endothelial dysfunction (29,30). It is unclear to what extent the components of this syndrome develop independently of each other or spring from "common soil" genetic abnormalities (31). Due to the frequent coexistence of these abnormalities, the syndrome has become a major clinical and public health problem.

VARIOUS DEFINITIONS OF METABOLIC SYNDROME

The World Health Organization (WHO) and the National Cholesterol Education Program Adult Treatment Panel III (NCEP ATP III) have attempted to define the syndrome for clinicians (Table 1) (35). Subjects identified using these clinical definitions have been shown to be at increased risk for CVD. Obesity is an independent risk factor for CVD, and is associated with elevated levels of several proinflammatory cytokines such as interleukin-6, interleukin-8, and C-reactive protein, a marker of inflammation (29). Markers of low-grade inflammation are positively associated with endothelial dysfunction in human obesity (36).

The term "metabolic syndrome" has been defined and institutionalized, principally by the WHO (32) and the Third Report of the NCEP ATP III (33,37), albeit with different definitions. In addition, other organizations including International Diabetes Federation (IDF) have developed similar, but again not identical, definitions (34,38,39). WHO, NCEP ATP III, and IDF definitions of the metabolic syndrome are listed in Table 1 (32–34). Lakka et al. (40), in a study conducted in men with the metabolic syndrome, showed that CVD and overall mortality was more consistently increased using a waist circumference criterion of 102 cm rather than 94 cm. Other investigators (41) found that reducing the

Table 1   Criteria for the Diagnosis of the Metabolic Syndrome

WHO criteria (32)	NCEP ATP III[a] criteria (33)	IDF criteria (34)
1) Hypertension: BP > 140/90 mmHg and/or on antihypertensive medication	1) Hypertension: BP ≥130/85 mmHg or on medication	1) Hypertension: BP ≥ 130/85 mmHg or on antihypertensive medication
2) Dyslipidemia: plasma triglycerides ≥(150 mg/dL (1.7 mmol/L) and/or HDL-cholesterol <35 mg/dL (0.9 mmol/L) in men and <39 mg/dL (<1.0 mmol/L) in women	2) Dyslipidemia: plasma triglycerides ≥(150 mg/dL (1.7 mmol/L), or on triglyc-erides-lowering medication; 3) HDL-cholesterol <40 mg/dL (1.03 mmol/L) in men and <50 mg/dL (1.13 mmol/L) in women, or on HDL-raising medication	2) Dyslipidemia: plasma triglycerides >150 mg/dL (1.7 mmol/L), or on triglycerides-lowering medica-tion), HDL-cholesterol <40 mg/dL (0.9 mmol/L) in males and <50 mg/dL (1.1 mmol/L) in females, or on HDL-raising medication
3) Obesity:BMI > 30 kg/m² and/or waist hip ratio >0.90 in males and >0.85 in females	4) Obesity: waist circumference ≥(102 cm (≥40 inches) in men; ≥88 cm (35 inches) in women	3) Obesity: waist circumference ≥94 cm (European men) and (80 cm (European women); ethnicity-specific values for other groups
4) Microalbuminuria (overnight urinary albumin excretion rate >20 mg/min)	5) FPG ≥ 100 mg/dL (5.6 mmol/L) or on antidiabetic therapy	4) FPG ≥100 mg/dL (5.6 mmol/L), or previously diagnosed Type 2 diabetes
WHO requires a person to have T2DM or IGT and any two of the above criteria; a person with normal glucose tolerance must demonstrate insulin resistance	NCEP requires any three of the above five criteria to be met	IDF requires a person to have: central obesity plus any two of the above four factors

[a]This later revison of the NCEP ATP III criteria is sometimes referred to as the AHA/NHLBI definition.
Abbreviations: WHO, World Health Organization; NCEP ATP III, National Cholesterol Education Program, Adult Treatment Panel III; IDF, International Diabetes Federation; HDL, high-density lipoprotein; BMI, body mass index; FPG, fasting plasma glucose; T2DM, Type 2 diabetes mellitus; IGT, impaired glucose tolerance.

threshold for impaired fasting glucose from 6.1 to 5.6 mmol/L did not materially change the hazard ratio for risk of CHD in the individuals identified. Other components of the syndrome show a continuous relationship with CVD risk (42). Although the thresholds defining the syndrome are generally derived from other well-established guidelines, we found no study that systematically examined the impact of all the metabolic syndrome thresholds on the risk of CVD, nor did we find a study that sought to optimize the positive predictive value of the definition by changing the cut points of the risk factors. Some of the criteria (e.g., waist circumference, HDL cholesterol) have sex-specific cut points, implying that the relationship between the risk factor level and outcomes differs between the sexes. However, we found no evidence that warrants establishing the sex-specific cut points used in the criteria as they relate to CVD risk. It is, for example, not known whether the same intra-abdominal fat mass carries a different risk in men than in women. An analogous argument can be made regarding whether cut points should vary according to race and ethnic groups. There is ample evidence to show that CVD risk is a function of the criteria cited in the definitions of the metabolic syndrome, but it is unjustified to assume that the optimal predictive power would be obtained by arbitrary dichotomies. Risk is a progressive function of, for example, hyperglycemia and hypertension and cannot simply be regarded as present or absent, depending on whether thresholds are exceeded or not.

Although the WHO and ATP III definitions generally identify the same individuals, important differences have been found (43,44). Ford and Giles (44) showed that in the National Health And Nutrition Examination Survey (NHANES), in a representative sample of the adult U.S. population, about the same proportions were identified as having the syndrome by the WHO or ATP III criteria (25.1% vs. 23.9%, respectively). However, 15% to 20% of individuals were classified as having the syndrome by one definition but not the other, with equal discordance. Meigs et al. (43) determined the prevalence of the syndrome, defined by ATP III or WHO criteria, in a population of non-Hispanic whites and Mexican American subjects in San Antonio and in subjects participating in the Framingham Offspring Study. Although the syndrome was common in these populations (affecting 20–30%), more Mexican American men were classified as having the syndrome using the WHO definition, whereas the ATP III criteria classified more Mexican American women. Depending on the sex and ethnicity of the populations, the prevalence of metabolic syndrome varied up to 24% between the two definitions.

Many studies have shown that patients diagnosed with the metabolic syndrome, by either the ATP III or WHO definition (or by their modifications), have an increased risk of CVD (28,40,44–48). There are three notable exceptions to the large body of evidence documenting the adverse impact of the metabolic syndrome. One is a study by Bruno et al. (49) conducted in 1565 elderly diabetic subjects from the Italian town of Casale Monferrato, who were followed for a median of eight years. At baseline, the prevalence of the metabolic syndrome was 76%, and those with the syndrome had hazard ratios for all-cause and CVD mortality that were no different from those of subjects without the syndrome. With frank diabetes of long duration, the incremental risk attributable, for example, to raised triglycerides or low HDL-cholesterol, is likely to be "swamped" by the presence of diabetes itself (50). The fact that subjects were, on average, much older (mean age at baseline: 69 years) than in virtually all other studies and that hypertension was highly prevalent in the cohort may have masked the detrimental effects of the syndrome. Another study was conducted in nondiabetic American Indians (51) and showed a nonsignificant hazard ratio for risk of CVD in those with the syndrome. The small number of events that occurred during the follow-up period, as well as several other factors reviewed by the authors, could have contributed to their borderline results. Finally, the presence of the metabolic syndrome in a cohort of women with suspected CVD who had no angiographically significant CHD did not result in an increased four-year risk of CVD, whereas the presence of the syndrome resulted in a significantly higher risk in those who were angiographically positive (52).

The IDF proposed a new definition of the metabolic syndrome in April 2005 (34). The IDF definition emphasizes central adiposity as determined by ethnic group–specific thresholds of waist circumference. Based on the IDF definition, the unadjusted prevalence of the metabolic syndrome was 39.0 ± 1.1% among all participants, 39.9 ± 1.7% among men, and 38.1 ± 1.2% among women. When the NCEP definition was applied to the study-population instead of the IDF definition, higher prevalence estimates for metabolic syndrome were observed. This increased prevalence was evident in all demograpic groups, especially among Mexican American men. Both IDF and NCEP definitions similarly, classified ~93% of the participants as having or not having the metabolic syndrome.

VARIOUS DEFINITIONS AND PREDICTIVE POWER FOR CVD

Three studies have examined whether the difference in prevalence between the two definitions affects the predictive power for subsequent development of CVD (40,43,46). Two of these found the ATP III definition to be a slightly better predictor of all-cause and cardiovascular mortality (46) or CHD (43), whereas one (40) showed that the WHO definition more consistently predicted CVD and all-cause mortality. The fact that all three studies made modifications to one or both of the definitions, and that they included populations with dissimilar baseline characteristics, precludes drawing any conclusions as to which definition is superior.

METABOLIC SYNDROME, DIABETES, AND CVD

The above points notwithstanding, individuals with metabolic syndrome, however it is defined, have a much higher CVD risk than subjects without the syndrome. This conclusion is not surprising, since the individual components of the syndrome have long been known to be major cardiovascular risk factors (54–59). Thus when they occur simultaneously, it is logical that adverse outcomes should be more likely (60,61).

Metabolic Syndrome Risk Factors: Are We Missing Something?

ATP III uses the term "metabolic syndrome" to imply that certain risk factors are associated with each other, and that insulin resistance is the primary cause (37,62). They identify six components of the metabolic syndrome as "underlying," "major," and "emerging" CVD risk factors (62). However, some risk factors associated with insulin resistance in each of those categories are not included in the definition of the syndrome. For example, physical inactivity is omitted as an underlying risk factor, while obesity is included. Family history, sex, and age are major CVD risk factors that do not enter into the definition, but hypertension is included. Some emerging risk factors associated with insulin resistance, e.g., certain proinflammatory and prothrombotic markers, are not included, but elevated triglycerides and glucose intolerance are. Interestingly, although all four were designated "metabolic risk factors" and a "component of the metabolic syndrome," only elevated triglycerides and glucose intolerance are included in the official list of components (62). The lack of any standardized methodology or rationale for how the definition was constructed, or can be modified, hampers its optimization and utility.

It is not known whether the substitution or addition of any other well-known, conventional CVD risk factor(s) would improve the predictive value of the syndrome. In studies demonstrating that metabolic syndrome was associated with higher CVD risk (28,40,46,50,63–72), this excess risk remained after adjustment for other conventional risk factors. This would suggest that if other risk factors are included in the definition, the predictive value of the syndrome may improve. However, we found no study that examined the impact of substituting another CVD risk factor for one already included in the definition. The issue of whether the risk factors act synergistically has also not been analyzed. Malik et al. (50) reported that, compared with individuals with no risk factors, those with one to two metabolic syndrome risk factors had a hazard ratio of 2.1 for CHD mortality and 3.5 if they had the full syndrome (i.e., three to five risk factors). Other investigators (41,73,74) also found that the risk for CVD increased with the number of factors present. Other studies, using multivariate analysis, have shown that the individual risk factors comprising the syndrome each carried a different odds ratio for predicting prevalent CHD, incident CHD, or CVD mortality. In addition to hyperglycemia, low HDL-cholesterol levels and hypertension usually conferred a significantly greater risk compared with the presence of obesity or high triglycerides (46,72), although McNeill et al. (41) found that only an elevated blood pressure and low HDL-cholesterol were significantly associated with CHD. Golden et al. (75) assessed carotid intima-medial thickness related to 57 combinations of six factors related to insulin resistance. In their analysis, 29 of the 57 groupings were associated with excess carotid intima-medial thickness. The difference in excess intima-medial thickness between individuals with two, three, or four factors was minimal, but those with five or six factors showed an appreciable increase in excess intima-medial thickness. Hypertension and hypertriglyceridemia were the two factors that most contributed to the excess intima-medial thickness. Taken together, these studies suggest that not all combinations that lead to the diagnosis of the syndrome convey equal risk, although the actual hierarchy of risk predictability for each of the syndrome combinations remains unknown.

Diabetes: Not All Risk Factors Are Created Equal

Both the ATP III and WHO definitions weigh each risk component equally, yet it is clear that some risk factors included in the definition have greater CVD predictive importance than others. Malik et al. (50) in their study on NHANES II participants observed that diabetes alone conveyed a much greater risk of CHD (hazard ratio = 5.02), CVD (hazard ratio = 3.6), or overall mortality (hazard ratio = 2.1) than the presence of the metabolic syndrome (3.5, 2.7, and 1.5, respectively) according to definitions that included subjects with and without impaired fasting glucose/impaired glucose tolerance (IGT)/diabetes. Adding preexisting CVD to diabetes was an even more powerful predictor of mortality (11.3, 7.9, and 2.9, respectively) over the 13-year follow-up period. Similarly, Stern et al. (76) showed that, among patients with prevalent CVD, the excess risk for all-cause and CVD mortality associated with the metabolic syndrome was entirely driven by the inclusion of diabetes in the definition, and once diabetes was controlled for, the presence of the metabolic syndrome no longer conferred excess risk. Finally, Hunt et al. (46) also showed that the presence of impaired fasting glucose alone was a stronger predictor of CVD or all-cause mortality in a general population than either the syndrome as a whole or any of its individual components. These reports raise the question of why glucose intolerance (particularly diabetes) is included in the definition of the metabolic syndrome, since it appears to account for most, if not all, of the CVD predictive value. Since the metabolic syndrome does not include all known CVD factors, it should convey risk independently of other conventional risk factors [e.g., low-density lipoproteins (LDLs), age, smoking, family history]; however, the proportion of the global CVD risk captured by the syndrome is unknown. It would be invaluable to know, from a list of all known CVD risk factors, the hierarchy of combinations with the highest predictive value. Then, a true comparison between the metabolic syndrome and other models using different risk factors (74,77) or perhaps some new combination would tell us what is the best CVD predictive model.

Metabolic Syndrome: Is the Whole Greater Than Its Parts?

Another important question is the degree to which the presence of the syndrome in itself adds to CVD prediction beyond the contribution of the component risk factors. At least five studies address this issue. One is the study by Golden et al. (75) reviewed above, which examined all possible combinations of six factors related to insulin resistance. Individuals with any four-, five-, or six-component groupings had no greater excess intima-medial thickness than the sum of the same factors taken separately. The cross-sectional studies by Alexander et al. (72) and Yarnell et al. (78) showed that the impact of the syndrome on CVD was greatly attenuated in a multivariate analysis by controlling for certain of its components, thereby suggesting that the whole is not greater than its parts. Also, in a prospective study of diabetic and nondiabetic subjects free of CVD and followed for an average of 11 years, the risk of incident CHD associated with the syndrome was no greater than that explained by the presence of its components (41). Finally, in the secondary analysis of the prospective WOSCOPS (West of Scotland Coronary Prevention Study), Sattar et al. (74) showed that the metabolic syndrome was not a significant predictor of CHD when adjusted for its component factors in a multivariate model. Thus, these studies suggest that the syndrome itself conveys no greater information than the sum of its component risk factors.

METABOLIC SYNDROME AND INSULIN RESISTANCE

Although many nondiabetic adult subjects with a wide range of age and body mass are hyperinsulinemic and insulin resistant (50%), 25% are insulin resistant but without hyperinsulinemia and the same proportion are hyperinsulinemic but without insulin resistance (79). The relationship between insulin resistance and hyperinsulinemia, reviewed in detail by Ferrannini and Balkau (79), is complex, and although both parameters will capture individuals with the metabolic syndrome, each makes an independent contribution to the clinical findings associated with the syndrome (80,81). Thus, hyperinsulinemia and insulin resistance each partially identify different groups of individuals, they each cluster with various CVD risk factors, and individuals with the metabolic syndrome may have either, both, or none of these "insulin-related" abnormalities.

Even though most people who have the metabolic syndrome are insulin resistant, as discussed earlier, this is probably due to the fact that almost all people with an elevated blood glucose value (the most prevalent characteristic among those with the syndrome) are insulin resistant. Conversely, many studies have shown that only a minority of nondiabetic individuals with insulin resistance (but who may have impaired fasting glucose or IGT) will have the metabolic syndrome. In a study of 260 nondiabetic, overweight/obese individuals, McLaughlin et al. (82) found that 78% of those with the metabolic syndrome were insulin resistant, but only 48% with insulin resistance had metabolic syndrome. Liao et al. (83) reported that 39% of 74 overweight/obese nondiabetic adults were insulin resistant, and 31% with insulin resistance met ATP III criteria. Moreover, the ATP III–negative/insulin-resistant individuals had cardiovascular risk factor profiles that were significantly worse than the ATP III–negative/insulin-sensitive group, implying that many presumably high-risk individuals will be not be identified by screening for the metabolic syndrome. Also, they found that the sensitivity, specificity, and positive predictive value for predicting insulin resistance in nondiabetic individuals with three or more metabolic syndrome traits were 20%, 92%, and 50%, respectively, denoting poor clinical utility

Cheal et al. (84) determined that 16% of 443 healthy, nondiabetic subjects were insulin resistant and/or positive for the metabolic syndrome, with a sensitivity, specificity, and positive predictive value for the metabolic syndrome as a predictor of insulin resistance of 46%, 93%, and 76%, respectively. This study also showed that very few of the possible three-, four-, or five-factor combinations occurred in the nondiabetic patients classified with the syndrome. As noted above, most investigators use the phrase "insulin resistance" to describe the hallmark of the metabolic syndrome, even though insulin resistance or hyperinsulinemia may not be present in subjects with the syndrome. Furthermore, the extent to which an elevated risk of CVD is due to insulin resistance itself, versus isolated hyperinsulinemia, or versus some other related factor, is still unclear.

Laws and Reaven (85) showed that a high triglyceride and low HDL-cholesterol concentration is a strong indicator of insulin resistance, and when expressed as a ratio (82), the optimal cut points in overweight/obese individuals resulted in a sensitivity, specificity, and positive predictive value for insulin resistance of 64%, 68%, and 67%, respectively. The addition of extra measurements, i.e., blood glucose, blood pressure, body mass index (BMI), was less sensitive (52%) but more specific (85%) in predicting insulin resistance. Thus, both the metabolic syndrome and this abbreviated index have only a moderate likelihood of identifying the person with insulin resistance. More recently, Stern et al. (42) collected euglycemic clamp (widely regarded as the gold standard for measuring insulin resistance) data from >2000 lean and overweight or obese individuals and used a decision tree classification scheme to develop decision rules for identifying insulin-resistant individuals based on common clinical measurements. In their study, decision rules based on either homeostasis model assessment of insulin resistance and BMI, or BMI and family history of diabetes had sensitivities and specificities in the range of 80%. Thus, if the aim is to identify insulin resistance in either lean or overweight/obese subjects, there are simpler ways to do so than by identifying those with the metabolic syndrome.

Over the last couple of decades, a variety of therapeutic interventions have been developed to treat insulin resistance. The most successful of these has been the peroxisome proliferator–activated receptor-γ (PPAR-γ) agonists such as the thiazolidinediones (TZDs), also known as glitazones. Although these drugs are approved only for the treatment of diabetes, they have attracted much attention to their potential for reducing cardiovascular events. This is due to the fact that they improve insulin sensitivity and directly or indirectly improve a wide array of cardiovascular risk factors, many of which may be pathogenic in inducing vascular events (38). Studies have suggested that TZDs can improve glycemic control, reduce the magnitude of several CVD risk factors, and generally result in a less unfavorable cardiovascular risk profile (86–92). However, much of this data comes from animal studies and small human studies. Several such trials have been initiated, using PPAR-γ agonists in a variety of settings from prediabetes to late-stage diabetes, to examine their role in primary as well as secondary prevention of cardiovascular events (93). The first of these was the PROactive study, which recently reported its results and is therefore being viewed with considerable interest (94). PROactive was a prospective, randomized, controlled trial in 5238 patients with Type 2 diabetes who had evidence of clinically overt CVD. The patients were randomized to pioglitazone, titrated to 45 mg daily or matching placebo. Importantly, the study drug was taken in addition to patients' usual glucose-lowering medications and therefore this study was designed to assess the pure effect of pioglitazone; however, there was an absolute reduction by 0.5% of hemoglobin A1c in the pioglitazone-treated group compared to placebo independent from any of its effects on lowering blood glucose. The results of the study show that pioglitazone had only a modest, and not statistically significant, 10% reduction in the risk of the primary composite endpoint, which consisted of all-cause mortality, nonfatal myocardial infarction (MI), stroke, acute coronary syndrome, and revascularization or amputation. However, the "main secondary endpoint," consisting only of certain of the primary outcome measures, namely all-cause mortality, MI, and stroke was significantly reduced by 16%.

TYPE 2 DIABETES MELLITUS

There are 18.2 million people in the United States, or 6.3% of the population, with diabetes (95). Every year 1.3 million adults over the age of 20 years are diagnosed with diabetes (95). The incidence of diabetes has increased by nearly 50% in just a decade (95). Diabetes and obesity are both associated with excess cardiovascular morbidity and mortality, the exact cause of which is unknown but is likely to be multifactorial, as discussed above and in other chapters (96). Impaired endothelial function assessed by flow-mediated dilatation is a common and early abnormality associated with obesity (26) and diabetes mellitus (97).

Prevalence and Impact of the Metabolic Syndrome in Patients with Diabetes and Prediabetes

Hyperinsulinemia is a marker of insulin resistance, a correlate of the metabolic syndrome, and an established precursor of Type 2 diabetes. The NHANES data from 1999 to 2002 of 3601 men and women aged greater than or equal to 20 years were analyzed by Ford (53). The objective of this study was to estimate the prevalence of this syndrome using the IDF definition among U.S. adults and to compare it with the prevalence estimated using the definition of the NCEP. Based on the NCEP definition, the unadjusted prevalence of the metabolic syndrome was about 34.5 ± 0.9% (percentage ± SE) among all participants, 33.7 ± 1.6% among men, and 35.4 ± 1.2% among women. Based on the IDF definition, the unadjusted prevalence of the metabolic syndrome was 39.0 ± 1.1% among all participants, 39.9 ± 1.7% among men, and 38.1 ± 1.2% among women (53). In the United States, 61% of the adult population is overweight or obese (98).

Effect of Ethnicity

The increase in the prevalence of obesity over the last few decades is well documented, with the increase in obesity prevalence occurring in all age and racial groups (99). Health statistics in the United States show that between 1963 and 2000, the prevalence of overweight adolescent children (12–19 years) increased from 5% to 15.5% (100). However, the increases were markedly greater in non-Hispanic blacks (13.4–23.6%) and Mexican Americans (13.8–23.4%) (101).

Among adults, the prevalence of obesity has increased in both men and women and in each racial group between the NHANES III 1988–1994 and NHANES 1999–2000. Although the increases have been statistically significant in all racial and sex groups (101), the longitudinal data on the development of obesity indicates that the rise in obesity rates in women has been greatest in African American women, followed by Hispanic women, and then white women. By the age of 39 years, the mean BMI of African American women was greater than 30 kg/m², which is at the WHO cut-off point for obesity. Similar trends were observed in men; however, for African American men, the acceleration in weight gain did not occur until after the age of 30 years (102).

EFFECT OF GENES ON METABOLIC SYNDROME AND DIABETES MELLITUS

Insulin resistance appears to be the best predictor of the development of diabetes in the children of patients with Type 2 diabetes mellitus, but the mechanism responsible is unknown. Recently, Petersen et al. (103) performed hyperinsulinemic–euglycemic clamp studies in combination with infusions of $[6,6-^2H_2]$glucose in healthy, young, lean, insulin-resistant offspring of patients with Type 2 diabetes and insulin-sensitive control subjects matched for age, height, weight, and physical activity to assess the sensitivity of liver and muscle to insulin. Proton (^1H) magnetic resonance spectroscopy studies were performed to measure intramyocellular lipid and intrahepatic triglyceride content. Rates of whole-body and subcutaneous fat lipolysis were assessed by measuring the rates of $[^2H_5]$glycerol turnover in combination with microdialysis measurements of glycerol release from subcutaneous fat. ^{31}P magnetic resonance spectroscopy studies were performed to assess the rates of mitochondrial oxidative-phosphorylation activity in muscle. The insulin-stimulated rate of glucose uptake by muscle was approximately 60% lower in the insulin-resistant subjects than in the insulin-sensitive control subjects ($P < 0.001$) and was associated with an increase of approximately 80% in the intramyocellular lipid content ($P = 0.005$). This increase in intramyocellular lipid content was most likely attributable to mitochondrial dysfunction, as reflected by a reduction of approximately 30% in mitochondrial phosphorylation ($P = 0.01$ for the comparison with controls), since there were no significant differences in systemic or localized rates of lipolysis or plasma concentrations of tumor necrosis factor-α, interleukin-6, resistin, or adiponectin. These data support the hypothesis that insulin resistance in the skeletal muscle of insulin-resistant offspring of patients with Type 2 diabetes is associated with dys-regulation of intramyocellular fatty acid metabolism, possibly because of an inherited defect in mitochondrial oxidative phosphorylation (103).

A case–control study in the outpatient setting was conducted by Pimenta et al. (104) to assess if insulin resistance precedes impaired insulin secretion in individuals genetically predisposed to Type 2 diabetes mellitus. One hundred volunteers of European ancestry having normal glucose tolerance, 50 with and 50 without a first-degree Type 2 diabetes mellitus relative, matched for age, sex, and degree of obesity, were enrolled. Insulin secretion and insulin sensitivity were assessed by hyperglycemic ($N = 100$) and euglycemic–hyperinsulinemic ($N = 62$) clamp experiments. The individuals with a first-degree Type 2 diabetes mellitus relative had reduced first- and second-phase insulin responses (mean $\pm$ standard error, 939 ± 68 vs. 1209 ± 82 pmol/L, and 322 ± 19 vs. 407 ± 24 pmol/L, respectively, $P = 0.001$ and 0.01), but their insulin sensitivity (148 ± 6 and 92 ± 6 nmol.kg^{-1}.min^{-1}/pmol.L^{-1} in hyperglycemic and euglycemic clamp studies) did not differ from that of the control group (126 ± 5 and 81 ± 7 nmol.kg^{-1}.min^{-1}/pmol.L^{-1}, in hyperglycemic and euglycemic clamp studies, $P = 0.07$ and 0.24, respectively). In some individuals only first- or only second-phase insulin responses were reduced. In this study-population, heterogeneous defects in insulin secretion were demonstrated, while defects in insulin sensitivity were not evident. It was concluded that since the earliest defects identified in a group genetically at high risk of developing Type 2 diabetes are those related to insulin secretion, defects in insulin secretion rather than insulin sensitivity are likely the major genetic factor predisposing to development of Type 2 diabetes (104).

INSULIN RESISTANCE AS A COMMON PRECURSOR AND PREDICTOR OF THE METABOLIC SYNDROME AND TYPE 2 DIABETES: THE COMMON SOIL HYPOTHESIS

Unlike classical microvascular complications, large-vessel atherosclerosis can precede the development of diabetes, suggesting that rather than atherosclerosis being a complication of diabetes, both conditions have common genetic and envi-ronmental antecedents, i.e., they spring from a "common soil" (31). It is now known that adverse environmental conditions, perhaps related to less-than-optimal nutrition, in fetal and early life are associated with an enhanced risk of both dia-betes and CVD many decades later. These same adverse environmental condi-tions are also associated with the development in adult life of abdominal obesity and the insulin resistance syndrome. The insulin resistance syndrome consists of glucose intolerance, hyperinsulinemia, dyslipidemia (high triglycerides and low levels of HDL-cholesterol), and hypertension. Although the mechanism underlying this cluster is controversial, the statistical association is well established. All the elements of the syndrome have been documented as risk factors for Type 2 diabetes. Some, but not all, of these elements are also CVD risk factors, in particular, hypertension and low HDL-cholesterol. Other factors associated with insulin resistance that may enhance cardiovascular risk are plasminogen activator inhibitor-1 (PAI-1) and small, dense LDL particles.

Whether insulin itself is a risk factor remains controversial, but recent epidemiological evidence has been mostly negative. This question has marked clinical relevance because if the insulin resistance syndrome enhances cardiovascular risk by virtue of its concomitant factors and not the hyperinsulinemia per se, this would tend to alleviate concerns that intensive treatment with exogenous insulin could enhance the risk of large-vessel atherosclerosis. Clinical trials are urgently needed to settle this point.

Many of the features of insulin resistance that are present before the onset of hyperglycemia remain operative during the natural history of the diabetes mellitus and contribute greatly to atherosclerosis and associated comorbidities (105,106).

The NCEP ATP III recently recognized the metabolic syndrome as a secondary therapeutic target for the prevention of CVD (37). Patients who have the metabolic syndrome meet at least three of the following criteria: triglycerides are greater than 150 mg/dL, HDL is less than 40 mg/dL (<2.22 mmol/L), blood pressure is greater than 130/85 mmHg, fasting blood glucose is greater than 110 mg/dL (>6.11 mmol/L), and waist circumference is greater than 40 cm in men and 50 cm in women (37).

ROLE OF ADIPOCYTOKINES IN THE PATHOGENESIS OF METABOLIC SYNDROME AND TYPE 2 DIABETES MELLITUS

There is a strong and consistent inverse association between circulating levels of adiponectin and both insulin resistance and inflammation (107–109). In addition, adiponectin is also inversely associated with other cardiovascular risk factors such as blood pressure, LDL-cholesterol levels, and triglycerides (110,111). Moreover, several studies have shown adiponectin to be a strong, inverse, and independent risk factor for CVD (112–115).

Adiponectin-1 is an adipocyte-derived peptide that has anti-inflammatory and insulin-sensitizing properties. In a nested case–control study, plasma adiponectin concentrations [mean ± standard deviation (SD)] at baseline were lower among individuals who later developed Type 2 diabetes than among controls (5.34 ± 3.49 μg/mL vs. 6.87 ± 4.58 μg/mL, $P < 0.0001$). High concentrations of adiponectin were associated with a substantially reduced relative risk of Type 2 diabetes after adjustment for age, sex, waist-to-hip ratio, BMI, smoking, exercise, alcohol consumption, education, and hemoglobin A_{1c} [odds ratio fourth vs. first quartile 0.3 (95% confidence interval [CI] 0.2–0.7, $P = 0.0051$)]. The study investigators concluded that adiponectin is independently associated with a reduced risk of Type 2 diabetes in apparently healthy individuals (116).

Adiponectin (117) is exclusively and abundantly expressed in white adipose tissue and has been shown to have insulin-sensitizing and anti-inflammatory properties (118,119). A diabetes susceptibility locus has been mapped to human chromosome 3q27, where the adiponectin gene is located. Thus, both genetic and functional data suggest that adiponectin could be involved in the pathogenesis of Type 2 diabetes. Additionally, decreased concentrations of adiponectin have been shown to precede the onset of disease in an animal model of diabetes. Alternatively, high concentrations of adiponectin might prevent the onset of Type 2 diabetes. In a prospective, nested case–control study within the population-based EPIC (European Prospective Investigation into Cancer and Nutrition) Potsdam cohort, which includes 27,548 individuals, baseline concentrations of adiponectin in plasma were measured. The purpose was to assess whether adiponectin levels independently modify the risk of Type 2 diabetes in apparently healthy individuals. Among this cohort, 192 individuals with medically confirmed incident Type 2 diabetes mellitus were identified; these subjects were matched with 384 controls. The mean adiponectin concentration was significantly lower in individuals with incident Type 2 diabetes mellitus than in controls. Increasing concentrations of adiponectin were associated with a lower risk of subsequent Type 2 diabetes in apparently healthy individuals, suggesting that adiponectin has a substantial role in the pathogenesis of Type 2 diabetes mellitus, and that adiponectin could be used as an indicator of risk in addition to the established risk factors such as obesity and physical activity levels.

Although adiponectin seems to be implicated in the development of insulin resistance and β-cell function, explicit mechanisms linking adiponectin and incident Type 2 diabetes remain speculative (119,120). Genetic polymorphisms might be involved in the regulation of adiponectin concentrations in plasma, especially taking into account the existing linkage in the region of the adiponectin gene with Type 2 diabetes mellitus. Unfortunately, information about family history of diabetes, which would reflect genetic influence, was not available in our cohort. Furthermore the precise time-course of adiponectin concentrations in plasma during development of Type 2 diabetes remains to be elucidated. These results accord with those of a study in Pima Indians (121). Both observations, combined with emerging functional and genetic evidence, support the concept that adiponectin has a central role in the development of Type 2 diabetes.

ENDOTHELIAL DYSFUNCTION, METABOLIC SYNDROME, AND DIABETES

The endothelium is important in the maintenance of vascular health. It is a critical determinant of vascular tone and patency, reactivity, inflammation, vascular remodeling, and blood fluidity. The importance of endothelial dysfunction in the pathogenesis of CVD in diabetes has only recently been recognized (122).

Nitric oxide (NO) is the most potent known vasodilator and is secreted by the endothelium. It is synthesized from L-arginine by the endothelial enzyme NO synthase (e-NOS). The bioavailability of NO can be decreased by various mechanisms—decreased production by e-NOS and enhanced NO breakdown due to increased oxidative stress, in isolation or in combination. e-NOS deactivation is often associated with an increase in plasma levels of its endogenous inhibitor, asymmetric dimethyl-L-arginine (123).

It has become clear that in addition to its many metabolic and growth-promoting actions, insulin is a vasoactive hormone (26,124–127). The action of insulin on endothelial NO–dependent vasodilatation is physiologic and dose-dependent (128). Insulin has been shown to induce the expression of the e-NOS (129), and this effect is inhibited by cytokines important in the pathogenesis of insulin resistance (130). Importantly, the effect of insulin on NO synthase is mediated through the same intracellular signaling pathway as insulin's effects on glucose metabolism (131). Thus insulin resistance in glucose metabolism and in the vasculature can be explained on the basis of a single defect. Recent data suggest that insulin's metabolic and vascular actions are closely linked. Insulin-resistant states exhibit diminished insulin-mediated glucose uptake into peripheral tissues as well as impaired insulin-mediated vasodilatation and impaired endothelium-dependent vasodilatation to the muscarinic receptor agonist acetylcholine. Thus, insulin action in peripheral tissues may be linked to its action on the endothelium.

Newer Markers of Inflammation in the Pathogenesis of Metabolic Syndrome and Diabetes

Numerous studies suggest that some relatively new indexes related to both insulin resistance and CVD may also be useful predictive tools (or useful additions to the syndrome definition). Since it is now well accepted that inflammation plays a major role in atherogenesis (132), it is not surprising that markers of inflammation might be used to predict cardiovascular events. There is also an association between other markers of inflammation and insulin resistance/hyperinsulinemia (77,108), as well as inflammation and obesity (133–135), leading some investigators to conclude that inflammation is integrally related to the components of the metabolic syndrome (135–137). C-reactive protein is also strongly associated with adipose-derived cytokines including interleukin-6 and tumor necrosis factor-α (138), and is more likely to be elevated in obese insulin-resistant, but not obese insulin-sensitive, subjects (139). Because obesity (particularly in the visceral compartment) is associated with insulin resistance, and these adipose-derived inflammatory markers have been linked to dyslipidemia, hypertension, and insulin action (77,108), there is a heightened interest in markers from adipose tissue that are predictive of CVD (138).

C-Reactive Protein

One of the aforementioned markers, C-reactive protein, has been studied in great detail in recent years. C-reactive protein has been found to be an independent risk marker for CVD (140–144) and an independent marker of insulin resistance (77,108,139,145). Three large population studies examined the relationship between C-reactive protein, the metabolic syndrome, and incident cardiovascular events (74,140,146). In all three, C-reactive protein was a strong independent predictor of events, and its predictive value was equal to that of the metabolic syndrome. In the two studies (74,140) that dichotomized C-reactive protein levels [above and below 3.0 mg/dL (0.167 mmol/L)], the age-adjusted relative risk of future events was no different in subjects with high C-reactive protein but without the metabolic syndrome from that in subjects with low C-reactive protein and with the metabolic syndrome. However, in subjects with high C-reactive protein levels plus the metabolic syndrome, the relative risk of events virtually doubled from that found with either parameter alone, indicating that C-reactive protein might be a valuable addition to the definition of the syndrome. Rutter et al. (146) also found that C-reactive protein and the metabolic syndrome were independent risk factors, but in contrast to the other two reports, combining C-reactive protein and metabolic syndrome did not improve the predictive value of either used alone. Reilly et al. (147) also found that C-reactive protein did not add significantly to the metabolic syndrome, but their study did not include CVD outcomes. It is unclear why some studies show great value when C-reactive protein is added while others do not. The discrepant results have not, however, deterred some investigators from advocating that C-reactive protein be included in the definition of the metabolic syndrome (137).

PAI-1 and Fibrinogen

Several other molecules have also been found to be closely associated with insulin resistance, metabolic syndrome risk factors, and risk of CVD. These include PAI (148–150) and fibrinogen (148,149,151,152).

PREVENTION AND TREATMENT OF METABOLIC SYNDROME AND TYPE 2 DIABETES

Several epidemiologic studies have shown that endogenous hyperinsulinemia is an independent risk factor for CVD (153). Correction of insulin resistance is clearly important in the management of Type 2 diabetes mellitus and may decrease the risk for CVD. In the UK Prospective Diabetes Study (UKPDS), patients with Type 2 diabetes mellitus treated with metformin, a relatively weak insulin sensitizer that decreases hyperinsulinemia and insulin resistance, had a 30% reduction in cardiovascular events and mortality compared with those treated with conventional treatment (92). TZDs improve insulin sensitivity and may exert numerous nonglycemic effects in patients with Type 2 diabetes (154,155). Additional clinical trials are currently being conducted to evaluate whether the treatment of diabetes mellitus with agents that reduce insulin resistance, such as TZDs, is superior to treatment with agents that stimulate insulin secretion, such as the sulfonylureas.

Few long-term studies comparing the effects of secretagogues with sensitizers on cardiovascular outcomes have been conducted. Sulfonylureas are effective pancreatic insulin secretagogues and rapidly improve glycemic control (93). Improved blood glucose control decreases the progression of diabetic microvascular disease, but the effect on macrovascular complications is unclear. This is particularly true when older sulfonylureas are used to treat hyperglycemia. Previously, there was concern that sulfonylureas may increase cardiovascular mortality in patients who have Type 2 diabetes mellitus and that high insulin concentrations may enhance atheroma formation. In the UKPDS trial, however, the effects of intensive blood glucose control, with either sulfonylurea or insulin and conventional treatment, on the risk of microvascular and macrovascular complications in patients who had Type 2 diabetes mellitus were compared in a randomized, controlled trial (156). When compared with conventional therapy, intensive treatment was associated with a decreased risk of predominantly microvascular complications, including a 12% reduction in any diabetes-related endpoint ($P = 0.03$) and a 25% reduction in all microvascular endpoints ($P < 0.001$). There was no significant effect on diabetes-related death or on all-cause mortality, however, and there only was a trend toward a small effect on the risk of MI ($P = 0.05$). Overall, there were no significant differences between subjects treated with sulfonylurea and those treated with insulin. It was concluded that improved glycemic control from sulfonylureas alone is not enough to decrease macrovascular risk. In contrast, obese patients who were randomized to metformin had a reduction in MI and cardiovascular mortality. Therefore the jury is still out on whether sulfonylureas have beneficial effects on macrovascular complications.

Lifestyle Modification

Weight reduction, diet, and exercise are important modifiers of insulin resistance and they have been identified as key elements in the treatment of the metabolic syndrome (37,157,158). However, they are also key elements in the treatment of all components of the syndrome when they occur in isolation (37,159,160). Indeed, only recently the IDF developed yet another new definition that suggests that the key element is central obesity (34).

The role of diet and exercise in the prevention of Type 2 diabetes mellitus has been prospectively evaluated in several studies. In the six-year Malmö feasibility study (161), 41 subjects with early-stage Type 2 diabetes and 181 subjects with IGT were selected for prospective study and to test the feasibility aspect of long-term intervention with an emphasis on lifestyle changes. A five-year protocol, including an initial six-month (randomized) pilot study, consisting of dietary treatment and/or increase of physical activity or training with annual check-ups, was completed by 90% of subjects. Body weight was reduced by 2.3% to 3.7% among participants, whereas values increased by 0.5% to 1.7% in nonintervened subjects with IGT in normal control subjects ($P < 0.0001$); maximal oxygen uptake (mL.min^{-1}.kg^{-1}) was increased by 10% to 14% and decreased by 5% to

9%, respectively ($P < 0.0001$). Glucose tolerance was normalized in greater than 50% of subjects with IGT, the accumulated incidence of diabetes was 10.6%, and more than 50% of the diabetic patients were in remission after a mean follow-up of six years (161).

In the Da Qing study, 110,660 men and women from 33 healthcare clinics in the city of Da Qing, China, were screened for IGT and Type 2 diabetes. Of these individuals, 577 were classified as having IGT. Subjects were randomized by clinic into a clinical trial, either to a control group or to one of three active treatment groups: diet only, exercise only, or diet plus exercise. Follow-up evaluation examinations were conducted at two-year intervals over a six-year period to identify subjects who developed Type 2 diabetes. The cumulative incidence of diabetes at six years was 67.7% (95% CI, 59.8–75.2) in the control group compared with 43.8% (95% CI 35.5–52.3) in the diet group, 41.1% (33.4–49.4) in the exercise group, and 46.0% (37.3–54.7) in the diet plus exercise group ($P < 0.05$). Diet and/or exercise interventions led to a significant decrease in the incidence of diabetes over a six-year period among those with IGT (162).

In the Finnish Diabetes Prevention Study (163), 522 middle-aged, overweight subjects (172 men and 350 women; mean age 55 years; mean BMI 31 kg/m^2) with IGT were randomized to either an intervention group or a control group. Each subject in the intervention group received individualized counseling aimed at reducing weight, total intake of fat, and intake of saturated fat and increasing intake of fiber and physical activity. An oral glucose-tolerance test was performed annually; the diagnosis of diabetes was confirmed by a second test. The mean duration of follow-up was 3.2 years. The mean (±SD) weight loss between baseline and the end of year 1 was 4.2 ± 5.1 kg in the intervention group and 0.8 ± 3.7 kg in the control group; the net loss by the end of year 2 was 3.5 ± 5.5 kg in the intervention group and 0.8 ± 4.4 kg in the control group ($P < 0.001$ for both comparisons between the groups). The cumulative incidence of diabetes after four years was 11% (95% CI 6–15) in the intervention group and 23% (95% CI 17–29) in the control group. During the trial, the risk of diabetes was reduced by 58% ($P < 0.001$) in the intervention group. The reduction in the incidence of diabetes was directly associated with changes in lifestyle.

The Diabetes Prevention Program (DPP), which included a successful intensive multifactorial lifestyle intervention in 3234 high-risk subjects with glucose intolerance, is considered in detail in the next section (88). It can be concluded from these studies that Type 2 diabetes mellitus can be prevented, or its development deferred, by changes in the lifestyles of high-risk subjects, at least in the setting of clinical trials.

The effect of intensive lifestyle intervention versus metformin therapy in a group of obese subjects with glucose intolerance was prospectively evaluated in the aforementioned DPP (164). The DPP was designed to quantify means of preventing or delaying the onset of Type 2 diabetes in high-risk subjects (88). The study was a U.S. multicenter, randomized, controlled clinical trial of participants who had IGT, defined according to WHO criteria, plus fasting plasma glucose level greater than 95 mg/dL (5.3 mmol/L). The participants were followed for a mean of 3.2 years after random assignment to intensive lifestyle intervention, metformin therapy, or placebo. Subjects received metformin, 850 mg twice daily, or intensive lifestyle intervention designed to achieve and maintain a 7% weight loss and 150 minutes of exercise/week. The metabolic syndrome was defined as having three or more risk factors including elevated waist circumference, high blood pressure, and low levels of HDL-cholesterol, hypertriglycerdemia, and/or elevated fasting plasma glucose concentration as defined by the aforementioned NCEP ATP III publication. According to this definition, the metabolic syndrome was present in half of the participants in the DPP at baseline. The incidence of the syndrome was reduced by 41% in the lifestyle group ($P < 0.001$) and by 17% in the metformin group ($P = 0.03$), compared with placebo. Three-year cumulative incidences were 51%, 45%, and 34% in the placebo, metformin, and lifestyle groups, respectively. Both lifestyle intervention and metformin therapy reduced the development of the metabolic syndrome in the remaining participants compared to placebo treatment, the former being the more effective intervention. This mirrored the impact of the interventions on the development of Type 2 diabetes, the reduction in new-onset diabetes being reduced by 58% (95% CI 48–66) by the lifestyle interventions, and by 31% (95% CI 17–43) by metformin, as compared with placebo (88).

Metformin

Metformin (dimethylbiguanide) is an orally administered drug used to lower blood glucose concentrations in patients with Type 2 diabetes (165). It improves aspects of insulin action and thus decreases the insulin resistance that is prevalent among patients with Type 2 diabetes. The glucose-lowering effect of metformin is attributed mainly to decreased hepatic glucose output and, to a lesser extent, enhanced peripheral glucose uptake. The efficacy of glycemic control achieved with metformin is broadly similar to that achieved with sulfonylureas, although their modes of action differ. Metformin can be used either as initial therapy or as an additional drug when sulfonylurea therapy alone is inadequate.

Participants with IGT have an enhanced risk of atherosclerotic CVD. This is thought to reflect the increased number and severity of classic and nontraditional CVD risk factors. Ratner et al. (166) analyzed the impact of the DPP on hypertension, dyslipidemia, and cardiovascular events. Annual assessment of blood pressure, lipids, electrocardiogram, and cardiovascular events was performed. Hypertension was defined as blood pressure greater than or equal to 140/90 mmHg or the use of antihypertensive medication. Hypertension was present in 30% of participants at study entry, the prevalence increasing with time in the placebo and metformin groups. In contrast, the intensive lifestyle modification group had no significant change in hypertension prevalence, accompanied by significantly decreased lower systolic and diastolic blood pressures, compared with that in the other treatment groups ($P < 0.001$). The use of antihypertensive medications at baseline was 17% in all treatment groups. At three years, the point prevalence of antihypertensive pharmacologic therapy is significantly lower (by 27–28%) in the lifestyle group (23%) compared with that in the placebo (31%) and metformin (32%) groups (*P* < 0.001). Lifestyle intervention improved CVD risk factor status compared with placebo and metformin therapy. Although no differences in cardiovascular events were noted after three years, the achieved risk factor modifications suggested that a longer intervention period may lead to reduced CVD event rates.

Thiazolidinediones

The TZDs are a relatively new class of compounds for the treatment of Type 2 diabetes. The TZDs have emerged as an important class in the management of Type 2 diabetes, and their efficacy in lowering plasma glucose is now well established although they are not generally more impressive than the other major oral antidiabetic agents (167–172). The glucose-lowering effects of the TZDs are mediated primarily by decreasing insulin resistance in muscle and fat and thereby increasing glucose uptake (155,173). TZDs increase insulin-mediated glucose disposal and reduce hepatic glucose production (174). The actions of the TZDs are achieved through binding and activation of the PPAR-γ receptor, a nuclear receptor that has a regulatory role in differentiation of cells, particularly adipocytes. This receptor is also expressed in several other tissues, including vascular tissue (175). In addition, TZDs lower plasma concentrations of free (nonesterified) fatty acids (FFAs); this may indirectly improve insulin sensitivity in glucose metabolism by reducing substrate competition in the glucose–FFA cycle originally described by Randle et al. (176). Elevated plasma FFA levels are strongly implicated in the pathogenesis of the dyslipidemia of Type 2 diabetes and can also have deleterious effects on the vasculature (chapter 5) (124). Thus, a reduction in plasma FFAs may have a beneficial effect on CVD via a multiplicity of biochemical mechanisms. Thus, TZDs have the potential to alter intermediary metabolism beyond reducing levels of glycemia (154). Because the TZDs target insulin resistance, these agents can improve many of the risk factors associated with the insulin resistance syndrome, albeit at the expense of some unwanted effects.

Impact of Thiazolidinediones on Cardiovascular Outcomes

Additional outcome data on the impact of the TZDs on cardiovascular outcomes is eagerly awaited (177). On the basis of the effects of these drugs on cardiovascular risk profiles, it seems reasonable to believe that occlusive cardiovascular events might be reduced and this hypothesis is being tested in clinical trials. However, the first of these to be published was the PROactive trial that compared effects of pioglitazone with placebo. The PROactive trial produced a somewhat mixed picture In PROactive, pioglitazone significantly reduced the incidence of cardiovascular events by 16% (*P* < 0.027); however, this was seen only in the main secondary outcome. Differences in the primary composite outcome, which included peripheral arterial revascularization along with all-cause mortality, non-fatal MI, and other events, were less dramatic and inconclusive (10% reduction vs. placebo, $P = 0.92$) (94,178,179). Moreover, there was an excess of episodes identified as heart failure in the PROactive study (94,178).

Impact of Thiazolidinediones on Lipid Abnormalities

Both pioglitazone and rosiglitazone raise HDL-cholesterol levels, although only pioglitazone has been shown to consistently lower plasma triglycerides (172,180,181). Pioglitazone and rosiglitazone both raise LDL-cholesterol levels, although this increase is predominantly in the larger, buoyant particles of LDL-cholesterol, which are regarded as being less atherogenic (87,90,176). Concomitantly, the small, dense LDL-cholesterol particles (pattern B) have been shown to decrease with TZD therapy (90,182).

Impact of Thiazolidinediones on Blood Pressure

If indeed insulin resistance causes or contributes to hypertension (Chapter 8), then improving insulin sensitivity should have the potential to lower systemic blood pressure. The effects of TZDs on blood pressure have been examined in several different experimental and clinical settings. A study of 24 nondiabetic hypertensive patients treated with rosiglitazone demonstrated that rosiglitazone treatment added onto the patient's usual antihypertensive medication resulted in a decline in both systolic and diastolic blood pressures along with improvements in insulin resistance (183). In another study of 203 patients with Type 2 diabetes mellitus, treatment with rosiglitazone significantly reduced ambulatory blood pressure (184). Scherbaum and Goke also reported decreases in systolic blood pressure by pioglitazone in normotensive and hypertensive patients with diabetes (185).

Raji et al. examined the effect of rosiglitazone on insulin resistance and blood pressure in patients with essential hypertension. There were significant decreases in mean 24-hour systolic blood pressure, and the decline in systolic blood pressure was correlated with the improvement in insulin sensitivity. Rosiglitazone treatment of nondiabetic hypertensive patients improves insulin sensitivity, reduces systolic and diastolic blood pressures, and induces favorable changes in markers of cardiovascular risk. In the Piogliatazone In Prevention of Diabetes (PIPOD) study, improvements in blood pressure may have contributed to the reduction in cardiovascular events with pioglitazone therapy (94).

Impact of Thiazolidinediones on Albuminuria

Urinary microalbuminuria is routinely monitored in clinical practice and is recognized as a marker of CVD and diabetic nephropathy (186,187). Current methods of reducing microalbuminuria include strict glycemic control and use of angiotensin-converting enzyme (ACE) inhibitors. In a 52-week open trial of patients with Type 2 diabetes mellitus given either rosiglitazone or glyburide, patients treated with rosiglitazone had a significant reduction in urinary albumin creatinine ratio compared with baseline (184). Similar results were shown by Lebovitz et al. as well (87). However, in the PROactive study, non-significant changes in microalbuminuria were observed between the pioglitazone and placebo groups (94).

Impact of Thiazolidinediones on Body Weight

Clinical trials suggest that TZDs often increase body weight; however, the weight gain is accompanied by improvement in glycemic control and may, at least in part, be secondary to fluid retention (188,189). Stimulation of adipogenesis through PPAR-γ is another potential mechanism for weight gain although prefer-ential effects on subcutaneous versus visceral adipocytes may explain the improved insulin action (190). The clinical significance of increased body weight with the TZDs is unclear. Studies have attempted to elucidate the mechanisms behind the apparent paradox of TZDs improving insulin sensitivity while causing weight gain. Data indicate that with TZD treatment, there is a favorable shift in fat distribution from visceral to subcutaneous adipose depots, which is associated with improvements in hepatic and peripheral tissue sensitivity to insulin (191). Weight gain in other settings usually increases the level of insulin resistance, which in turn tends to lead to increases in plasma glucose concentrations.

Role of Thiazolidinediones in Prevention of the Metabolic Syndrome

Buchanan et al. (192) investigated whether troglitazone could preserve pancreatic β-cell function and thereby delay or prevent the onset of Type 2 diabetes in high-risk Hispanic women. In the Troglitazone In Prevention Of Diabetes (TRIPOD) study, women with a history of gestational diabetes were randomized to placebo ($N = 133$) or troglitazone (400 mg/d; $N = 133$) in a double-blind fashion. Fasting plasma glucose was measured every three months, and oral glucose tolerance tests (OGTTs) were performed annually to detect diabetes. Intravenous glucose tolerance tests (IVGTTs) were performed at baseline and three months later to identify early metabolic changes associated with any protection from diabetes. Women who did not develop diabetes during the trial returned for OGTTs and IVGTTs eight months after study medications were stopped. During a median follow-up of 30 months on blinded medication, average annual diabetes incidence rates in the 236 women who returned for at least one follow-up visit were 12.1% and 5.4% in women assigned to placebo and troglitazone, respectively ($P < 0.01$). Protection from diabetes in the troglitazone group was closely related to the degree of reduction in endogenous insulin requirements three months after ran-domization, persisted eight months after study medications were stopped, and was associated with improved preservation of β-cell compensation for insulin resistance. In summary, the TRIPOD study showed that treatment with troglita-zone can reduce or delay the incidence of diabetes by 55% in Hispanic women with a history of gestational diabetes (192).

    The Pioglitazone In Prevention Of Diabetes (PIPOD) study was conducted to evaluate β-cell function, insulin resistance, and the incidence of diabetes during treatment with pioglitazone in Hispanic women with prior gestational diabetes who had completed participation in the TRIPOD study (193). Women who completed the TRIPOD study were offered participation in the PIPOD study for a planned three years of drug treatment and six months of postdrug washout. OGTTs were performed annually on pioglitazone and at the end of the postdrug washout. IVGTTs for assessment of insulin sensitivity and β-cell function were conducted at baseline, after one year on pioglitazone, and at the end of the postdrug washout. Of 95 women who were not diabetic at the end of the TRIPOD study, 89 enrolled in the PIPOD study, 86 completed at least one follow-up visit, and 65 completed all study visits, including the postdrug tests. Comparison of changes in β-cell compensation for insulin resistance across the TRIPOD and PIPOD studies revealed that pioglitazone stopped the decline in β-cell function that occurred during placebo treatment in the TRIPOD study and maintained the stability of β-cell function that had occurred during troglitazone treatment in the TRIPOD study. The risk of diabetes, which occurred at an average rate of 4.6% per year, was lowest in women with the largest reduction in total IVGTT insulin area after one year of treatment. The similarity of findings between the PIPOD and TRIPOD studies support a class effect of TZD drugs to enhance insulin sensitivity, reduce insulin secretory demands, and preserve pancreatic β-cell function, all in association with a relatively low rate of Type 2 diabetes, in Hispanic women with prior gestational diabetes.

Troglitazone has been withdrawn from the market. It is assumed that rosiglitazone shares the same diabetes prevention properties. However, to date no prospective studies have been concluded that validate their effects in this regard. Ongoing clinical trials are evaluating newer pharmacotherapies, including ACE inhibitors, angiotensin receptor antagonists, and metglitinides, to prevent both Type 2 diabetes mellitus and cardiovascular events (194). These drugs are considered in more detail in other chapters.

Most recently released (European Association for the Study of Diabetes, Copenhagen, September 2006) were the results of the Diabetes REduction Assessment with Ramipril and Rosiglitazone Medication (DREAM) study involving 5,269 persons with prediabetes randomized to rosiglitazone (8 mg daily) versus placebo and ramipril versus placebo. After treatment for an average of 3 years, 10.6% of those on rosiglitazone progressed to Type 2 diabetes versus 25% on placebo, representing a 62% risk reduction ($P < 0.0001$), with a similar 60% reduction in the primary endpoint of development of diabetes or death from any cause. There was a higher rate of new heart failure in the rosiglitazone (0.5%) versus placebo (0.1%) arm, however. This study supports the role of thiazolidinediones for the prevention of new diabetes onset in those with prediabetes or the metabolic syndrome (195).

Acarbose

Acarbose is an oral antidiabetic which helps to counter postprandial hyperglycemia by inhibiting the enzyme α-glucosidase in the brush border of the upper intestinal villi. When taken just before eating, acarbose retards the breakdown of complex carbohydrates thereby reducing the rise in systemic plasma glucose after meals. Limited evidence suggests that acarbose can improve peripheral insulin sensitivity and/or increase insulin secretion (196). The Study to Prevent Noninsulin Dependent Diabetes Mellitus (STOP-NIDDM) was a multicenter, placebo-controlled, randomized trial conducted to assess the effect of acarbose in preventing or delaying conversion of IGT to Type 2 diabetes mellitus. Patients with IGT were randomly allocated to 100 mg acarbose or placebo three times daily. The primary endpoint was development of diabetes on the basis of a yearly OGTT. A total of 714 patients with IGT were randomized to acarbose and 715 to placebo. Of these, 221 (32%) patients randomized to acarbose and 285 (42%) randomized to placebo developed diabetes [relative hazard 0.75 (95% CI 0.63–0.90); $P = 0.0015$]. Also, acarbose significantly increased the reversion of IGT to normal glucose tolerance ($P < 0.0001$). At the end of the study, treatment with placebo for three months was associated with an increase in conversion of IGT to diabetes. In conclusion, the STOP-NIDDM trial showed that acarbose could be used either as an alternative or in addition to changes in lifestyle, to delay development of Type 2 diabetes in patients with IGT (197). Associated reductions in new-onset hypertension, acute coronary events, and carotid intima media thickness require further study (198).

Orlistat

Orlistat decreases the absorption of dietary triglycerides by inhibiting intestinal lipases. Orlistat therapy is associated with a greater decline in plasma LDL-cholesterol concentrations than that expected from weight loss alone. Orlistat inhibits dietary cholesterol absorption, which may have beneficial effects on lipoprotein metabolism in obese subjects that are independent of weight loss itself (199). In the XENical in the prevention of Diabetes in Obese Subjects (XEN-DOS) (chapter 7) study, 3305 patients were randomized to lifestyle changes plus either orlistat 120 mg. Participants had a BMI greater than or equal to 30 kg/m^2 and either normal glucose tolerance (79%) or IGT (21%). Primary endpoints were time to onset of Type 2 diabetes and change in body weight. Of the orlistat-treated patients, 52% completed treatment compared with 34% of those who received placebo ($P < 0.0001$). After four years of treatment, the cumulative incidence of diabetes was 9.0% with placebo and 6.2% with orlistat, corresponding to a risk reduction of 37.3% ($P = 0.0032$). Exploratory analyses indicated that the preventive effect was explained by the difference between orlistat and placebo in subjects with IGT. Mean weight loss after four years was significantly greater with orlistat (5.8 vs. 3.0 kg with placebo; $P < 0.001$) and similar between orlistat recipients with impaired (5.7 kg) or normal glucose tolerance (5.8 kg) at baseline. Compared with lifestyle changes alone, orlistat plus lifestyle changes resulted in a greater reduction in the incidence of Type 2 diabetes over four years and produced greater weight loss in a clinically representative obese population. In summary, the XENDOS trial showed that among an obese population on intensive lifestyle modification program, the addition of orlistat was associated with a 37% reduced incidence of diabetes compared to placebo (200). As with acarbose and metformin, however, gastrointestinal side-effects often lead to problems with compliance (201).

Certain antihypertensives medications that block the renin–angiotensin system may also reduce the risk of Type 2 diabetes melluite and cardiovascular events. This topic is discussed in more detail in Chapter 8.

SUMMARY

The metabolic syndrome is a common state of insulin resistance characterized by clustering of cardiovascular risk factors. Affected individuals, who are often but not invariably obese, are at increased risk of developing atherosclerotic CVD and/or Type 2 diabetes. Hyperinsulinemia is a marker of insulin resistance, a correlate of the metabolic syndrome, and a precursor of Type 2 diabetes mellitus. Many of the features of insulin resistance are present before the onset of hyperglycemia; these contribute greatly to the development of atherosclerosis and associated comorbidities. These findings suggest that rather than atherosclerosis being a complication of diabetes, both conditions have common genetic and environmental antecedents; i.e., they spring from a "common soil." Higher plasma concentrations of adiponectin are associated with a lower risk of developing Type 2 diabetes in apparently healthy individuals, suggesting that adiponectin plays a substantial role in the pathogenesis of Type 2 diabetes mellitus. Newer markers of inflammation such as C-reactive protein, PAI-1, and fibrinogen are useful predictors of cardiovascular risk. Correction of insulin resistance is clearly important in the management of Type 2 diabetes mellitus and/or the metabolic syndrome and may decrease the risk of CVD. Prevention and treatment of the metabolic syndrome and Type 2 diabetes mellitus include lifestyle modifications such as weight loss, diet, and physical exercise. Pharmacological agents such as metformin, TZDs, acarbose, and orlistat have also been shown to be effective in selected high-risk subjects. In combination with lifestyle modification wherever possible, these therapies offer hope for effective prevention of Type 2 diabetes mellitus and its consequences in high-risk patients.

REFERENCES

1. Avogaro P, CGEGT. SAssociazione di iperlidemia, diabete mellito e obesita di medio grado. Acto Diabetol Lat 1967; 4:36–41.
2. Singer P. Diagnosis of primary hyperlipoproteinemias. Z Gesamte Inn Med 1977; 32(8):128.
3. Haller H. Epidermiology and associated risk factors of hyperlipoproteinemia. Z Gesamte Inn Med 1977; 32(8):124–128.
4. Himsworth H. Diabetes mellitus: a differentiation into insulin-sensitive and insulin-insensitive types. Lancet 1936; 1:127–130.

5. Ginsberg H, Kimmerling G, Olefsky JM, Reaven GM. Demonstration of insulin resistance in untreated adult onset diabetic subjects with fasting hyperglycemia. J Clin Invest 1975; 55(3):454–461.

6. Shen SW, Reaven GM, Farquhar JW. Comparison of impedance to insulin-mediated glucose uptake in normal subjects and in subjects with latent diabetes. J Clin Invest 1970; 49(12):2151–2160.

7. Orchard TJ, Becker DJ, Bates M, Kuller LH, Drash AL. Plasma insulin and lipoprotein concentrations: an atherogenic association? Am J Epidemiol 1983; 118(3):326–337.

8. Olefsky JM, Farquhar JW, Reaven GM. Reappraisal of the role of insulin in hypertriglyceridemia. Am J Med 1974; 57(4):551–560.

9. Reaven GM, Lerner RL, Stern MP, Farquhar JW. Role of insulin in endogenous hypertriglyceridemia. J Clin Invest 1967; 46(11):1756–1767.

10. Haffner SM, Fong D, Hazuda HP, Pugh JA, Patterson JK. Hyperinsulinemia, upper body adiposity, and cardiovascular risk factors in non-diabetics. Metabolism 1988; 37(4):338–345.

11. Modan M, Halkin H, Almog S, et al. Hyperinsulinemia. A link between hypertension obesity and glucose intolerance. J Clin Invest 1985; 75(3):809–817.

12. Stern MP, Haffner SM. Body fat distribution and hyperinsulinemia as risk factors for diabetes and cardiovascular disease. Arteriosclerosis 1986; 6(2):123–130.

13. Olefsky JM, Kolterman OG, Scarlett JA. Insulin action and resistance in obesity and noninsulin-dependent Type II diabetes mellitus. Am J Physiol 1982; 243(1):E15–E30.

14. Ferrannini E, Buzzigoli G, Bonadonna R, et al. Insulin resistance in essential hypertension. N Engl J Med 1987; 317(6):350–357.

15. Wingard DL, Barrett-Connor E, Criqui MH, Suarez L. Clustering of heart disease risk factors in diabetic compared to nondiabetic adults. Am J Epidemiol 1983; 117(1):19–26.

16. Reaven GM. Banting lecture 1988. Role of insulin resistance in human disease. Diabetes 1988; 37(12):1595–1607.

17. Liese AD, Mayer-Davis EJ, Haffner SM. Development of the multiple metabolic syndrome: an epidemiologic perspective. Epidemiol Rev 1998; 20(2):157–172.

18. Meigs JB, D'Agostino RB Sr, Wilson PW, Cupples LA, Nathan DM, Singer DE. Risk variable clustering in the insulin resistance syndrome. The Framingham Offspring Study. Diabetes 1997; 46(10):1594–1600.

19. Schmidt MI, Watson RL, Duncan BB, et al. Clustering of dyslipidemia, hyperuricemia, diabetes, and hypertension and its association with fasting insulin and central and overall obesity in a general population. Atherosclerosis Risk in Communities Study Investigators. Metabolism 1996; 45(6):699–706.

20. Laakso M, Sarlund H, Mykkanen L. Insulin resistance is associated with lipid and lipoprotein abnormalities in subjects with varying degrees of glucose tolerance. Arteriosclerosis 1990; 10(2):223–231.

21. Schmidt MI, Duncan BB, Watson RL, Sharrett AR, Brancati FL, Heiss G. A metabolic syndrome in whites and African Americans. The Atherosclerosis Risk in Communities baseline study. Diabetes Care 1996; 19(5):414–418.

22. Mykkanen L, Kuusisto J, Pyorala K, Laakso M. Cardiovascular disease risk factors as predictors of Type 2 (non-insulin-dependent) diabetes mellitus in elderly subjects. Diabetologia 1993; 36(6):553–559.

23. Haffner SM, Valdez RA, Hazuda HP, Mitchell BD, Morales PA, Stern MP. Prospective analysis of the insulin-resistance syndrome (syndrome X). Diabetes 1992; 41(6):715–722.

24. Ferrannini E, Haffner SM, Mitchell BD, Stern MP. Hyperinsulinaemia: the key feature of a cardiovascular and metabolic syndrome. Diabetologia 1991; 34(6):416–422.

25. Zavaroni I, Bonora E, Pagliara M, et al. Risk factors for coronary artery disease in healthy persons with hyperinsulinemia and normal glucose tolerance. N Engl J Med 1989; 320(11):702–706.

26. Steinberg HO, Chaker H, Leaming R, Johnson A, Brechtel G, Baron AD. Obesity/insulin resistance is associated with endothelial dysfunction. Implications for the syndrome of insulin resistance. J Clin Invest 1996; 97(11):2601–2610.

27. McFarlane SI, Banerji M, Sowers JR. Insulin resistance and cardiovascular disease. J Clin Endocrinol Metab 2001; 86(2):713–718.

28. Pyorala M, Miettinen H, Halonen P, Laakso M, Pyorala K. Insulin resistance syndrome predicts the risk of coronary heart disease and stroke in healthy middle-aged men: the 22-year follow-up results of the Helsinki Policemen Study. Arterioscler Thromb Vasc Biol 2000; 20(2):538–544.

29. Fonseca V, DeSouza C, Asnani S, Jialal I. Nontraditional risk factors for cardiovascular disease in diabetes. Endocr Rev 2004; 25(1):153–175.

30. Fonseca VA. Risk factors for coronary heart disease in diabetes. Ann Intern Med 2000; 133(2):154–156.

31. Stern MP. Diabetes and cardiovascular disease. The "common soil" hypothesis. Diabetes 1995; 44(4):369–374.

32. Alberti KG, Zimmet PZ. Definition, diagnosis and classification of diabetes mellitus and its complications. Part 1: diagnosis and classification of diabetes mellitus provisional report of a WHO consultation. Diabet Med 1998; 15(7):539–553.

33. Grundy SM, Cleeman JI, Daniels SR, et al. Diagnosis and management of the metabolic syndrome: an American Heart Association/National Heart, Lung, and Blood Institute Scientific Statement. Circulation 2005; 112(17):2735–2752.

34. International Diabetes Federation. The IDF Consensus worldwide definition of the metabolic syndrome [article online]. International Diabetes Federation . 2-8-2006, www.idf.org. Ref Type: Internet Communication

35. http://www.nhlbi.nih.gov/guidelines/cholesterol/atp_iii.html.

36. Ziccardi P, Nappo F, Giugliano G, et al. Reduction of inflammatory cytokine concentrations and improvement of endothelial functions in obese women after weight loss over one year. Circulation 2002; 105(7):804–809.

37. Expert Panel on the Detection EaToHBCA. Executive Summary of The Third Report of The National Cholesterol Education Program (NCEP) Expert Panel on Detection, Evaluation, And Treatment of High Blood Cholesterol In Adults (Adult Treatment Panel III). JAMA 2001; 285(19):2486–2497.

38. Balkau B, Charles MA, Drivsholm T, et al. Frequency of the WHO metabolic syndrome in European cohorts, and an alternative definition of an insulin resistance syndrome. Diabetes Metab 2002; 28(5):364–376.

39. Einhorn D, Reaven GM, Cobin RH, et al. American College of Endocrinology position statement on the insulin resistance syndrome. Endocr Pract 2003; 9(3):237–252.

40. Lakka HM, Laaksonen DE, Lakka TA, et al. The metabolic syndrome and total and cardiovascular disease mortality in middle-aged men. JAMA 2002; 288(21):2709–2716.

41. McNeill AM, Rosamond WD, Girman CJ, et al. The metabolic syndrome and 11-year risk of incident cardiovascular disease in the atherosclerosis risk in communities study. Diabetes Care 2005; 28(2):385–390.
42. Stern SE, Williams K, Ferrannini E, DeFronzo RA, Bogardus C, Stern MP. Identification of individuals with insulin resistance using routine clinical measurements. Diabetes 2005; 54(2):333–339.
43. Meigs JB, Wilson PW, Nathan DM, D'Agostino RB Sr, Williams K, Haffner SM. Prevalence and characteristics of the metabolic syndrome in the San Antonio Heart and Framingham Offspring Studies. Diabetes 2003; 52(8):2160–2167.
44. Ford ES, Giles WH. A comparison of the prevalence of the metabolic syndrome using two proposed definitions. Diabetes Care 2003; 26(3):575–581.
45. Malik S, Wong ND, Franklin S, Pio J, Fairchild C, Chen R. Cardiovascular disease in U.S. patients with metabolic syndrome, diabetes, and elevated C-reactive protein. Diabetes Care 2005; 28(3):690–693.
46. Hunt KJ, Resendez RG, Williams K, Haffner SM, Stern MP. National Cholesterol Education Program versus World Health Organization metabolic syndrome in relation to all-cause and cardiovascular mortality in the San Antonio Heart Study. Circulation 2004; 110(10):1251–1257.
47. Girman CJ, Dekker JM, Rhodes T, et al. An exploratory analysis of criteria for the metabolic syndrome and its prediction of long-term cardiovascular outcomes: the Hoorn study. Am J Epidemiol 2005; 162(5):438–447.
48. Ford ES. Risks for all-cause mortality, cardiovascular disease, and diabetes associated with the metabolic syndrome: a summary of the evidence. Diabetes Care 2005; 28(7):1769–1778.
49. Bruno G, Merletti F, Biggeri A, et al. Metabolic syndrome as a predictor of all-cause and cardiovascular mortality in Type 2 diabetes: the Casale Monferrato Study. Diabetes Care 2004; 27(11):2689–2694.
50. Malik S, Wong ND, Franklin SS, et al. Impact of the metabolic syndrome on mortality from coronary heart disease, cardiovascular disease, and all causes in United States adults. Circulation 2004; 110(10):1245–1250.
51. Resnick HE, Jones K, Ruotolo G, et al. Insulin resistance, the metabolic syndrome, and risk of incident cardiovascular disease in nondiabetic American Indians: the Strong Heart Study. Diabetes Care 2003; 26(3):861–867.
52. Marroquin OC, Kip KE, Kelley DE, et al. Metabolic syndrome modifies the cardiovascular risk associated with angiographic coronary artery disease in women: a report from the Women's Ischemia Syndrome Evaluation. Circulation 2004; 109(6):714–721.
53. Ford ES. Prevalence of the metabolic syndrome defined by the International Diabetes Federation among adults in the U.S. Diabetes Care 2005; 28(11):2745–2749.
54. Lewington S, Clarke R, Qizilbash N, Peto R, Collins R. Age-specific relevance of usual blood pressure to vascular mortality: a meta-analysis of individual data for one million adults in 61 prospective studies. Lancet 2002; 360(9349):1903–1913.
55. Deckert T, Feldt-Rasmussen B, Borch-Johnsen K, Jensen T, Kofoed-Enevoldsen A. Albuminuria reflects widespread vascular damage. The Steno hypothesis. Diabetologia 1989; 32(4):219–226.
56. Keys A, Aravanis C, Blackburn H, et al. Coronary heart disease: overweight and obesity as risk factors. Ann Intern Med 1972; 77(1):15–27.

57. Miller GJ, Miller NE. Plasma-high-density-lipoprotein concentration and development of ischaemic heart-disease. Lancet 1975; 1(7897):16–19.

58. Lippel K, Tyroler H, Eder H, Gotto A Jr, Vahouny G. Relationship of hypertriglyceridemia to atherosclerosis. Arteriosclerosis 1981; 1(6):406–417.

59. Fuller JH, Shipley MJ, Rose G, Jarrett RJ, Keen H. Coronary-heart-disease risk and impaired glucose tolerance. The Whitehall study. Lancet 1980; 1(8183):1373–1376.

60. Stamler J, Vaccaro O, Neaton JD, Wentworth D. Diabetes, other risk factors, and 12-yr cardiovascular mortality for men screened in the Multiple Risk Factor Intervention Trial. Diabetes Care 1993; 16(2):434–444.

61. Kannel WB, McGee DL. Diabetes and cardiovascular risk factors: the Framingham study. Circulation 1979; 59(1):8–13.

62. Grundy SM, Brewer HB Jr, Cleeman JI, Smith SC Jr, Lenfant C. Definition of metabolic syndrome: report of the National Heart, Lung, and Blood Institute/American Heart Association conference on scientific issues related to definition. Circulation 2004; 109(3):433–438.

63. Scuteri A, Najjar SS, Morrell CH, Lakatta EG. The metabolic syndrome in older individuals: prevalence and prediction of cardiovascular events: the Cardiovascular Health Study. Diabetes Care 2005; 28(4):882–887.

64. Onat A, Ceyhan K, Basar O, Erer B, Toprak S, Sansoy V. Metabolic syndrome: major impact on coronary risk in a population with low cholesterol levels—a prospective and cross-sectional evaluation. Atherosclerosis 2002; 165(2):285–292.

65. Lempiainen P, Mykkanen L, Pyorala K, Laakso M, Kuusisto J. Insulin resistance syndrome predicts coronary heart disease events in elderly nondiabetic men. Circulation 1999; 100(2):123–128.

66. Kuusisto J, Lempiainen P, Mykkanen L, Laakso M. Insulin resistance syndrome predicts coronary heart disease events in elderly Type 2 diabetic men. Diabetes Care 2001; 24(9):1629–1633.

67. Kekalainen P, Sarlund H, Pyorala K, Laakso M. Hyperinsulinemia cluster predicts the development of Type 2 diabetes independently of family history of diabetes. Diabetes Care 1999; 22(1):86–92.

68. Katzmarzyk PT, Church TS, Blair SN. Cardiorespiratory fitness attenuates the effects of the metabolic syndrome on all-cause and cardiovascular disease mortality in men. Arch Intern Med 2004; 164(10):1092–1097.

69. Isomaa B, Almgren P, Tuomi T, et al. Cardiovascular morbidity and mortality associated with the metabolic syndrome. Diabetes Care 2001; 24(4):683–689.

70. Girman CJ, Rhodes T, Mercuri M, et al. The metabolic syndrome and risk of major coronary events in the Scandinavian Simvastatin Survival Study (4S) and the Air Force/Texas Coronary Atherosclerosis Prevention Study (AFCAPS/TexCAPS). Am J Cardiol 2004; 93(2):136–141.

71. Ford ES. The metabolic syndrome and mortality from cardiovascular disease and all-causes: findings from the National Health and Nutrition Examination Survey II Mortality Study. Atherosclerosis 2004; 173(2):309–314.

72. Alexander CM, Landsman PB, Teutsch SM, Haffner SM. NCEP-defined metabolic syndrome, diabetes, and prevalence of coronary heart disease among NHANES III participants age 50 years and older. Diabetes 2003; 52(5):1210–1214.

73. Klein BE, Klein R, Lee KE. Components of the metabolic syndrome and risk of cardiovascular disease and diabetes in beaver dam. Diabetes Care 2002; 25(10):1790–1794.

74. Sattar N, Gaw A, Scherbakova O, et al. Metabolic syndrome with and without C-reactive protein as a predictor of coronary heart disease and diabetes in the West of Scotland Coronary Prevention Study. Circulation 2003; 108(4): 414–419.

75. Golden SH, Folsom AR, Coresh J, Sharrett AR, Szklo M, Brancati F. Risk factor groupings related to insulin resistance and their synergistic effects on subclinical atherosclerosis: the atherosclerosis risk in communities study. Diabetes 2002; 51(10):3069–3076.

76. Stern MP, Williams K, Hunt KJ. Impact of diabetes/metabolic syndrome in patients with established cardiovascular disease. Atheroscler Suppl 2005; 6(2):3–6.

77. Festa A, D'Agostino R Jr, Howard G, Mykkanen L, Tracy RP, Haffner SM. Chronic subclinical inflammation as part of the insulin resistance syndrome: the Insulin Resistance Atherosclerosis Study (IRAS). Circulation 2000; 102(1):42–47.

78. Yarnell JW, Patterson CC, Bainton D, Sweetnam PM. Is metabolic syndrome a discrete entity in the general population? Evidence from the Caerphilly and Speedwell population studies. Heart 1998; 79(3):248–252.

79. Ferrannini E, Balkau B. Insulin: in search of a syndrome. Diabet Med 2002; 19(9):724–729.

80. Weyer C, Hanson RL, Tataranni PA, Bogardus C, Pratley RE. A high fasting plasma insulin concentration predicts Type 2 diabetes independent of insulin resistance: evidence for a pathogenic role of relative hyperinsulinemia. Diabetes 2000; 49(12):2094–2101.

81. Mykkanen L, Haffner SM, Ronnemaa T, Bergman RN, Laakso M. Low insulin sensitivity is associated with clustering of cardiovascular disease risk factors. Am J Epidemiol 1997; 146(4):315–321.

82. McLaughlin T, Abbasi F, Cheal K, Chu J, Lamendola C, Reaven G. Use of metabolic markers to identify overweight individuals who are insulin resistant. Ann Intern Med 2003; 139(10):802–809.

83. Liao Y, Kwon S, Shaughnessy S, et al. Critical evaluation of adult treatment panel III criteria in identifying insulin resistance with dyslipidemia. Diabetes Care 2004; 27(4):978–983.

84. Cheal KL, Abbasi F, Lamendola C, McLaughlin T, Reaven GM, Ford ES. Relationship to insulin resistance of the adult treatment panel III diagnostic criteria for identification of the metabolic syndrome. Diabetes 2004; 53(5):1195–1200.

85. Laws A, Reaven GM. Evidence for an independent relationship between insulin resistance and fasting plasma HDL-cholesterol, triglyceride and insulin concentrations. J Intern Med 1992; 231(1):25–30.

86. Shadid S, Jensen MD. Effects of pioglitazone versus diet and exercise on metabolic health and fat distribution in upper body obesity. Diabetes Care 2003; 26(11):3148–3152.

87. Lebovitz HE, Dole JF, Patwardhan R, Rappaport EB, Freed MI. Rosiglitazone monotherapy is effective in patients with Type 2 diabetes. J Clin Endocrinol Metab 2001; 86(1):280–288.

88. Knowler WC, Barrett-Connor E, Fowler SE, et al. Reduction in the incidence of Type 2 diabetes with lifestyle intervention or metformin. N Engl J Med 2002; 346(6):393–403.

89. Haffner SM, Greenberg AS, Weston WM, Chen H, Williams K, Freed MI. Effect of rosiglitazone treatment on nontraditional markers of cardiovascular disease in patients with Type 2 diabetes mellitus. Circulation 2002; 106(6):679–684.

90.   Freed MI, Ratner R, Marcovina SM, et al. Effects of rosiglitazone alone and in combination with atorvastatin on the metabolic abnormalities in Type 2 diabetes mellitus. Am J Cardiol 2002; 90(9):947–952.

91.   Aronoff S, Rosenblatt S, Braithwaite S, Egan JW, Mathisen AL, Schneider RL. Pioglitazone hydrochloride monotherapy improves glycemic control in the treatment of patients with Type 2 diabetes: a 6-month randomized placebo-controlled dose-response study. The Pioglitazone 001 Study Group. Diabetes Care 2000; 23(11):1605–1611.

92.   Effect of intensive blood-glucose control with metformin on complications in overweight patients with Type 2 diabetes (UKPDS 34). UK Prospective Diabetes Study (UKPDS) Group. Lancet 1998; 352(9131):854–865.

93.   Jawa AA, Fonseca VA. Role of insulin secretagogues and insulin sensitizing agents in the prevention of cardiovascular disease in patients who have diabetes. Cardiol Clin 2005; 23(2):119–138.

94.   Xiang AH, Peters RK, Kjos SL, et al. Effect of pioglitazone on Pancreatic (beta) cell function and diabetes risk in hispanic women with prior gestational diabetes. Diabetes 2006; 55(2):517–522.

95.   American Diabetes Association. All About Diabetes. American Diabetes Association . 2005 Last accessed February 8, 2006, www.idf.org.

96.   Colwell JA. Vascular thrombosis in Type II diabetes mellitus. Diabetes 1993; 42(1):8–11.

97.   Saenz dT I, Goldstein I, Azadzoi K, Krane RJ, Cohen RA. Impaired neurogenic and endothelium-mediated relaxation of penile smooth muscle from diabetic men with impotence. N Engl J Med 1989; 320(16):1025–1030.

98.   Keller KB, Lemberg L. Obesity and the metabolic syndrome. Am J Crit Care 2003; 12(2):167–170.

99.   Cossrow N, Falkner B. Race/ethnic issues in obesity and obesity-related comorbidities. J Clin Endocrinol Metab 2004; 89(6):2590–2594.

100. Falkner B. Obesity: clinical impact and interventions that work: an update. Ethn Dis 2003; 13(3 suppl 3):S3-30–31.

101. Flegal KM, Carroll MD, Ogden CL, Johnson CL. Prevalence and trends in obesity among US adults, 1999–2000. JAMA 2002; 288(14):1723–1727.

102. McTigue KM, Garrett JM, Popkin BM. The natural history of the development of obesity in a cohort of young U.S. adults between 1981 and 1998. Ann Intern Med 2002; 136(12):857–864.

103. Petersen KF, Dufour S, Befroy D, Garcia R, Shulman GI. Impaired mitochondrial activity in the insulin-resistant offspring of patients with Type 2 diabetes. N Engl J Med 2004; 350(7):664–671.

104. Pimenta W, Korytkowski M, Mitrakou A, et al. Pancreatic beta-cell dysfunction as the primary genetic lesion in NIDDM. Evidence from studies in normal glucose-tolerant individuals with a first-degree NIDDM relative. JAMA 1995; 273(23):1855–1861.

105. Brunzell JD, Hokanson JE. Dyslipidemia of central obesity and insulin resistance. Diabetes Care 1999; 22(suppl 3):C10–C13.

106. Ginsberg HN, Huang LS. The insulin resistance syndrome: impact on lipoprotein metabolism and atherothrombosis. J Cardiovasc Risk 2000; 7(5):325–331.

107. Weyer C, Funahashi T, Tanaka S, et al. Hypoadiponectinemia in obesity and Type 2 diabetes: close association with insulin resistance and hyperinsulinemia. J Clin Endocrinol Metab 2001; 86(5):1930–1935.

108. Yudkin JS, Stehouwer CD, Emeis JJ, Coppack SW. C-reactive protein in healthy subjects: associations with obesity, insulin resistance, and endothelial dysfunction: a potential role for cytokines originating from adipose tissue? Arterioscler Thromb Vasc Biol 1999; 19(4):972–978.

109. Chandran M, Phillips SA, Ciaraldi T, Henry RR. Adiponectin: more than just another fat cell hormone? Diabetes Care 2003; 26(8):2442–2450.

110. Kazumi T, Kawaguchi A, Sakai K, Hirano T, Yoshino G. Young men with high-normal blood pressure have lower serum adiponectin, smaller LDL size, and higher elevated heart rate than those with optimal blood pressure. Diabetes Care 2002; 25(6):971–976.

111. Matsubara M, Maruoka S, Katayose S. Decreased plasma adiponectin concentrations in women with dyslipidemia. J Clin Endocrinol Metab 2002; 87(6):2764–2769.

112. Pischon T, Girman CJ, Hotamisligil GS, Rifai N, Hu FB, Rimm EB. Plasma adiponectin levels and risk of myocardial infarction in men. JAMA 2004; 291(14):1730–1737.

113. Zoccali C, Mallamaci F, Tripepi G, et al. Adiponectin, metabolic risk factors, and cardiovascular events among patients with end-stage renal disease. J Am Soc Nephrol 2002; 13(1):134–141.

114. Kojima S, Funahashi T, Sakamoto T, et al. The variation of plasma concentrations of a novel, adipocyte derived protein, adiponectin, in patients with acute myocardial infarction. Heart 2003; 89(6):667.

115. Kumada M, Kihara S, Sumitsuji S, et al. Association of hypoadiponectinemia with coronary artery disease in men. Arterioscler Thromb Vasc Biol 2003; 23(1):85–89.

116. Spranger J, Kroke A, Mohlig M, et al. Adiponectin and protection against Type 2 diabetes mellitus. Lancet 2003; 361(9353):226–228.

117. Scherer PE, Williams S, Fogliano M, Baldini G, Lodish HF. A novel serum protein similar to C1q, produced exclusively in adipocytes. J Biol Chem 1995; 270(45):26746–26749.

118. Ouchi N, Kihara S, Arita Y, et al. Adiponectin, an adipocyte-derived plasma protein, inhibits endothelial NF-kappaB signaling through a cAMP-dependent pathway. Circulation 2000; 102(11):1296–1301.

119. Berg AH, Combs TP, Du X, Brownlee M, Scherer PE. The adipocyte-secreted protein Acrp30 enhances hepatic insulin action. Nat Med 2001; 7(8):947–953.

120. Kubota N, Terauchi Y, Yamauchi T, et al. Disruption of adiponectin causes insulin resistance and neointimal formation. J Biol Chem 2002; 277(29):25863–25866.

121. Lindsay RS, Funahashi T, Hanson RL, et al. Adiponectin and development of Type 2 diabetes in the Pima Indian population. Lancet 2002; 360(9326):57–58.

122. Calles-Escandon J, Cipolla M. Diabetes and endothelial dysfunction: a clinical perspective. Endocr Rev 2001; 22(1):36–52.

123. Theuma P, Fonseca VA. Novel cardiovascular risk factors and macrovascular and microvascular complications of diabetes. Curr Drug Targets 2003; 4(6):477–486.

124. Steinberg HO, Paradisi G, Hook G, Crowder K, Cronin J, Baron AD. Free fatty acid elevation impairs insulin-mediated vasodilation and nitric oxide production. Diabetes 2000; 49(7):1231–1238.

125. Baron AD. Insulin and the vasculature—old actors, new roles. J Investig Med 1996; 44(8):406–412.

126. Baron AD, Steinberg HO. Endothelial function, insulin sensitivity, and hypertension. Circulation 1997; 96(3):725–726.

127. Baron AD. Insulin resistance and vascular function. J Diabetes Complications 2002; 16(1):92–102.

128. Grover A, Padginton C, Wilson MF, Sung BH, Izzo JL Jr, Dandona P. Insulin attenuates norepinephrine-induced venoconstriction. An ultrasonographic study. Hypertension 1995; 25(4 Pt 2):779–784.

129. Aljada A, Dandona P. Effect of insulin on human aortic endothelial nitric oxide synthase. Metabolism 2000; 49(2):147–150.

130. Aljada A, Ghanim H, Assian E, Dandona P. Tumor necrosis factor-alpha inhibits insulin-induced increase in endothelial nitric oxide synthase and reduces insulin receptor content and phosphorylation in human aortic endothelial cells. Metabolism 2002; 51(4):487–491.

131. Zeng G, Quon MJ. Insulin-stimulated production of nitric oxide is inhibited by wortmannin. Direct measurement in vascular endothelial cells. J Clin Invest 1996; 98(4):894–898.

132. Ross R. Atherosclerosis—an inflammatory disease. N Engl J Med 1999; 340(2):115–126.

133. Wellen KE, Hotamisligil GS. Obesity-induced inflammatory changes in adipose tissue. J Clin Invest 2003; 112(12):1785–1788.

134. Xu H, Barnes GT, Yang Q, et al. Chronic inflammation in fat plays a crucial role in the development of obesity-related insulin resistance. J Clin Invest 2003; 112(12):1821–1830.

135. Yudkin JS, Kumari M, Humphries SE, Mohamed-Ali V. Inflammation, obesity, stress and coronary heart disease: is interleukin-6 the link? Atherosclerosis 2000; 148(2):209–214.

136. Pearson TA, Mensah GA, Alexander RW, et al. Markers of inflammation and cardiovascular disease: application to clinical and public health practice. A statement for healthcare professionals from the Centers for Disease Control and Prevention and the American Heart Association. Circulation 2003; 107(3):499–511.

137. Ridker PM, Wilson PW, Grundy SM. Should C-reactive protein be added to metabolic syndrome and to assessment of global cardiovascular risk? Circulation 2004; 109(23):2818–2825.

138. Kershaw EE, Flier JS. Adipose tissue as an endocrine organ. J Clin Endocrinol Metab 2004; 89(6):2548–2556.

139. McLaughlin T, Abbasi F, Lamendola C, et al. Differentiation between obesity and insulin resistance in the association with C-reactive protein. Circulation 2002; 106(23):2908–2912.

140. Ridker PM, Buring JE, Cook NR, Rifai N. C-reactive protein, the metabolic syndrome, and risk of incident cardiovascular events: an 8-year follow-up of 14719 initially healthy American women. Circulation 2003; 107(3):391–397.

141. Ridker PM, Cannon CP, Morrow D, et al. C-reactive protein levels and outcomes after statin therapy. N Engl J Med 2005; 352(1):20–28.

142. Ridker PM. Clinical application of C-reactive protein for cardiovascular disease detection and prevention. Circulation 2003; 107(3):363–369.

143. Ridker PM, Hennekens CH, Buring JE, Rifai N. C-reactive protein and other markers of inflammation in the prediction of cardiovascular disease in women. N Engl J Med 2000; 342(12):836–843.

144. Danesh J, Collins R, Appleby P, Peto R. Association of fibrinogen, C-reactive protein, albumin, or leukocyte count with coronary heart disease: meta-analyses of prospective studies. JAMA 1998; 279(18):1477–1482.

145. Pradhan AD, Cook NR, Buring JE, Manson JE, Ridker PM. C-reactive protein is independently associated with fasting insulin in nondiabetic women. Arterioscler Thromb Vasc Biol 2003; 23(4):650–655.

146. Rutter MK, Meigs JB, Sullivan LM, D'Agostino RB Sr, Wilson PW. C-reactive protein, the metabolic syndrome, and prediction of cardiovascular events in the Framingham Offspring Study. Circulation 2004; 110(4):380–385.

147. Reilly MP, Wolfe ML, Rhodes T, Girman C, Mehta N, Rader DJ. Measures of insulin resistance add incremental value to the clinical diagnosis of metabolic syndrome in association with coronary atherosclerosis. Circulation 2004; 110(7):803–809.

148. Festa A, D'Agostino R Jr, Mykkanen L, et al. Relative contribution of insulin and its precursors to fibrinogen and PAI-1 in a large population with different states of glucose tolerance. The Insulin Resistance Atherosclerosis Study (IRAS). Arterioscler Thromb Vasc Biol 1999; 19(3):562–568.

149. Haffner SM, D'Agostino R Jr, Mykkanen L, et al. Insulin sensitivity in subjects with Type 2 diabetes. Relationship to cardiovascular risk factors: the Insulin Resistance Atherosclerosis Study. Diabetes Care 1999; 22(4):562–568.

150. Potter van Loon BJ, Kluft C, Radder JK, Blankenstein MA, Meinders AE. The cardiovascular risk factor plasminogen activator inhibitor Type 1 is related to insulin resistance. Metabolism 1993; 42(8):945–949.

151. Imperatore G, Riccardi G, Iovine C, Rivellese AA, Vaccaro O. Plasma fibrinogen: a new factor of the metabolic syndrome. A population-based study. Diabetes Care 1998; 21(4):649–654.

152. Ernst E, Resch KL. Fibrinogen as a cardiovascular risk factor: a meta-analysis and review of the literature. Ann Intern Med 1993; 118(12):956–963.

153. Despres JP, Lamarche B, Mauriege P, et al. Hyperinsulinemia as an independent risk factor for ischemic heart disease. N Engl J Med 1996; 334(15):952–957.

154. Parulkar AA, Pendergrass ML, Granda-Ayala R, Lee TR, Fonseca VA. Nonhypoglycemic effects of thiazolidinediones. Ann Intern Med 2001; 134(1):61–71.

155. Martens FM, Visseren FL, Lemay J, de Koning EJ, Rabelink TJ. Metabolic and additional vascular effects of thiazolidinediones. Drugs 2002; 62(10):1463–1480.

156. Intensive blood-glucose control with sulphonylureas or insulin compared with conventional treatment and risk of complications in patients with Type 2 diabetes (UKPDS 33). UK Prospective Diabetes Study (UKPDS) Group. Lancet 1998; 352(9131):837–853.

157. Grundy SM, Hansen B, Smith SC Jr, Cleeman JI, Kahn RA. Clinical management of metabolic syndrome: report of the American Heart Association/National Heart, Lung, and Blood Institute/American Diabetes Association conference on scientific issues related to management. Circulation 2004; 109(4):551–556.

158. Wilson PW, Grundy SM. The metabolic syndrome: practical guide to origins and treatment: part I. Circulation 2003; 108(12):1422–1424.

159. Chobanian AV, Bakris GL, Black HR, et al. Seventh report of the Joint National Committee on prevention, detection, evaluation, and treatment of high blood pressure. Hypertension 2003; 42(6):1206–1252.

160. Smith SC Jr, Jackson R, Pearson TA, et al. Principles for national and regional guidelines on cardiovascular disease prevention: a scientific statement from the World Heart and Stroke Forum. Circulation 2004; 109(25):3112–3121.

161. Eriksson KF, Lindgarde F. Prevention of Type 2 (non-insulin-dependent) diabetes mellitus by diet and physical exercise. The 6-year Malmo feasibility study. Diabetologia 1991; 34(12):891–898.

162. Pan XR, Li GW, Hu YH, et al. Effects of diet and exercise in preventing NIDDM in people with impaired glucose tolerance. The Da Qing IGT and Diabetes Study. Diabetes Care 1997; 20(4):537–544.

163. Tuomilehto J, Lindstrom J, Eriksson JG, et al. Prevention of Type 2 diabetes mellitus by changes in lifestyle among subjects with impaired glucose tolerance. N Engl J Med 2001; 344(18):1343–1350.

164. Orchard TJ, Temprosa M, Goldberg R, et al. The effect of metformin and intensive lifestyle intervention on the metabolic syndrome: the Diabetes Prevention Program randomized trial. Ann Intern Med 2005; 142(8):611–619.

165. Bailey CJ, Turner RC. Metformin. N Engl J Med 1996; 334(9):574–579.

166. Ratner R, Goldberg R, Haffner S, et al. Impact of intensive lifestyle and metformin therapy on cardiovascular disease risk factors in the diabetes prevention program. Diabetes Care 2005; 28(4):888–894.

167. Yamasaki Y, Kawamori R, Wasada T, et al. Pioglitazone (AD-4833) ameliorates insulin resistance in patients with NIDDM. AD-4833 Glucose Clamp Study Group, Japan. Tohoku J Exp Med 1997; 183(3):173–183.

168. Scheen AJ, Lefebvre PJ. Troglitazone: antihyperglycemic activity and potential role in the treatment of Type 2 diabetes. Diabetes Care 1999; 22(9):1568–1577.

169. Raskin P, Rappaport EB, Cole ST, Yan Y, Patwardhan R, Freed MI. Rosiglitazone short-term monotherapy lowers fasting and post-prandial glucose in patients with Type II diabetes. Diabetologia 2000; 43(3):278–284.

170. Prigeon RL, Kahn SE, Porte D Jr. Effect of troglitazone on B cell function, insulin sensitivity, and glycemic control in subjects with Type 2 diabetes mellitus. J Clin Endocrinol Metab 1998; 83(3):819–823.

171. Nolan JJ, Ludvik B, Beerdsen P, Joyce M, Olefsky J. Improvement in glucose tolerance and insulin resistance in obese subjects treated with troglitazone. N Engl J Med 1994; 331(18):1188–1193.

172. Ghazzi MN, Perez JE, Antonucci TK, et al. Cardiac and glycemic benefits of troglitazone treatment in NIDDM. The Troglitazone Study Group. Diabetes 1997; 46(3):433–439.

173. Wagstaff AJ, Goa KL. Rosiglitazone: a review of its use in the management of Type 2 diabetes mellitus. Drugs 2002; 62(12):1805–1837.

174. Inzucchi SE, Maggs DG, Spollett GR, et al. Efficacy and metabolic effects of metformin and troglitazone in Type II diabetes mellitus. N Engl J Med 1998; 338(13):867–872.

175. Kersten S, Desvergne B, Wahli W. Roles of PPARs in health and disease. Nature 2000; 405(6785):421–424.

176. Olefsky JM. Treatment of insulin resistance with peroxisome proliferator-activated receptor gamma agonists. J Clin Invest 2000; 106(4):467–472.

177. Viberti G, Kahn SE, Greene DA, et al. A diabetes outcome progression trial (ADOPT): an international multicenter study of the comparative efficacy of

rosiglitazone, glyburide, and metformin in recently diagnosed Type 2 diabetes. Diabetes Care 2002; 25(10):1737–1743.

178. Yki-Jarvinen H. The Proactive study: some answers, many questions. Lancet 2005; 366(9493):1241–1242.

179. Fonseca V, Jawa A, Asnani S. The proactive study: the glass is half full. J Clin Endocrinol Metab 2005.

180. Rosenblatt S, Miskin B, Glazer NB, Prince MJ, Robertson KE. The impact of pioglitazone on glycemic control and atherogenic dyslipidemia in patients with Type 2 diabetes mellitus. Coron Artery Dis 2001; 12(5):413–423.

181. Suter SL, Nolan JJ, Wallace P, Gumbiner B, Olefsky JM. Metabolic effects of new oral hypoglycemic agent CS-045 in NIDDM subjects. Diabetes Care 1992; 15(2):193–203.

182. Tack CJ, Smits P, Demacker PN, Stalenhoef AF. Troglitazone decreases the proportion of small, dense LDL and increases the resistance of LDL to oxidation in obese subjects. Diabetes Care 1998; 21(5):796–799.

183. Raji A, Seely EW, Bekins SA, Williams GH, Simonson DC. Rosiglitazone improves insulin sensitivity and lowers blood pressure in hypertensive patients. Diabetes Care 2003; 26(1):172–178.

184. Bakris G, Viberti G, Weston WM, Heise M, Porter LE, Freed MI. Rosiglitazone reduces urinary albumin excretion in Type II diabetes. J Hum Hypertens 2003; 17(1):7–12.

185. Scherbaum WA, Goke B. Metabolic efficacy and safety of once-daily pioglitazone monotherapy in patients with Type 2 diabetes: a double-blind, placebo-controlled study. Horm Metab Res 2002; 34(10):589–595.

186. Mattock MB, Morrish NJ, Viberti G, Keen H, Fitzgerald AP, Jackson G. Prospective study of microalbuminuria as predictor of mortality in NIDDM. Diabetes 1992; 41(6):736–741.

187. Imano E, Kanda T, Nakatani Y, et al. Effect of troglitazone on microalbuminuria in patients with incipient diabetic nephropathy. Diabetes Care 1998; 21(12):2135–2139.

188. Patel J, Anderson RJ, Rappaport EB. Rosiglitazone monotherapy improves glycaemic control in patients with Type 2 diabetes: a twelve-week, randomized, placebo-controlled study. Diabetes Obes Metab 1999; 1(3):165–172.

189. Fonseca V, Rosenstock J, Patwardhan R, Salzman A. Effect of metformin and rosiglitazone combination therapy in patients with Type 2 diabetes mellitus: a randomized controlled trial. JAMA 2000; 283(13):1695–1702.

190. Spiegelman BM. PPAR-gamma: adipogenic regulator and thiazolidinedione receptor. Diabetes 1998; 47(4):507–514.

191. Fonseca V. Effect of thiazolidinediones on body weight in patients with diabetes mellitus. Am J Med 2003; 115(suppl 8A):42S–48S.

192. Buchanan TA, Xiang AH, Peters RK, et al. Preservation of pancreatic beta-cell function and prevention of Type 2 diabetes by pharmacological treatment of insulin resistance in high-risk hispanic women. Diabetes 2002; 51(9):2796–2803.

193. Xiang AH, Peters RK, Kjos SL, et al. Effect of pioglitazone on pancreatic {beta}-cell function and diabetes risk in hispanic women with prior gestational diabetes. Diabetes 2006; 55(2):517–522.

194. Petersen JL, McGuire DK. Impaired glucose tolerance and impaired fasting glucose—a review of diagnosis, clinical implications and management. Diab Vasc Dis Res 2005; 2(1):9–15.

195. The DREAM (Diabetes REduction Assessment with ramipril and rosiglitazone Medication) investigators. Effect of rosiglitazone on the frequency of diabetes in patients with impaired glucose tolerance or impaired fasting glucose: a randomised controlled trial. Lancet 2006; 368:1096–1105.

196. Delgado H, Lehmann T, Bobbioni-Harsch E, Ybarra J, Golay A. Acarbose improves indirectly both insulin resistance and secretion in obese Type 2 diabetic patients. Diabetes Metab 2002; 28(3):195–200.

197. Chiasson JL, Josse RG, Gomis R, Hanefeld M, Karasik A, Laakso M. Acarbose for prevention of Type 2 diabetes mellitus: the STOP-NIDDM randomised trial. Lancet 2002; 359(9323):2072–2077.

198. Delorme S, Chiasson JL. Acarbose in the prevention of cardiovascular disease in subjects with impaired glucose tolerance and Type 2 diabetes mellitus. Curr Opin Pharmacol 2005; 5(2):184–189.

199. Mittendorfer B, Ostlund RE Jr, Patterson BW, Klein S. Orlistat inhibits dietary cholesterol absorption. Obes Res 2001; 9(10):599–604.

200. Torgerson JS, Hauptman J, Boldrin MN, Sjostrom L. XENical in the prevention of diabetes in obese subjects (XENDOS) study: a randomized study of orlistat as an adjunct to lifestyle changes for the prevention of Type 2 diabetes in obese patients. Diabetes Care 2004; 27(1):155–161.

201. Krentz AJ, Bailey CJ. Oral antidiabetic agents: current role in Type 2 diabetes mellitus. Drugs 2005; 65(3):385–411.

4

Vascular Biology of the Metabolic Syndrome

Justin M. S. Lee and Robin P. Choudhury

Department of Cardiovascular Medicine, University of Oxford, John Radcliffe Hospital, Oxford, U.K.

SUMMARY

- Incidence of the metabolic syndrome is increasing across all age groups.
- The presence of the syndrome significantly increases the risk of cardiovascular events such as myocardial infarction and stroke.
- Features of the syndrome including obesity, dyslipidemia, hypertension, and hyperglycemia act synergistically to promote the development of atherosclerosis.
- The mechanisms by which atherosclerosis is accelerated include impairment of endothelial function and increased oxidative stress and inflammation, and thrombosis.
- A better appreciation of the molecular and cellular events involved will allow the development of more effective therapies.

INTRODUCTION

The metabolic syndrome was initially recognized by the tendency for certain cardiovascular risk factors—hypertension, glucose intolerance, and dyslipidemia—to cluster together. Subsequently a metabolic "syndrome X" was described by Reaven (1), who proposed insulin resistance as the central pathogenic feature. Over the last few years, various organizations have proposed diagnostic criteria including the World Health Organization (WHO), International Diabetes

Federation (IDF), and the National Cholesterol Education Program Adult Treatment Panel III (NCEP ATP III). The ATP III and IDF definitions are very similar and hold a practical advantage over the WHO criteria in that they do not require formal assessment of insulin resistance. The ATP III definition was most recently updated in 2005 (2) and defines the metabolic syndrome as the presence of three or more of the following five features:

1. Central obesity—waist >102 cm (M) or >88 cm (F).
2. Triglycerides (TGs) ≥150 mg/dL (1.7 mmol/L) or treatment for raised TGs.
3. High-density lipoprotein cholesterol (HDL-C) <40 mg/dL (1.03 mmol/L) in males or <50 mg/dL (1.29 mmol/L) in females or treatment for low HDL.
4. Blood pressure (BP) systolic ≥130 mmHg or diastolic ≥85 mmHg or treatment for hypertension.
5. Fasting glucose ≥100 mg/dL (5.6 mmol/L) or treatment for raised plasma glucose concentration.

According to recent estimates, over a third of the U.S. adult population fulfils these criteria (3), and the situation will likely worsen as the incidence appears to

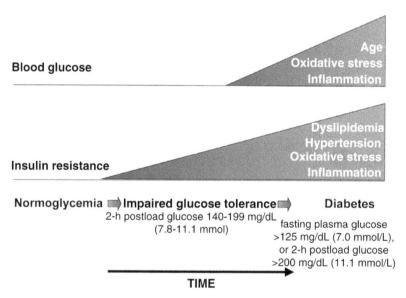

Figure 1   Schematic of the temporal relationship between the metabolic syndrome and Type 2 diabetes. The metabolic syndrome is associated with glucose intolerance and a constellation of vasculopathic features. Over time, a proportion of patients will develop Type 2 diabetes, which is associated with additional mechanisms of vascular damage, in particular those related to hyperglycemia and its consequences. *Abbreviation*: AGE, advanced glycation endproducts.

be increasing, including in adolescents (4). Likely causative factors include a sedentary lifestyle and an excessively calorific diet that is rich in carbohydrate and saturated fat. Individuals with the metabolic syndrome are at risk of developing Type 2 diabetes (5). The increased risk of vascular disease associated with diabetes is well established, and it is now clear that the metabolic syndrome itself carries a two- to threefold increased risk of cardiovascular disease (6,7). As insulin resistance and glucose tolerance worsen, there is an associated increase in the frequency of the other metabolic risk factors, e.g., hypertension and dyslipidemia (Fig. 1) (8). Each of these is associated with increased cardiovascular risk, but occurring together, the risk is further increased (7). Thus, it is not surprising that vascular disease often accompanies the metabolic syndrome and is actually present before the development of overt Type 2 diabetes (9). The burden of mortality and morbidity due to vascular disease in the metabolic syndrome arises largely from "macrovascular disease," i.e., atherosclerosis of the coronary, cerebral, and peripheral circulations (Fig. 2), although long-term microvascular complications affecting the nerves, kidney, and retina also occur if circulating glucose levels reach the diabetic range.

Increasingly, we understand better the molecular mechanisms through which vascular disease occurs as a consequence of the metabolic syndrome. In the first part of this chapter, the pathogenesis of vascular disease, in particular atherosclerosis, will be reviewed with particular reference to the specific features of the metabolic syndrome that accelerate the atherogenesis. The second part will

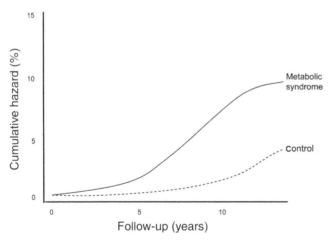

Figure 2 Deaths attributable to CVD and all-cause mortality are increased in men with the metabolic syndrome, even in the absence of baseline CVD and diabetes. In this Finnish study, men with the metabolic syndrome as defined by the NCEP were 2.9 times more likely to die of CAD after adjustment for conventional cardiovascular risk factors. *Abbreviations*: CVD, cardiovascular disease; CAD, coronary artery disease; NCEP, National Cholesterol Education Program. *Source:* From Ref. 10.

consider how specific current and emerging treatments can target these processes and retard the progression of, or potentially regress, this disease.

ENDOTHELIAL FUNCTION

The endothelium is central to vascular homeostasis, overseeing a complex array of vascular processes. It comprises a cellular monolayer on the innermost aspect of blood vessels and has multiple dynamic functions. In fact, it serves as a selective interface between the intravascular and extravascular compartments. The endothelium also regulates inflammation and coagulation and influences the tone of vascular smooth muscle and as a consequence exerts local control over blood vessel size and flow. Furchgott and Zawadzki (11) initially demonstrated that the vasodilator response to infusion of acetylcholine depends on a vessel having intact endothelium and postulated the existence of an endothelium-derived relaxing factor—later identified as nitric oxide (NO). We now know that the endothelium produces a number of vasodilator substances including prostacyclin and NO and that, in health, they balance the action of vasoconstrictors such as endothelin and angiotensin II (Fig. 3). An analogous balance exists between procoagulant and anticoagulant factors. Prostacyclin and NO also function as inhibitors of platelet aggregation (12), thereby antagonizing the action of endothelium-derived prothrombotic factors such as von Willebrand factor (Fig. 3) (13).

The endothelial response to "injury" includes an inflammatory reaction that results in the recruitment of inflammatory cells. A variety of insults can affect

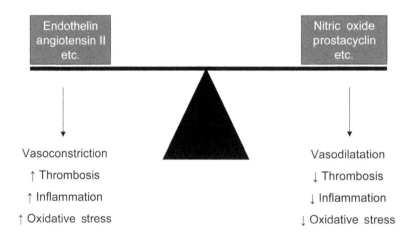

Figure 3   Equilibrium of endothelial function. In health, normal vascular function reflects homeostasis due to balance between pro- and anticoagulant, vasorelaxant, and vasoconstrictor tendencies. Adverse conditions, e.g., dyslipidemia and hyperglycemia, impair protective mechanisms, shifting the balance toward endothelial dysfunction and vascular damage.

normal endothelial function, including hemodynamic factors, hyperglycemia, and dyslipidemia. If the insult is sustained, the inflammatory process will be prolonged, eventually damaging the vessel. Diabetes is thought to cause endothelial dysfunction partly through increased oxidative stress (14). Insulin resistance is also associated with increased asymmetric dimethylarginine (15), an endogenous inhibitor of endothelial NO synthase (e-NOS)—the enzyme responsible for NO synthesis in healthy vessels (16). Loss of vascular homeostasis shifts the balance in favor of vasoconstriction and thrombosis. A dysfunctional endothelium is thought to be one of the earliest events in atherogenesis. Clinically, this is detectable by a loss of or reduction in vasodilator function, though other endothelial functions including the capacity to act as selective barrier are also affected. Endothelial dysfunction is likely to be important at all the stages of atherogenesis right through to the advanced disease and acute plaque events.

A large body of evidence has been established linking clinical measures of endothelial dysfunction and risk of vascular events. Noninvasive imaging with ultrasound (17) and, more recently, magnetic resonance imaging (MRI) (18) have shown changes in endothelium-dependent flow-mediated vasodilatation in patients with risk factors for vascular disease; indeed even children with hyperlipidemia can show impaired endothelial function (17). Both coronary (19) and systemic (20) endothelial dysfunction predict adverse cardiovascular events. It is not surprising then that the metabolic syndrome, given the increased cardiovascular risk, is also strongly associated with endothelial dysfunction (21).

ATHEROSCLEROSIS

Atherosclerosis usually develops over decades and is characterized by the accumulation of lipid-rich and inflammatory material within the walls of arteries (22). This process is accelerated in the metabolic syndrome—early atherosclerosis measured by carotid artery intima media thickness (IMT) is increased in individuals with the metabolic syndrome, and furthermore IMT increases with the presence of each component of the syndrome (23,24). Atherosclerosis usually becomes clinically apparent only when a substantial burden of disease has developed—progressive narrowing of the vessel lumen results in ischemia of the vascular territory downstream of the stenosis. In addition, acute vascular syndromes may develop as a result of thrombotic occlusion of a vessel at the site of plaque rupture or erosion. Various factors including composition, physical properties, and inflammation determine the behavior or "stability" of plaques. This section (Fig. 4) comprises an overview of atherogenesis, from endothelial dysfunction through to plaque formation, with an emphasis on the features that can be influenced by the metabolic syndrome.

The earliest visible change in atherosclerosis appears to be the deposition of small lipoprotein particles within the subendothelial space (25). This tends to occur in locations that do not experience smooth laminar blood flow, such as at

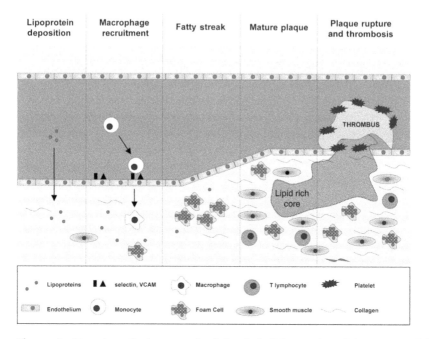

Figure 4   Overview of atherogenesis. Subendothelial retention of Apo-B–containing lipoproteins contributes to endothelial dysfunction and inflammation. Monocytes are recruited through the expression of endothelial cell adhesion molecules and through the secretion of chemokines. Uptake of oxLDL by macrophages results in the formation of foam cells. As inflammation continues, plaques become more complex with smooth muscle, connective tissue, and necrotic elements. Rupture of a plaque exposes thrombogenic constituents, which can lead to vascular occlusion. *Abbreviations*: LDL, low-density lipoprotein; VCAM, vascular cell adhesion molecule.

arterial branch points (26). Here, increased permeability resulting from endothelial dysfunction allows lipoproteins to cross the endothelium. Lipoproteins are then retained in the subendothelial space, because of interactions between arterial wall proteoglycans and apolipoprotein B (Apo-B) on the lipoprotein particle surface (27,28). Subsequently, lipoproteins undergo oxidative modification that renders them susceptible to uptake by macrophages. A local inflammatory reaction is characterized by the expression or upregulation of cell adhesion molecules including P-selectin and E-selectin, vascular cell adhesion molecule-1, and intercellular adhesion molecule-1. These bind to ligands expressed by mononuclear leukocytes in the blood with the result that the cells selectively become adherent to the endothelium. Under the influence of chemokines, e.g., monocyte chemottractant protein-1 (MCP-1), more inflammatory cells cross the endothelium and enter the subendothelial space. There the monocytes differentiate into macrophages, which play a key role in atherogenesis.

Macrophages take up lipoproteins through several different types of receptors. Uptake of nonmodified low-density lipoprotein (LDL) via the LDL-receptor is not deleterious, because there is a negative feedback loop controlling this process. However lipoproteins that have undergone oxidative modification are taken up by the CD36 and macrophage scavenger receptors (SR), which are not subject to regulation. The result is progressive accumulation of cholesterol within the macrophage. Conversion to cholesteryl ester then results in visible fatty droplets—hence these are termed "foam cells." Collections of foam cells form macroscopically visible "fatty streaks."

In addition, macrophages also produce cytokines such as interferon-γ, interleukin (IL)-1, and tumor necrosis factor (TNF), which further drive the inflammatory process by recruiting more macrophages and T-lymphocytes. Thereafter, continued cell influx and proliferation leads to the formation of more advanced lesions. Coalescence of lipids due to foam cell death contributes to the formation of a lipid-rich necrotic core, while peptide growth factors produced by macrophages and other cells promote smooth muscle cell proliferation and generation of a collagen and proteoglycan-based extracellular matrix. The fibrous elements confine the lipid-rich necrotic core within the vessel wall and away from blood in the vessel lumen.

As a result of enzymatic degradation and mechanical forces, plaque rupture or erosion of the fibrous cap may occur, with exposure of prothrombotic material of the necrotic core. Phospholipids, tissue factor, and components of the extracellular matrix provoke the formation of a thrombus that can obstruct the vessel lumen. Plaque ruptures tend to occur at sites of mechanical weakness where the fibrous cap is thin. Inflammation plays a role in determining plaque stability, because inflammatory cells produce proteolytic enzymes, e.g., matrix metalloproteinases (MMPs) that erode the fibrous cap.

Although often seen as progressive and relentless, the development of atherosclerotic plaque probably reflects the net effect of dynamic processes, including the deposition and removal of cholesterol. There is accumulating evidence that cholesterol can be removed from the macrophages via the adenosine triphosphate (ATP)-binding cassette (ABC) proteins (29), which transfer cholesterol to Apo-AI, the main apolipooprotein found in HDL particles. Similarly, macrophages appear to exit plaque under appropriate conditions (30). Individual features of the metabolic syndrome that accelerate development of atherosclerosis will be discussed first, then targeted therapies to stabilize and regress atherosclerosis will be discussed in detail in the section "Current and Emerging Treatment Targets."

VASCULAR EFFECTS OF THE METABOLIC SYNDROME

The following section considers how features of the metabolic syndrome can accelerate atherogenesis. Wherever possible, discussion relates directly to the metabolic syndrome; however, when specific data are not available, the effects of Type 2 diabetes mellitus are considered. This is justifiable because diabetes forms

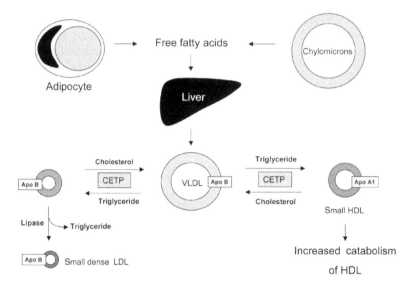

Figure 5 Dyslipidemia in the metabolic syndrome is characterized by low HDL-C, high TGs, and LDL cholesterol, which is typically not greatly elevated, but which comprises small, dense, atherogenic LDL particles. Increased fatty acid flux to the liver causes overproduction of TG-rich VLDL, which in turn increases catabolism of HDL and leads to generation of small dense LDL. *Abbreviations*: HDL, high-density lipoprotein; LDL, low-density lipoprotein; VLDL, very low–density lipoprotein; CETP, cholesteryl ester transfer protein; Apo-B, apolipoprotein B.

part of the "spectrum" of the metabolic syndrome and also serves to highlight areas for future investigation.

Dyslipidemia

Lipids within blood are carried in complex lipoprotein particles. The general structure of these particles is a core of TGs and cholesteryl esters, encapsulated within a monolayer of phospholipids, unesterified cholesterol, and protein (e.g., Apo-B-100 in LDL). The particles are classified according to their density due to differential composition. In broad terms, very low–density lipoprotein (VLDL) and LDL are atherogenic, while HDLs are protective. The metabolic syndrome is associated with low levels of HDL-C, elevated TGs, and abnormal LDL particles, which tend to be smaller and denser than normal (see below).

In the metabolic syndrome, adipocytes are resistant to the action of insulin, and lipolysis continues unchecked. Increased release of free (i.e., nonesterified) fatty acids from adipocytes and their delivery to the liver provide additional substrate for hepatic production of TG-rich VLDL. Another source of free fatty acids for hepatic VLDL synthesis is the hydrolysis of TG-containing chylomicrons particles derived from the gastrointestinal tract. Exchange of TG from VLDL particles for cholesterol HDL (and LDL) particles by the action of cholesteryl ester transfer protein (CETP) results in cholesterol-depleted HDL and TG-rich LDL (31,32). The action of hepatic lipase on TG-rich LDL particles produces "small dense LDL" (sdLDL) particles (33), which are particularly atherogenic and characteristic of the metabolic syndrome. TG-rich HDL particles also become smaller due to the action of hepatic lipase, which renders them easier to catabolize (34).

Thus, the metabolic syndrome has a lipid profile characterized by low HDL and elevated TGs (VLDL), which contributes to the susceptibility to atherosclerotic disease. LDL-cholesterol (LDL-C) itself may not be particularly raised, but as discussed in the following section, it becomes more atherogenic. (See Fig. 5 for an overview of dyslipidemia in this context.)

Small, Dense LDL Particles

The metabolic syndrome is characterized by smaller, denser LDL particles. The greatly increased cardiovascular risk due to the effect of small LDL particle size in association with insulin resistance was demonstrated in the Quebec study of nondiabetic men (35). Although LDL-C is strongly associated with cardiovascular disease, blood levels of LDL-C are not particularly raised in the metabolic syndrome. However, because each LDL particle contains one molecule of Apo-B, plasma Apo-B is equivalent to the total atherogenic particle number. As the LDL particles tend to be smaller, for the same amount of LDL-C, the total number of atherogenic particles is actually increased in the metabolic syndrome. Accordingly, measurement of Apo-B may allow better, more direct estimation of risk than measurement of LDL-C (36,37). At present, however, measurement of Apo-B is not widely available to clinicians. The high atherogenicity of small, dense LDL particles is accounted for by many factors. It has a lower binding affinity for the LDL receptor (38), resulting in prolonged plasma half-life and more opportunities to enter the vessel wall. Aortic perfusion experiments have shown a relatively greater penetration into the subendothelial space, possibly due to smaller particle size (39). Once in the subendothelial space, binding to arterial wall proteoglycans (40) is higher for sdLDL than for larger LDL particles. In vitro sdLDL more readily undergoes oxidative modification (41).

Oxidized LDL-C

The metabolic syndrome is associated with increased oxidative stress (42). Modification of lipoproteins to generate oxidized LDL (oxLDL) is a key step in atherogenesis. The presence of markers of LDL oxidation including circulating oxLDL (43) and autoantibodies to oxLDL (44) appear to predict atherosclerotic disease. In vitro, oxLDL has been shown to promote many of the steps involved in atherogenesis. OxLDL promotes expression of endothelial cell adhesion molecules (45) and inflammatory cell chemoattractants (46); indeed oxLDL itself is a chemoattractant (47). OxLDL is also toxic (48) and promotes cell death, contributing to the formation of the necrotic core of the mature plaque. Finally, oxLDL increases the expression of tissue factor (49) and plasminogen activator inhibitor-1 (PAI-1) (50), known prothrombotic factors (below).

Very Low–Density Lipoproteins

High levels of TG-rich lipoproteins (VLDL and chylomicrons) are a notable feature of the dyslipidemia of the metabolic syndrome and are an independent predictor of cardiovascular disease (51). Plasma levels of TGs are actually dynamic, with postprandial peaks, the magnitude of which varies between individuals. Postprandial lipemia has been shown to correlate with carotid intima thickness, an early measure of atherosclerosis, independent of LDL cholesterol and fasting TGs (52). The magnitude of postprandial lipemia following a single fatty meal is negatively related to measures of vascular function (53) and associated with a transient increase in the concentrations of proinflammatory cytokines and soluble adhesion molecules (54). It is possible that repeated postprandial exposure of the blood vessel wall to the activities of proinflammatory cytokines and pro-oxidants may damage the vascular endothelium and promote atherogenesis. Lipoproteins actually vary greatly in size, and while it is thought that the larger VLDL and chylomicron particles probably cannot penetrate the arterial wall, smaller "remnant" particles can. Remnant lipoproteins predict impaired vasomotor function and presence of coronary artery disease (CAD) in the metabolic syndrome (55). Furthermore, chylomicron remnants contain a truncated Apo, Apo-B48, rather than Apo-B100 found in VLDL and LDL, and appear to be more avidly retained in the vascular wall (56). Interestingly, it has also been observed that postprandial levels of chylomicron remnants, in particular, are associated with greater progression of coronary artery lesions on angiography (57).

High-Density Lipoprotein

As outlined in the section "Dyslipidemia," a low circulating concentration of HDL is often encountered in the metabolic syndrome. Epidemiological data suggest that HDL cholesterol exerts a stronger influence on risk than LDL-C (58). Each percentage reduction in LDL-C is associated with approximately a 1% reduction in risk, while each percentage increase in HDL-C is associated with up to a 3% reduction in risk. Low HDL-C levels are particularly prevalent in the metabolic syndrome wherein they represent a strong predictor of risk (59). HDL has multiple functions that may contribute to its beneficial effects in vivo. "Reverse cholesterol transport" is the most well-known function of HDL (Fig. 7) and describes the process whereby cholesterol is removed from cells, e.g., macrophage foam cells (60) and delivered to the liver for disposal. HDL particles acquire cholesterol via ABC proteins, e.g., ABCA-1. Cholesterol can then be removed by two routes. The first is direct uptake of HDL-C by scavenger receptor B1 (SR-B1) found in the liver. The second is transfer of cholesterol ester to LDL by CETP and subsequent uptake of LDL-C, primarily by the liver. In addition, protein components of HDL, specifically apoAI (61), paraoxonase (62), and platelet-activating factor acetyl hydrolase (63) confer antioxidant properties that may inhibit oxidation of LDL (64,65). Anti-inflammatory effects of HDL were initially demonstrated in vitro where HDL can prevent TNF-α- or C-reactive protein (CRP)-induced expression of cell adhesion molecules on vascular endothelium (66,67). In vivo infusions of reconstituted HDL prevented both cell adhesion molecule expression in a porcine model (68) and the arterial response to injury in a rabbit model (69). In patients, short-term infusion of reconstituted HDL particles has shown improvements in endothelial function (70,71).

Inflammation and the Role of Obesity

The involvement of inflammation in atherosclerosis is well recognized (22)—from lesion initiation and progression through to atherosclerotic plaque rupture. An increased adipose tissue mass, in particular intra-abdominal adiposity (72), is regarded by some investigators as being central to the pathogenesis of the metabolic syndrome (73). Adipose tissue is highly metabolically active and produces a large number of signaling molecules collectively termed "adipocytokines." These have a broad range of functions and can modulate appetite, insulin sensitivity, and inflammation. Examples of adipocyte-secreted factors with particular vascular relevance include TNF-α, CRP, and adiponectin.

C-Reactive Protein

CRP is produced from the liver and adipose tissue mainly under the influence of IL-6. Recently, Ridker et al. have shown the potential for the use of CRP as a marker of risk in cardiovascular disease in the metabolic syndrome, noting that, in a large sample of women, CRP levels were directly associated with the number of metabolic syndrome risk factors, and among those with the metabolic syndrome, prognosis was worse for those with higher CRP levels (74). It also appears that CRP may be directly involved in the development of atherosclerotic disease. In vitro experiments have demonstrated that CRP downregulates e-NOS expression (75) and induces the expression of cell adhesion molecules (76). CRP also has direct proatherogenic effects in vascular smooth muscle cells, directly upregulating the angiotensin Type 1 receptor (77), which stimulates smooth muscle proliferation and reactive oxygen species (ROS) production. CRP may play a role in acute plaque events by upregulating the expression of MMPs (78) and impairing fibrinolysis by promoting the synthesis of PAI-1 (79). Furthermore, CRP upregulates nuclear factor-κB (NF-κB), a transcription factor that controls a broad range of inflammatory genes, and inhibits bone marrow–derived endothelial progenitor cell survival and differentiation (80). The clinical relevance of these observations remains uncertain.

Adipocytokines

Other products of adipose tissue that exert a negative influence on the vasculature include leptin, TNF-α, and resistin (73). Adiponectin is also produced by adipose tissue; however, by contrast with most other "adipocytokines," plasma levels are negatively correlated with obesity, and adiponectin appears to have beneficial vascular effects. For instance, adiponectin inhibits NF-κB signaling to reduce inflammation (81). In a mouse model, expression of human adiponectin reduced atherosclerosis (82), while in a case–control study, lower adiponectin levels were associated with increased CAD (83). It has also been proposed that the visceral fat adjacent to blood vessels may play an important paracrine role in the development of vascular disease. Yudkin et al. have hypothesized that impaired NO-mediated dilatation observed in obese rat arterioles might be due to TNF-α secreted by such deposits of fat (84).

Hyperglycemia

Patients with the metabolic syndrome will commonly have either frank diabetes or a prediabetic state. Hyperglycemia is more closely associated with the development of microvascular complications of diabetes than macrovascular disease; accordingly, studies to date that have examined the impact of intensive control of hyperglycemia in patients with diabetes have shown a greater effect on microvascular than macrovascular complications (85). However, exposure of vascular tissues to chronic hyperglycemia can still exacerbate atherosclerosis through mechanisms that will be described (see below). Certainly, by the time Type 2 diabetes has developed, substantial damage may have already accrued in the vasculature during the long prediabetic state when cardiovascular risk factors were operative, often in combination (Fig. 1).

Advanced Glycation Endproducts

Chronically elevated blood glucose levels result in nonenzymatic modification of proteins and other macromolecules. "Advanced glycation endproducts" (AGE) is a broad term applied to a range of such products. Figure 6 illustrates the formation of AGE initially through a reversible reaction between glucose and a protein amino to form a Schiff base, which subsequently undergoes irreversible rearrangement to form an Amadori product. Probably the best-known example of an Amadori product is glycated hemoglobin (HbA$_{1c}$). Further modification including crosslinking results in AGE, examples of which include pentosidine and N-carboxymethyllysine. Factors that influence the rate of formation of AGE include the time of exposure and concentration of glucose, as well as oxidative stress; thus, it is unsurprising that higher levels of HbA$_1$C are found in individuals with features of the metabolic syndrome (86,87).

AGE cause damage by two principal mechanisms. First, structural modification of proteins perturbs their normal function. For instance, the glycosylation of LDL renders it more prone to oxidative modification (88). In the vessel wall, AGE formation in the basement membrane may affect permeability, while crosslinking of collagen contributes to increased vascular stiffening. Second, AGEs are ligands for the receptor for AGE (RAGE), a member of the immunoglobulin superfamily, which is found on macrophages and endothelial and smooth muscle cells (89). This multiligand receptor also binds other non-AGE ligands. Ligand-binding to RAGE results in multiple proinflammatory effects. There is increased oxidative stress as well as activation of the transcription factor NF-κB (90). Activation of NF-κB results in increased expression of inflammatory cytokines such as IL-6 and TNF-α and chemokines such as MCP-1 and increased expression of cell adhesion molecules. RAGE binding also promotes cellular proliferation by stimulation of platelet-derived growth factor and insulin-like growth factor release from monocytes. In humans, RAGE expression in carotid plaques is associated with increased inflammatory cells and metalloproteinase expression (91).

Reverse cholesterol transport (see section "High-Density Lipoprotein") mediated by ABCA-1 also appears to be impaired in the presence of AGE (92). Impaired reverse cholesterol transport from macrophages may accelerate foam cell formation and atherogenesis.

Protein Kinase-C and Hexosamine Pathway

Protein kinase-C (PKC) is a signal transduction system located in all cells. Hyperglycemia can activate PKC signaling through increased production of diacylglycerol from glycolysis. Chronic activation of PKC increases expression of transforming growth factor-β (TGF-β), which leads to basement membrane thickening, which is particularly harmful in the renal glomerulus (94). PKC signaling also increases endothelial permeability (95) and leads to increased oxidative stress (96).

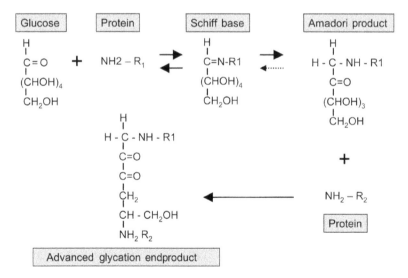

Figure 6   Illustration of the pathways by which hyperglycemia leads to formation of AGE via Schiff base and Amadori product intermediates. The initial chemical reactions are reversible, culminating in a final largely irreversible step. Modification of proteins in this way can lead to alteration in function and to the activation of specific AGE receptors and is the target of a number of therapeutic approaches. *Abbreviation*: AGE, advanced glycation endproducts.

The hexosamine pathway uses fructose derived from glycolysis to combine *N*-acetylglucosamine with the serine/threonine residues of proteins. Many proteins including e-NOS are dependent on serine phosphorylation for activation. Hyperglycemia thus increases hexosamine flux, preventing phosphorylation and activation of e-NOS (97). A similar mechanism is responsible for hyperglycemia-induced increases in TGF-β (98) and PAI-1 (99).

Oxidative Stress and Nitric Oxide

ROS are highly bioactive substances, the best-known example of which is superoxide. In health, production of ROS by vascular tissue is balanced by antioxidant systems. Oxidative stress has been implicated at all stages of atherogenesis. The metabolic syndrome is associated with decreased antioxidant systems and increased oxidative stress (100,101). The oxidative modification of LDL has already been discussed. In addition, ROS induce inflammation and endothelial dysfunction and promote vascular smooth muscle cell proliferation (102), MMP expression (103), apoptosis, and platelet aggregation (104). Macrophages, endothelial cells, and smooth muscle cells all contain multiple enzyme systems implicated in the production of ROS. Probably the best characterized is nicotinamide adenine dinucleotide oxidase found on the cell membrane. Additional sources of ROS include the mitochondrial electron transport chain and xanthine oxidase (105), and, under certain circumstances, e-NOS.

As discussed above, NO is a key mediator of vascular health, promoting smooth muscle relaxation and exerting anti-inflammatory and antithrombotic influences. Under normal conditions, e-NOS transfers electrons to L-arginine to produce citrulline and NO. Decreased NO bioavailability has been observed in clinical studies of patients with insulin resistance (106,107). A potential mechanism for this could be selectively impaired insulin signaling. Insulin is thought to have both beneficial actions in increasing NO production and potentially harmful actions in increasing production of PAI-1. It has been demonstrated in vitro that insulin resistance reduces fibroblast production of NO but not PAI-1 (108). Similarly, decreased e-NOS expression and activity has also been demonstrated in arterial specimens obtained from patients with diabetes at the time of coronary artery bypass surgery (109). Tetrahydrobiopterin (BH4) is an essential cofactor for e-NOS (110). If there is a lack of BH4, e-NOS becomes "uncoupled" and instead transfers electrons to oxygen to form superoxide (111). Recent findings in a mouse model of diabetes demonstrated that BH4 promotes e-NOS dimerization and normal e-NOS function (112). Furthermore short-term administration of BH4 improved endothelial function in diabetic patients but not controls, suggesting that BH4 deficiency may be a particularly important mechanism of vascular dysfunction in insulin-resistant states (113).

Thrombosis

The acute thrombotic complications of atherosclerosis occur when plaque rupture or erosion exposes thrombogenic substances to the coagulation factors and platelets in blood. Platelets aggregate, and the activation of the coagulation cascade leads to the formation of a thrombus, which can occlude the vessel lumen (Fig. 4). These events may be clinically silent, followed by the organization of the thrombus and healing of the rupture site, but at the expense of significant progression in lesion size.

Compared to age- and sex-matched controls, patients with the metabolic syndrome have an increased incidence of acute vascular events (7). The latter are predictable from the increased presence of atherosclerotic plaque allied to enhanced blood coagulability. Plaques that are at risk of rupture, typically, have thin fibrous caps with a high lipid content (114) and marked inflammatory cell infiltrate. In a study of nondiabetic patients, using transesophageal echocardiography, insulin resistance was a predictor of the presence of complex (large, ulcerated) thoracic aortic plaques (115). Atherectomy specimens from diabetic patients also show features of vulnerability such as increased lipid content and macrophage infiltration compared to controls (116,117). Adventitial microvessels are also associated with plaque instability and are more common in diabetic atherosclerosis (118).

Upon exposure to a wide range of stimuli including thrombin, collagen, adenosine diphosphate, and thromboxan A2 platelets are activated, becoming adherent or "sticky" and expressing surface glycoproteins, e.g., Gp IIb/IIIa and Gp Ib. The aim is to plug vascular defects following injury, and, in health, this process must be kept in check to prevent platelet aggregation in normal vessels with negative feedback provided by both prostacyclin and NO derived from the endothelium. In the setting of endothelial dysfunction and diabetes, platelets become activated due to lack of NO (119). In a small study of CAD patients, measurement of coagulation using an ex vivo technique demonstrated that hyperglycemia was the strongest predictor of platelet aggregation (120).

Increased circulating levels of coagulation factors VII to IX as well as von Willebrand factor have been reported in the metabolic syndrome (121). Insulin resistance is also associated with increased fibrinogen and PAI-1, which further increase the risk of thrombosis (122). PAI-1 inhibits the activation of plasminogen, the main endogenous thrombolytic enzyme; hence raised levels of PAI-1 are associated with a increased potential for cardiovascular events (123).

Arterial Stiffness

Elastic central arteries, in particular the aorta, play an important role in buffering and cushioning the pulsatile cardiac output. Aortic stiffness is a key determinant of systolic BP and increases with age and disease states including the metabolic syndrome (124). Interest has increased in this parameter, because it can be measured noninvasively and is a marker of both the presence of atherosclerotic disease (125) and the risk of future cardiovascular events (126). Key determinants of stiffness include the ratio of rigid collagen versus elastin in the arterial wall, as well as the endothelial influence upon arterial tone. Factors accounting for increased arterial stiffness in the metabolic syndrome have been discussed above and include modification of collagen by AGE cross-linking.

CURRENT AND EMERGING TREATMENT TARGETS

Reversing Endothelial Dysfunction

Restoring endothelial function in susceptible individuals may prove to be an important treatment goal. Treating diabetic patients with angiotensin-converting enzyme inhibitors (127) or angiotensin receptor (subtype 1) blockers (128) can lead to improved endothelial function. Similarly, plasma HDL-C is cardioprotective (129,130), and elevation of HDL-C levels using fibrates is associated with improved endothelial function in patients with diabetes (131). It therefore seems possible that similar pharmacological approaches may improve reversing endothelial dysfunction in the metabolic syndrome. Rigorous clinical trials will be necessary to test this hypothesis.

Statins

Reduction of LDL-C levels with statins reduced cardiovascular mortality in studies examining both unselected patients (132) and patients with diabetes (133). Furthermore, subgroup analyses of two major statin trials—the Scandinavian Simvastatin Survival Study and West of Scotland Coronary Prevention Study demonstrated that metabolic syndrome patients benefit from statin treatment (134,135). Current opinion regarding targets for lowering LDL can be summarized as "lower is better" (136). In a subgroup analysis of the Myocardial Ischemia Reduction with Aggressive Cholesterol Lowering study, patients with the metabolic syndrome had an increased risk of recurrent events following an acute coronary syndrome, but the relative benefit from high-dose statin was similar to the unselected group (137). Statins may also extract benefit through noncholesterol related or "pleiotropic" effects—as suggested by rapid improvements in vascular function prior to a reduction in serum cholesterol, as well as reductions in CRP levels (138). Individual statins may also differ in their effects on individual components of the lipid profile such as HDL (139). Statins may improve endothelial function through a number of mechanisms, including by increasing expression of e-NOS. This involves both suppression of the inhibitory factor Rho (140) and increased activation of NOS by the PK-Akt. Accordingly, statin treatment slows down the progression of atherosclerosis, in studies of carotid IMT (141) and coronary angiography (142). High doses of statin have been shown to halt the progression of coronary atherosclerosis, as measured by intravascular ultrasound (143). Beneficial stabilizing effects have also been demonstrated on atherosclerotic plaque morphology ex vivo in carotid endarterectomy specimens following statin treatment (144). Another recent development is high-resolution MRI (Fig. 8), which can noninvasively assess plaque burden, composition, and response to treatment (145,146).

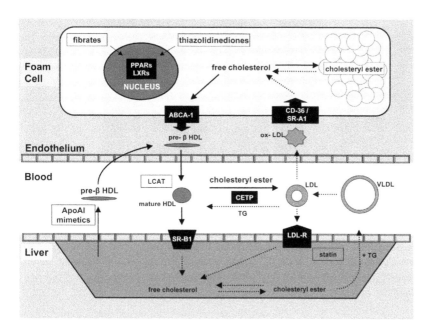

Figure 7 Schematic of cholesterol transport pathways and targets for therapeutic interventions. Excess free cholesterol is transferred from cells to nascent HDL particles by the ABC family of proteins. Free cholesterol is then esterified by the enzyme LCAT and sequestered in the core of the mature HDL particle. CETP exchanges cholesteryl ester from HDL with TG from Apo-B–containing lipoprotein particles. Alternatively HDL-C can be directly taken up by the liver via the SR-B1 receptor. Targets for therapeutic intervention are shown as solid black symbols. The molecules listed under the nuclear hormone receptors are some of their known ligands. *Abbreviations*: ABC, ATP-binding cassette; ATP, adenosine triphosphate; oxLDL, oxidized LDL; TG, triglyceride; LXR, liver X receptors; LCAT, lecithin cholesterol acyl transferase; CETP, cholesteryl ester transfer protein; SR-B1, scavenger receptor type B1; LDL, low-density lipoprotein; HDL, high-density lipoprotein; VLDL, very low–density lipoprotein; Apo-B, apolipoprotein B; Apo-AI, apolipoprotein AI; PPARs, peroxisome proliferator–activated receptors. *Source*: From Ref. 93.

HDL Elevation

HDL cholesterol, in particular reverse cholesterol transport, are potential targets for intervention (Fig. 7). Current options include fibrates or niacin, which can raise HDL by approximately 10% and 25% respectively. Niacin is a relatively old lipid-modifying agent that has gained renewed interest recently because of the discovery of adipocyte receptors for niacin (147) and the demonstration that niacin stimulates ABCA-mediated cholesterol efflux (148). Emerging HDL treatment strategies include increasing reverse cholesterol transport by recombinant

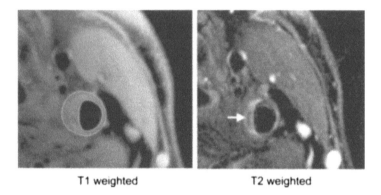

T1 weighted   T2 weighted

Figure 8   High-resolution magnetic resonance imaging of an eccentric plaque in the left common carotid artery at T1 and T2 weighting. In the T1 image, planimetry of vessel wall cross-sectional area can be measured; this might be used to evaluate response to antiatherosclerotic treatment. In the T2 image, a low-signal region (*arrow*) at the center of the plaque, which is not seen on the corresponding T1 image, represents the lipid-rich necrotic core.

apoAI-milano (149) or apoAI peptide mimetics such as D4F (150). Another novel class of agents that can substantially raise HDL are the inhibitors of CETP, such as torcetrapib (151).

Advanced Glycation Endproduct Inhibition

Of the various sequelae of hyperglycemia, AGEs are attracting particular attention as a potential target for intervention. There are several types of compounds under development, including inhibitors of AGE formation such as aminoguanidine (152) and cross-link breakers such as ALT-711 (153). Aminoguanidine is a hydrazine derivative that binds to the early glycation products, preventing progression to AGE formation. ALT-711 is able to cleave the cross-links formed between AGEs, which facilitates clearance of broken-down AGEs by the kidney and liver. Preliminary investigations using ALT-711 have shown decreases in arterial stiffening (154). Both agents have been tested in murine models of atherosclerosis, demonstrating reductions in size of plaque (155). A different strategy that has been applied is soluble receptors for AGE, which bind circulating AGE, preventing signal transduction via cell-bound receptors. Administration of a soluble RAGE receptor in order to block RAGE signaling inhibited atherogenesis in mice (156,157).

Peroxisome Proliferator–Activated Receptor Agonists

Peroxisome proliferator–activated receptors (PPARs) are members of a nuclear receptor superfamily responsible for controlling metabolism of lipids and other substrates, as well as inflammation. Genes regulated through these mechanisms appear to form functional groups. PPARs can influence vascular disease through systemic effects on lipid metabolism (especially TGs and VLDL) but may also influence plaque biology directly because they are expressed in endothelial cells, smooth muscle cells, and macrophages.

Ligands for PPAR-α include fatty acids, eicosanoids, and the fibrate drugs (e.g., gemfibrozil and fenofibrate), while oxidized fatty acids, prostaglandins, and the thiazolidinediones (e.g., rosiglitazone) activate PPAR-γ. Upon ligand activation, the PPARs regulate transcription through the formation of heterodimers with the retinoid X receptor, which in turn binds to nuclear response elements. In cultured macrophages, oxLDL activates PPAR-γ, resulting in upregulation of CD36 and enhanced foam cell formation (158,159). Chinetti et al. have found that while neither PPAR-α nor PPAR-γ activation affected the rate of foam cell formation, both induced the expression of the ABCA1 transporter and, furthermore, increased the rate of cholesterol efflux from these cells (160). In fact, cell culture studies have demonstrated several potentially atheroprotective effects including reduced cholesterol esterification (161), allowing more cholesterol to be exported through ABCA1; enhanced monocyte apoptosis through reduced NF-κB activity (162) and decreased promoter activity for genes such as MMP-9. Gene regulation by PPARs is clearly extremely complex, so it has been important to demonstrate beneficial effects of PPAR agonists in vivo. In LDL-receptor knockout mice, PPAR-α and PPAR-γ activation inhibited the progression of atherosclerosis (163).

Clinical trials of PPAR agonists have shown mixed results. The Veterans Affairs High-Density Lipoprotein Intervention Trial study (164) showed lower cardiovascular mortality in the gemfibrozil treatment arm, in particular the insulin-resistant subgroup (165), but a recent study of fenofibrate in Type 2 diabetes (the Fenofibrate Intervention and Event Lowering in Diabetes (FIELD) trial) did not show any significant benefit in its primary endpoint (166). Likewise, the recent Prospective Pioglitazone Clinical Trial in Macrovascular Events study of pioglitazone in Type 2 diabetes only showed significant improvement in the principal secondary endpoint of all-cause mortality, nonfatal myocardial infarction, and stroke (167).

Endocannabinoid System Blockade

The discovery of the endocannabinoid system and its involvement in central and peripheral control of energy balance via lipid and glucose metabolism has raised the possibility of direct targeting of obesity (168). The recent RIO-Europe study demonstrated that cannabonoid-1 receptor blockade using rimonabant resulted in significant decreases in weight (including central adiposity), TGs, and insulin resistance and increased HDL-C—all of which would suggest a reduction in cardiovascular risk (169). Further studies are required to examine the long-term efficacy and safety of interventions to this pathway.

SUMMARY AND CONCLUSIONS

The worldwide incidence of the metabolic syndrome is increasing due to adverse changes in diet and lifestyle, allied to aging populations. If this continues unchecked, a huge burden of cardiovascular mortality and morbidity will result. Unfavorable features of the metabolic syndrome, including the triad of dyslipidemia (sdLDL, low HDL, and raised TGs) and dysregulation of glucose homeostasis combine to damage the vasculature through multiple mechanisms. The clinical and biochemical manifestations of the metabolic syndrome have been related to molecular and cellular processes such as endothelial dysfunction, oxidative stress, and formation of AGE. Fortunately, increased understanding of these disease processes may enable the development of targeted therapies to retard the progression or even promote regression of vascular disease in the metabolic syndrome.

REFERENCES

1. Reaven GM. Banting lecture 1988. Role of insulin resistance in human disease. Diabetes 1988; 37:1595–1607.
2. Grundy SM, Cleeman JI, Daniels SR, et al. Diagnosis and management of the metabolic syndrome: An American Heart Association/National Heart, Lung, and Blood Institute scientific statement: executive summary. Circulation 2005; 112:e285–e290.
3. Ford ES. Prevalence of the metabolic syndrome defined by the International Diabetes Federation among adults in the U.S. Diabetes Care 2005; 28:2745–2749.
4. de Ferranti SD, Gauvreau K, Ludwig DS, Neufeld EJ, Newburger JW, Rifai N. Prevalence of the metabolic syndrome in American Adolescents: findings from the Third National Health and Nutrition Examination Survey. Circulation 2004; 110:2494–2497.
5. Laaksonen DE, Lakka HM, Niskanen LK, Kaplan GA, Salonen JT, Lakka TA. Metabolic syndrome and development of diabetes mellitus: application and validation of recently suggested definitions of the metabolic syndrome in a prospective cohort study. Am J Epidemiol 2002; 156:1070–1077.
6. Dekker JM, Girman C, Rhodes T, Nijpels G, Stehouwer CD, Bouter LM, Heine RJ. Metabolic syndrome and 10-year cardiovascular disease risk in the Hoorn Study. Circulation 2005; 112:666–673.
7. Isomaa B, Almgren P, Tuomi T, et al. Cardiovascular morbidity and mortality associated with the metabolic syndrome. Diabetes Care 2001; 24:683–689.
8. Meigs JB, Nathan DM, Wilson PW, Cupples LA, Singer DE. Metabolic risk factors worsen continuously across the spectrum of nondiabetic glucose tolerance. The Framingham Offspring Study. Ann Intern Med 1998; 128:524–533.
9. Hu FB, Stampfer MJ, Haffner SM, Solomon CG, Willett WC, Manson JE. Elevated risk of cardiovascular disease prior to clinical diagnosis of Type 2 diabetes. Diabetes Care 2002; 25:1129–1134.
10. Lakka HM, Laaksonen DE, Lakka TA, et al. The metabolic syndrome and total cardiovascular disease morality in middle-aged men. JAMA 2002; 288(21):2709–2716.
11. Furchgott RF, Zawadzki JV. The obligatory role of endothelial cells in the relaxation of arterial smooth muscle by acetylcholine. Nature 1980; 288:373–376.

12. Radomski MW, Palmer RM, Moncada S. Comparative pharmacology of endothelium-derived relaxing factor, nitric oxide and prostacyclin in platelets. Br J Pharmacol 1987; 92:181–187.
13. Ruggeri ZM, Zimmerman TS. von Willebrand factor and von Willebrand disease. Blood 1987; 70:895–904; erratum Blood 1988; 71(3):830.
14. Guzik TJ, Mussa S, Gastaldi D, et al. Mechanisms of increased vascular superoxide production in human diabetes mellitus: role of NAD(P)H oxidase and endothelial nitric oxide synthase. Circulation 2002; 105:1656–1662.
15. Stuhlinger MC, Abbasi F, Chu JW, et al. Relationship between insulin resistance and an endogenous nitric oxide synthase inhibitor. JAMA 2002; 287:1420–1426.
16. Vallance P, Leone A, Calver A, Collier J, Moncada S. Endogenous dimethylarginine as an inhibitor of nitric oxide synthesis. J Cardiovasc Pharmacol 1992; 20(suppl 12): S60–S62.
17. Celermajer DS, Sorensen KE, Gooch VM, et al. Non-invasive detection of endothelial dysfunction in children and adults at risk of atherosclerosis. Lancet 1992; 340:1111–1115.
18. Sorensen MB, Collins P, Ong PJ, et al. Long-term use of contraceptive depot medroxyprogesterone acetate in young women impairs arterial endothelial function assessed by cardiovascular magnetic resonance. Circulation 2002; 106:1646–1651.
19. Halcox JPJ, Schenke WH, Zalos G, et al. Prognostic Value of coronary vascular endothelial dysfunction. Circulation 2002; 106:653–658.
20. Heitzer T, Schlinzig T, Krohn K, Meinertz T, Munzel T. Endothelial dysfunction, oxidative stress, and risk of cardiovascular events in patients with coronary artery disease. Circulation 2001; 104:2673–2678.
21. Lteif AA, Han K, Mather KJ. Obesity, insulin resistance, and the metabolic syndrome: determinants of endothelial dysfunction in whites and blacks. Circulation 2005; 112:32–38.
22. Ross R. Atherosclerosis—an inflammatory disease. N Engl J Med 1999; 340:115–126.
23. Tzou WS, Douglas PS, Srinivasan SR, et al. Increased subclinical atherosclerosis in young adults with metabolic syndrome: the Bogalusa Heart Study. J Am Coll Cardiol 2005; 46:457.
24. Iannuzzi A, De Michele M, Bond MG, et al. Carotid artery remodeling in middle-aged women with the metabolic syndrome (from the "Progetto ATENA" Study). Am J Cardiol 2005; 96:1162.
25. Simionescu M, Simionescu N. Proatherosclerotic events: pathobiochemical changes occurring in the arterial wall before monocyte migration. FASEB J 1993; 7:1359–1366.
26. Malek AM, Alper SL, Izumo S. Hemodynamic shear stress and its role in atherosclerosis. JAMA 1999; 282:2035–2042.
27. Williams KJ, Tabas I. The response-to-retention hypothesis of early atherogenesis. Arterioscler Thromb Vasc Biol 1995; 15:551–561.
28. Skalen K, Gustafsson M, Rydberg EK, et al. Subendothelial retention of atherogenic lipoproteins in early atherosclerosis. Nature 2002; 417:750–754.
29. Oram JF, Lawn RM. ABCA1. The gatekeeper for eliminating excess tissue cholesterol. J Lipid Res 2001; 42:1173–1179.
30. Llodra J, Angeli V, Liu J, Trogan E, Fisher EA, Randolph GJ. Emigration of monocyte-derived cells from atherosclerotic lesions characterizes regressive, but not progressive, plaques. Proc Natl Acad Sci USA 2004; 101:11779–11784.

31. Murakami T, Michelagnoli S, Longhi R, et al. Triglycerides are major determinants of cholesterol esterification/transfer and HDL remodeling in human plasma. Arterioscler Thromb Vasc Biol 1995; 15:1819–1828.

32. Halle M, Berg A, Baumstark MW, Konig D, Huonker M, Keul J. Influence of mild to moderately elevated triglycerides on low density lipoprotein subfraction concentration and composition in healthy men with low high density lipoprotein cholesterol levels. Atherosclerosis 1999; 143:185–192.

33. Zambon A, Austin MA, Brown BG, Hokanson JE, Brunzell JD. Effect of hepatic lipase on LDL in normal men and those with coronary artery disease. Arterioscler Thromb 1993; 13:147–153.

34. Brinton EA, Eisenberg S, Breslow JL. Increased apo A-I and apo A-II fractional catabolic rate in patients with low high density lipoprotein-cholesterol levels with or without hypertriglyceridemia. J Clin Invest 1991; 87:536–544.

35. Lamarche B, Tchernof A, Mauriege P, et al. Fasting insulin and apolipoprotein B levels and low-density lipoprotein particle size as risk factors for ischemic heart disease. JAMA 1998; 279:1955–1961.

36. Yusuf S, Hawken S, Ounpuu S, et al. Effect of potentially modifiable risk factors associated with myocardial infarction in 52 countries (the INTERHEART study): case-control study. Lancet 2004; 364:937.

37. Sattar N, Williams K, Sniderman AD, D'Agostino R Jr, Haffner SM. Comparison of the associations of apolipoprotein B and non-high-density lipoprotein cholesterol with other cardiovascular risk factors in patients with the metabolic syndrome in the Insulin Resistance Atherosclerosis Study. Circulation 2004; 110:2687–2693.

38. Campos H, Arnold KS, Balestra ME, Innerarity TL, Krauss RM. Differences in receptor binding of LDL subfractions. Arterioscler Thromb Vasc Biol 1996; 16:794–801.

39. Bjornheden T, Babyi A, Bondjers G, Wiklund O. Accumulation of lipoprotein fractions and subfractions in the arterial wall, determined in an in vitro perfusion system. Atherosclerosis 1996; 123:43–56.

40. Anber V, Griffin BA, McConnell M, Packard CJ, Shepherd J. Influence of plasma lipid and LDL-subfraction profile on the interaction between low density lipoprotein with human arterial wall proteoglycans. Atherosclerosis 1996; 124:261.

41. Chait A, Brazg RL, Tribble DL, Krauss RM. Susceptibility of small, dense, low-density lipoproteins to oxidative modification in subjects with the atherogenic lipoprotein phenotype, pattern B. Am J Med 1993; 94:350–356.

42. Sigurdardottir V, Fagerberg B, Hulthe J. Circulating oxidized low-density lipoprotein (LDL) is associated with risk factors of the metabolic syndrome and LDL size in clinically healthy 58-year-old men (AIR study). J Intern Med 2002; 252:440–447.

43. Toshima S, Hasegawa A, Kurabayashi M, et al. Circulating oxidized low density lipoprotein levels: a biochemical risk marker for coronary heart disease. Arterioscler Thromb Vasc Biol 2000; 20:2243–2247.

44. Erkkila AT, Narvanen O, Lehto S, Uusitupa MIJ, Yla-Herttuala S. Autoantibodies against oxidized low-density lipoprotein and cardiolipin in patients with coronary heart disease. Arterioscler Thromb Vasc Biol 2000; 20:204–209.

45. Kume N, Cybulsky MI, Gimbrone MA Jr. Lysophosphatidylcholine, a component of atherogenic lipoproteins, induces mononuclear leukocyte adhesion molecules in

cultured human and rabbit arterial endothelial cells. J Clin Invest 1992; 90:1138–1144.

46. Cushing SD, Berliner JA, Valente AJ, et al. Minimally modified low density lipoprotein induces monocyte chemotactic protein 1 in human endothelial cells and smooth muscle cells. Proc Natl Acad Sci USA 1990; 87:5134–5138.

47. Quinn MT, Parthasarathy S, Fong LG, Steinberg D. Oxidatively modified low density lipoproteins: a potential role in recruitment and retention of monocyte/macrophages during atherogenesis. Proc Natl Acad Sci USA 1987; 84:2995–2998.

48. Hughes H, Mathews B, Lenz ML, Guyton JR. Cytotoxicity of oxidized LDL to porcine aortic smooth muscle cells is associated with the oxysterols 7-ketocholesterol and 7-hydroxycholesterol. Arterioscler Thromb 1994; 14:1177–1185.

49. Drake TA, Hannani K, Fei HH, Lavi S, Berliner JA. Minimally oxidized low-density lipoprotein induces tissue factor expression in cultured human endothelial cells. Am J Pathol 1991; 138:601–607.

50. Kugiyama K, Sakamoto T, Misumi I, et al. Transferable lipids in oxidized low-density lipoprotein stimulate plasminogen activator inhibitor-1 and inhibit tissue-type plasminogen activator release from endothelial cells. Circ Res 1993; 73:335–343.

51. Cullen P. Evidence that triglycerides are an independent coronary heart disease risk factor. Am J Cardiol 2000; 86:943.

52. Karpe F, de Faire U, Mercuri M, Gene Bond M, Hellenius M-L, Hamsten A. Magnitude of alimentary lipemia is related to intima-media thickness of the common carotid artery in middle-aged men. Atherosclerosis 1998; 141:307.

53. Vogel RA, Corretti MC, Plotnick GD. Effect of a single high-fat meal on endothelial function in healthy subjects. Am J Cardiol 1997; 79:350.

54. Nappo F, Esposito K, Cioffi M, et al. Postprandial endothelial activation in healthy subjects and in Type 2 diabetic patients: role of fat and carbohydrate meals. J Am Coll Cardiol 2002; 39:1145.

55. Nakamura T, Takano H, Umetani K, et al. Remnant lipoproteinemia is a risk factor for endothelial vasomotor dysfunction and coronary artery disease in metabolic syndrome. Atherosclerosis 2005; 181:321.

56. Proctor SD, Vine DF, Mamo JC. Arterial permeability and efflux of apolipoprotein B-containing lipoproteins assessed by in situ perfusion and three-dimensional quantitative confocal microscopy. Arterioscler Thromb Vasc Biol 2004; 24:2162–2167.

57. Karpe F, Steiner G, Uffelman K, Olivecrona T, Hamsten A. Postprandial lipoproteins and progression of coronary atherosclerosis. Atherosclerosis 1994; 106:83–97.

58. Gordon T, Castelli WP, Hjortland MC, Kannel WB, Dawber TR. High density lipoprotein as a protective factor against coronary heart disease. The Framingham Study. Am J Med 1977; 62:707–714.

59. Ninomiya JK, L'Italien G, Criqui MH, Whyte JL, Gamst A, Chen RS. Association of the metabolic syndrome with history of myocardial infarction and stroke in the Third National Health and Nutrition Examination Survey. Circulation 2004; 109:42–46.

60. Miyazaki A, Rahim AT, Ohta T, Morino Y, Horiuchi S. High density lipoprotein mediates selective reduction in cholesteryl esters from macrophage foam cells. Biochim Biophys Acta 1992; 1126:73.

61. Garner B, Waldeck AR, Witting PK, Rye K-A, Stocker R. Oxidation of high density lipoproteins. II. Evidence for direct reduction of lipid hydroperoxides by methionine residues of apolipoproteins AI and AII. J Biol Chem 1998; 273:6088–6095.

62. Mackness MI, Arrol S, Durrington PN. Paraoxonase prevents accumulation of lipoperoxides in low-density lipoprotein. FEBS Lett 1991; 286:152.
63. Kakafika AI, Xenofontos S, Tsimihodimos V, et al. The PON1 M55L gene polymorphism is associated with reduced HDL-associated PAF-AH activity. J Lipid Res 2003; 44:1919–1926.
64. Watson AD, Berliner JA, Hama SY, et al. Protective effect of high density lipoprotein associated paraoxonase. Inhibition of the biological activity of minimally oxidized low density lipoprotein. J Clin Invest 1995; 96:2882–2891.
65. Watson AD, Navab M, Hama SY, et al. Effect of platelet activating factor-acetylhydrolase on the formation and action of minimally oxidized low density lipoprotein. J Clin Invest 1995; 95:774–782.
66. Cockerill GW, Rye KA, Gamble JR, Vadas MA, Barter PJ. High-density lipoproteins inhibit cytokine-induced expression of endothelial cell adhesion molecules. Arterioscler Thromb Vasc Biol 1995; 15:1987–1994.
67. Wadham C, Albanese N, Roberts J, et al. High-density lipoproteins neutralize C-reactive protein proinflammatory activity. Circulation 2004; 109:2116.
68. Cockerill GW, Huehns TY, Weerasinghe A, et al. Elevation of plasma high-density lipoprotein concentration reduces interleukin-1-induced expression of E-selectin in an in vivo model of acute inflammation. Circulation (Online) 2001; 103:108–112.
69. Nicholls SJ, Dusting GJ, Cutri B, et al. Reconstituted high-density lipoproteins inhibit the acute pro-oxidant and proinflammatory vascular changes induced by a periarterial collar in normocholesterolemic rabbits. Circulation 2005; 111(12):1543–1550.
70. Bisoendial RJ, Hovingh GK, Levels JH, et al. Restoration of endothelial function by increasing high-density lipoprotein in subjects with isolated low high-density lipoprotein. Circulation 2003; 107:2944–2948.
71. Spieker LE, Sudano I, Hurlimann D, et al. High-density lipoprotein restores endothelial function in hypercholesterolemic men. Circulation 2002; 105:1399–1402.
72. Goodpaster BH, Krishnaswami S, Harris TB, et al. Obesity, regional body fat distribution, and the metabolic syndrome in older men and women. Arch Intern Med 2005; 165:777–783.
73. Lau DC, Dhillon B, Yan H, Szmitko PE, Verma S. Adipokines: molecular links between obesity and atheroslcerosis. Am J Physiol Heart Circ Physiol 2005; 288:H2031–H2041.
74. Ridker PM, Buring JE, Cook NR, Rifai N. C-reactive protein, the metabolic syndrome, and risk of incident cardiovascular events: an 8-year follow-up of 14 719 initially healthy American women. Circulation 2003; 107:391–397.
75. Verma S, Wang CH, Li SH. A self-fulfilling prophecy: C-reactive protein attenuates nitric oxide production and inhibits angiogenesis. Circulation 2002; 106:913–919.
76. Pasceri V, Willerson JT, Yeh ET. Direct proinflammatory effect of C-reactive protein on human endothelial cells. Circulation 2000; 102:2165–2168.
77. Wang CH, Li SH, Weisel RD, et al. C-reactive protein upregulates angiotensin Type 1 receptors in vascular smooth muscle. Circulation 2003; 107:1783–1790.
78. Williams TN, Zhang CX, Game BA, He L, Huang Y. C-reactive protein stimulates MMP-1 expression in U937 histiocytes through Fc[gamma]RII and extracellular signal-regulated kinase pathway: an implication of CRP involvement in plaque destabilization. Arterioscler Thromb Vasc Biol 2004; 24:61–66.

79. Devaraj S, Xu DY, Jialal I. C-reactive protein increases plasminogen activator inhibitor-1 expression and activity in human aortic endothelial cells: implications for the metabolic syndrome and atherothrombosis. Circulation 2003; 107:398–404.

80. Verma S, Kuliszewski MA, Li SH, et al. C-reactive protein attenuates endothelial progenitor cell survival, differentiation, and function: further evidence of a mechanistic link between C-reactive protein and cardiovascular disease. Circulation 2004; 109:2058–2067.

81. Ouchi N, Kihara S, Arita Y, et al. Adiponectin, an adipocyte-derived plasma protein, inhibits endothelial NF-kappaB signaling through a cAMP-dependent pathway. Circulation 2000; 102:1296–1301.

82. Okamoto Y, Kihara S, Ouchi N, et al. Adiponectin reduces atherosclerosis in apolipoprotein E-deficient mice. Circulation 2002; 106:2767–2770.

83. Ouchi N, Kihara S, Arita Y, et al. Novel modulator for endothelial adhesion molecules: adipocyte-derived plasma protein adiponectin. Circulation 1999; 100:2473–2476.

84. Yudkin JS, Eringa E, Stehouwer CD. "Vasocrine" signalling from perivascular fat: a mechanism linking insulin resistance to vascular disease. Lancet 2005; 365:1817–1820.

85. UK Prospective Diabetes Study G. Intensive blood-glucose control with sulphonylureas or insulin compared with conventional treatment and risk of complications in patients with Type 2 diabetes (UKPDS 33). Lancet 1998; 352:837.

86. Osei K, Rhinesmith S, Gaillard T, Schuster D. Is glycosylated hemoglobin A1c a surrogate for metabolic syndrome in nondiabetic, first-degree relatives of African American patients with Type 2 diabetes? J Clin Endocrinol Metab 2003; 88:4596–4601.

87. Williams DE, Cadwell BL, Cheng YJ, et al. Prevalence of impaired fasting glucose and its relationship with cardiovascular disease risk factors in US adolescents, 1999–2000. Pediatrics 2005; 116:1122–1126.

88. Bowie A, Owens D, Collins P, Johnson A, Tomkin GH. Glycosylated low density lipoprotein is more sensitive to oxidation: implications for the diabetic patient? Atherosclerosis 1993; 102:63–67.

89. Schmidt AM, Yan SD, Wautier JL, Stern D. Activation of receptor for advanced glycation end products: a mechanism for chronic vascular dysfunction in diabetic vasculopathy and atherosclerosis. Circ Res 1999; 84:489–497.

90. Wautier JL, Wautier MP, Schmidt AM, et al. Advanced glycation end products (AGEs) on the surface of diabetic erythrocytes bind to the vessel wall via a specific receptor inducing oxidant stress in the vasculature: a link between surface-associated AGEs and diabetic complications. Proc Natl Acad Sci USA 1994; 91:7742–7746.

91. Cipollone F, Iezzi A, Fazia M, et al. The Receptor RAGE as a progression factor amplifying arachidonate-dependent inflammatory and proteolytic response in human atherosclerotic plaques: role of glycemic control. Circulation 2003; 108:1070–1077.

92. Passarelli M, Tang C, McDonald TO, et al. Advanced glycation end product precursors impair ABCA1-dependent cholesterol removal from cells. Diabetes 2005; 54:2198–2205.

93. Lee JM, Choudhury RP. Prospects for atherosclerosis regression: HDL elevation and other emerging therapeutic technologies. Heart 2006; [EPub ahead of print-doi:10.1136/hrt.2005.066050].

94. Koya D, Jirousek MR, Lin YW, Ishii H, Kuboki K, King GL. Characterization of protein kinase C beta isoform activation on the gene expression of transforming growth factor-beta, extracellular matrix components, and prostanoids in the glomeruli of diabetic rats. J Clin Invest 1997; 100:115–126.

95. Yuan SY, Ustinova EE, Wu MH, et al. Protein kinase C activation contributes to microvascular barrier dysfunction in the heart at early stages of diabetes. Circ Res 2000; 87:412–417.

96. Brownlee M. Biochemistry and molecular cell biology of diabetic complications. Nature 2001; 414:813–820.

97. Du XL, Edelstein D, Dimmeler S, Ju Q, Sui C, Brownlee M. Hyperglycemia inhibits endothelial nitric oxide synthase activity by posttranslational modification at the Akt site. J Clin Invest 2001; 108:1341–1348.

98. Kolm-Litty V, Sauer U, Nerlich A, Lehmann R, Schleicher ED. High glucose-induced transforming growth factor beta1 production is mediated by the hexosamine pathway in porcine glomerular mesangial cells. J Clin Invest 1998; 101:160–169.

99. Du XL, Edelstein D, Rossetti L, et al. Hyperglycemia-induced mitochondrial superoxide overproduction activates the hexosamine pathway and induces plasminogen activator inhibitor-1 expression by increasing Sp1 glycosylation. Proc Natl Acad Sci USA 2000; 97:12222–12226.

100. Ford ES, Mokdad AH, Giles WH, Brown DW. The metabolic syndrome and antioxidant concentrations: findings from the Third National Health and Nutrition Examination Survey. Diabetes 2003; 52:2346–2352.

101. Hansel B, Giral P, Nobecourt E, et al. Metabolic syndrome is associated with elevated oxidative stress and dysfunctional dense high-density lipoprotein particles displaying impaired antioxidative activity. J Clin Endocrinol Metab 2004; 89:4963–4971.

102. Griendling KK, Ushio-Fukai M. Redox control of vascular smooth muscle proliferation. J Lab Clin Med 1998; 132:9–15.

103. Rajagopalan S, Meng XP, Ramasamy S, Harrison DG, Galis ZS. Reactive oxygen species produced by macrophage-derived foam cells regulate the activity of vascular matrix metalloproteinases in vitro. Implications for atherosclerotic plaque stability. J Clin Invest 1996; 98:2572–2579.

104. Yao SK, Ober JC, Gonenne A, Clubb FJ Jr, et al. Active oxygen species play a role in mediating platelet aggregation and cyclic flow variations in severely stenosed and endothelium-injured coronary arteries. Circ Res 1993; 73:952–967.

105. Madamanchi NR, Vendrov A, Runge MS. Oxidative stress and vascular disease. Arterioscler Thromb Vasc Biol 2005; 25:29–38.

106. Balletshofer BM, Rittig K, Enderle MD, et al. Endothelial dysfunction is detectable in young normotensive first-degree relatives of subjects with Type 2 diabetes in association with insulin resistance. Circulation 2000; 101:1780–1784.

107. Petrie JR, Ueda S, Webb DJ, Elliott HL, Connell JMC. Endothelial nitric oxide production and insulin sensitivity: a physiological link with implications for pathogenesis of cardiovascular disease. Circulation 1996; 93:1331–1333.

108. Pandolfi A, Solini A, Pellegrini G. Selective insulin resistance affecting nitric oxide release but not plasminogen activator inhibitor-1 synthesis in fibroblasts from insulin-resistant individuals. Arterioscler Thromb Vasc Biol 2005; 25:2392–2397.

109. Okon EB, Chung AWY, Rauniyar P, et al. Compromised arterial function in human Type 2 diabetic patients. Diabetes 2005; 54:2415–2423.

110. Cosentino F, Luscher TF. Tetrahydrobiopterin and endothelial nitric oxide synthase activity. Cardiovasc Res 1999; 43:274–278.
111. Vasquez-Vivar J, Kalyanaraman B, Martasek P, et al. Superoxide generation by endothelial nitric oxide synthase: the influence of cofactors. Proc Natl Acad Sci USA 1998; 95:9220–9225.
112. Cai S, Khoo J, Mussa S, Alp N, Channon K. Endothelial nitric oxide synthase dysfunction in diabetic mice: importance of tetrahydrobiopterin in eNOS dimerisation. Diabetologia 2005; 48:1933.
113. Heitzer T, Krohn K, Albers S, Meinertz T. Tetrahydrobiopterin improves endothelium-dependent vasodilation by increasing nitric oxide activity in patients with Type II diabetes mellitus. Diabetologia 2000; 43:1435–1438.
114. Burke AP, Farb A, Malcom GT, Liang YH, Smialek J, Virmani R. Coronary risk factors and plaque morphology in men with coronary disease who died suddenly. N Engl J Med 1997; 336:1276–1282.
115. Takahashi F, Hasebe N, Kawashima E, et al. Hyperinsulinemia is an independent predictor for complex atherosclerotic lesion of thoracic aorta in non-diabetic patients. Atherosclerosis. In press.
116. Moreno PR, Fuster V. New aspects in the pathogenesis of diabetic atherothrombosis. J Am Coll Cardiol 2004; 44:2293–2300.
117. Moreno PR, Murcia AM, Palacios IF, et al. Coronary composition and macrophage infiltration in atherectomy specimens from patients with diabetes mellitus. Circulation 2000; 102(18):2180–2184.
118. Hayden MR, Tyagi SC. Vasa vasorum in plaque angiogenesis, metabolic syndrome, Type 2 diabetes mellitus, and atheroscleropathy: a malignant transformation. Cardiovasc Diabetol 2004; 3:1.
119. Schafer A, Alp NJ, Cai S, et al. Reduced vascular NO bioavailability in diabetes increases platelet activation in vivo. Arterioscler Thromb Vasc Biol 2004; 24:1720–1726.
120. Shechter M, Bairey Merz CN, Paul-Labrador MJ, Kaul S. Blood glucose and platelet-dependent thrombosis in patients with coronary artery disease. J Am Coll Cardiol 2000; 35:300.
121. Wannamethee SG, Lowe GD, Shaper AG, Rumley A, Lennon L, Whincup PH. The metabolic syndrome and insulin resistance: relationship to haemostatic and inflammatory markers in older non-diabetic men. Atherosclerosis 2005; 181:101–108.
122. Sakkinen PA, Wahl P, Cushman M, Lewis MR, Tracy RP. Clustering of procoagulation, inflammation, and fibrinolysis variables with metabolic factors in insulin resistance syndrome. Am J Epidemiol 2000; 152:897–907.
123. Juhan-Vague I, Pyke SDM, Alessi MC, Jespersen J, Haverkate F, Thompson SG. Fibrinolytic factors and the risk of myocardial infarction or sudden death in patients with angina pectoris. Circulation 1996; 94:2057–2063.
124. Schram MT, Henry RM, van Dijk RA, et al. Increased central artery stiffness in impaired glucose metabolism and Type 2 diabetes: the Hoorn Study. Hypertension 2004; 43:176–181.
125. Weber T, Auer J, O'Rourke MF, et al. Arterial stiffness, wave reflections, and the risk of coronary artery disease. Circulation 2004; 109:184–189.
126. Sutton-Tyrrell K, Najjar SS, Boudreau RM, et al. Elevated aortic pulse wave velocity, a marker of arterial stiffness, predicts cardiovascular events in well-functioning older adults. Circulation 2005; 111:3384–3390.

127. O'Driscoll G, Green D, Maiorana A, Stanton K, Colreavy F, Taylor R. Improvement in endothelial function by angiotensin-converting enzyme inhibition in non-insulin-dependent diabetes mellitus. J Am Coll Cardiol 1999; 33:1506–1511.

128. Cheetham C, Collis J, O'Driscoll G, Stanton K, Taylor R, Green D. Losartan, an angiotensin Type 1 receptor antagonist, improves endothelial function in non-insulin-dependent diabetes. J Am Coll Cardiol 2000; 36:1461–1466.

129. Wilson PW, Abbott RD, Castelli WP. High density lipoprotein cholesterol and mortality. The Framingham Heart Study. Arteriosclerosis 1988; 8:737–741.

130. Lupattelli G, Marchesi S, Lombardini R, et al. Mechanisms of high-density lipoprotein cholesterol effects on the endothelial function in hyperlipemia. Metabolism 2003; 52:1191–1195.

131. Avogaro A, Miola M, Favaro A, et al. Gemfibrozil improves insulin sensitivity and flow-mediated vasodilatation in Type 2 diabetic patients. Eur J Clin Invest 2001; 31:603–609.

132. Heart Protection Study Collaborative Group. MRC/BHF Heart Protection Study of cholesterol lowering with simvastatin in 20536 high-risk individuals: a randomised placebo-controlled trial. Lancet 2002; 360:7–22.

133. Colhoun HM, Betteridge DJ, Durrington PN, et al. Primary prevention of cardiovascular disease with atorvastatin in Type 2 diabetes in the Collaborative Atorvastatin Diabetes Study (CARDS): multicentre randomised placebo-controlled trial. Lancet 2004; 364:685.

134. Sattar N, Gaw A, Scherbakova O, et al. Metabolic syndrome with and without c-reactive protein as a predictor of coronary heart disease and diabetes in the West of Scotland Coronary Prevention Study. Circulation 2003; 108:414–419.

135. Pyorala K, Ballantyne CM, Gumbiner B, et al. Reduction of cardiovascular events by simvastatin in nondiabetic coronary heart disease patients with and without the metabolic syndrome: subgroup analyses of the Scandinavian Simvastatin Survival Study (4S). Diabetes Care 2004; 27:1735–1740.

136. Cannon CP, Braunwald E, McCabe CH, et al. (The Pravastatin or Atorvastatin Evaluation and Infection Therapy-Thrombolysis in Myocardial Infarction 22 Investigators). Intensive versus moderate lipid lowering with statins after acute coronary syndromes. N Engl J Med 2004; 350:1495–1504.

137. Schwartz GG, Olsson AG, Szarek M, Sasiela WJ. Relation of characteristics of metabolic syndrome to short-term prognosis and effects of intensive statin therapy after acute coronary syndrome: an analysis of the Myocardial Ischemia Reduction with Aggressive Cholesterol Lowering (MIRACL) trial. Diabetes Care 2005; 28:2508–2513.

138. Tsunekawa T, Hayashi T, Kano H, et al. Cerivastatin, a hydroxymethylglutaryl coenzyme a reductase inhibitor, improves endothelial function in elderly diabetic patients within 3 days. Circulation 2001; 104:376–379.

139. Hunninghake DB, Ballantyne CM, Maccubbin DL, Shah AK, Gumbiner B, Mitchel YB. Comparative effects of simvastatin and atorvastatin in hypercholesterolemic patients with characteristics of metabolic syndrome. Clin Ther 2003; 25:1670.

140. Laufs U, Liao JK. Post-transcriptional regulation of endothelial nitric oxide synthase mRNA stability by Rho GTPase. J Biol Chem 1998; 273:24266–24271.

141. Taylor AJ, Kent SM, Flaherty PJ, Coyle LC, Markwood TT, Vernalis MN. ARBITER: arterial biology for the investigation of the treatment effects of reducing cholesterol: a randomized trial comparing the effects of atorvastatin and pravastatin on carotid intima medial thickness. Circulation 2002; 106:2055–2060.

142. Blankenhorn DH, Azen SP, Kramsch DM, et al. Coronary angiographic changes with lovastatin therapy. The Monitored Atherosclerosis Regression Study (MARS). Ann Intern Med 1993; 119:969–976.

143. Nissen SE, Tuzcu EM, Schoenhagen P, et al. Effect of intensive compared with moderate lipid-lowering therapy on progression of coronary atherosclerosis: a randomized controlled trial. JAMA 2004; 291:1071–1080.

144. Crisby M, Nordin-Fredriksson G, Shah PK, Yano J, Zhu J, Nilsson J. Pravastatin treatment increases collagen content and decreases lipid content, inflammation, metalloproteinases, and cell death in human carotid plaques: implications for plaque stabilization. Circulation 2001; 103:926–933.

145. Corti R, Fayad ZA, Fuster V, et al. Effects of lipid-lowering by simvastatin on human atherosclerotic lesions: a longitudinal study by high-resolution, noninvasive magnetic resonance imaging. Circulation 2001; 104:249–252.

146. Zhao X-Q, Yuan C, Hatsukami TS, et al. Effects of prolonged intensive lipid-lowering therapy on the characteristics of carotid atherosclerotic plaques in vivo by MRI: a case-control study. Arterioscler Thromb Vasc Biol 2001; 21:1623–1629.

147. Tunaru S, Kero J, Schaub A, et al. PUMA-G and HM74 are receptors for nicotinic acid and mediate its anti-lipolytic effect. Nat Med 2003; 9:352–355.

148. Rubic T, Trottmann M, Lorenz RL. Stimulation of CD36 and the key effector of reverse cholesterol transport ATP-binding cassette A1 in monocytoid cells by niacin. Biochem Pharmacol 2004; 67:411–419.

149. Nissen SE, Tsunoda T, Tuzcu EM, et al. Effect of recombinant ApoA-I Milano on coronary atherosclerosis in patients with acute coronary syndromes: a randomized controlled trial. JAMA 2003; 290:2292–2300.

150. Navab M, Anantharamaiah GM, Reddy ST, et al. Oral D-4F causes formation of pre-{beta} high-density lipoprotein and improves high-density lipoprotein-mediated cholesterol efflux and reverse cholesterol transport from macrophages in apolipoprotein E-null mice. Circulation 2004; 109:3215–3220.

151. Brousseau ME, Schaefer EJ, Wolfe ML, et al. Effects of an inhibitor of cholesteryl ester transfer protein on HDL cholesterol. N Engl J Med 2004; 350:1505–1515.

152. Brownlee M, Vlassara H, Kooney A, Ulrich P, Cerami A. Aminoguanidine prevents diabetes-induced arterial wall protein cross-linking. Science 1986; 232:1629–1632.

153. Vaitkevicius PV, Lane M, Spurgeon H, et al. A cross-link breaker has sustained effects on arterial and ventricular properties in older rhesus monkeys. Proc Natl Acad Sci USA 2001; 98:1171–1175.

154. Kass DA, Shapiro EP, Kawaguchi M, et al. Improved arterial compliance by a novel advanced glycation end-product crosslink breaker. Circulation 2001; 104:1464–1470.

155. Forbes JM, Yee LT, Thallas V, et al. Advanced glycation end product interventions reduce diabetes-accelerated atherosclerosis. Diabetes 2004; 53:1813–1823.

156. Park L, Raman KG, Lee KJ, et al. Suppression of accelerated diabetic atherosclerosis by the soluble receptor for advanced glycation endproducts. Nat Med 1998; 4:1025.

157. Bucciarelli LG, Wendt T, Qu W, et al. RAGE blockade stabilizes established atherosclerosis in diabetic apolipoprotein E-null mice. Circulation 2002; 106:2827–2835.

158. Nagy L, Tontonoz P, Alvarez JG, Chen H, Evans RM. Oxidized LDL regulates macrophage gene expression through ligand activation of PPARgamma. Cell 1998; 93:229–240.

159. Tontonoz P, Nagy L, Alvarez JG, Thomazy VA, Evans RM. PPARgamma promotes monocyte/macrophage differentiation and uptake of oxidized LDL. Cell 1998; 93:241–252.

160. Chinetti G, Lestavel S, Bocher V, et al. PPAR-alpha and PPAR-gamma activators induce cholesterol removal from human macrophage foam cells through stimulation of the ABCA1 pathway. Nat Med 2001; 7:53–58.

161. Chinetti G, Lestavel S, Fruchart JC, Clavey V, Staels B. Peroxisome proliferator-activated receptor alpha reduces cholesterol esterification in macrophages. Circ Res 2003; 92:212–217.

162. Chinetti G, Griglio S, Antonucci M, et al. Activation of proliferator-activated receptors alpha and gamma induces apoptosis of human monocyte-derived macrophages. J Biol Chem 1998; 273:25573–25580.

163. Li AC, Binder CJ, Gutierrez A, et al. Differential inhibition of macrophage foam-cell formation and atherosclerosis in mice by PPAR (alpha), (beta)/(delta), and (gamma). J Clin Invest 2004; 114:1564–1576.

164. Rubins HB, Robins SJ, Collins D, et al. The Veterans Affairs High-Density Lipoprotein Cholesterol Intervention Trial Study Group. Gemfibrozil for the secondary prevention of coronary heart disease in men with low levels of high-density lipoprotein cholesterol. N Engl J Med 1999; 341:410–418.

165. Rubins HB, Robins SJ, Collins D, et al. Diabetes, plasma insulin, and cardiovascular disease: subgroup analysis from the Department of Veterans Affairs High-Density Lipoprotein Intervention Trial (VA-HIT). Arch Intern Med 2002; 162:2597–2604.

166. Keech A, Simes RJ, Barter P, et al. (FIELD study investigators). Effects of long-term fenofibrate therapy on cardiovascular events in 9795 people with Type 2 diabetes mellitus (the FIELD study): randomised controlled trial. Lancet 2005; 366:1849.

167. Dormandy JA, Charbonnel B, Eckland DJA, et al. Secondary prevention of macrovascular events in patients with Type 2 diabetes in the PROACTIVE Study (PROspective pioglitAzone Clinical Trial In macroVascular Events): a randomised controlled trial. Lancet 2005; 366:1279.

168. Cota D, Marsicano G, Tschop M, et al. The endogenous cannabinoid system affects energy balance via central orexigenic drive and peripheral lipogenesis. J Clin Invest 2003; 112:423–431.

169. Van Gaal LF, Rissanen AM, Scheen AJ, Ziegler O, Rossner S. Effects of the cannabinoid-1 receptor blocker rimonabant on weight reduction and cardiovascular risk factors in overweight patients: 1-year experience from the RIO-Europe study. Lancet 2005; 365:1389–1397.

5

Vascular Disease in the Metabolic Syndrome: Mechanisms and Consequences

Andrew J. Krentz

Southampton University Hospitals, University of Southampton, Southampton, U.K.

Sarah Wild

Public Health Sciences, University of Edinburgh, Edinburgh, U.K.

Christopher D. Byrne

Endocrinology and Metabolism Unit, Southampton General Hospital, University of Southampton, Southampton, U.K.

SUMMARY

- The metabolic syndrome confers an increased risk of developing Type 2 diabetes and atherosclerotic cardiovascular disease (CVD).
- Lesser degrees of hyperglycemia are often accompanied by a clustering of cardiovascular risk factors associated with central obesity and insulin resistance.
- Risk factors for atherosclerosis, e.g., high blood pressure, dyslipidemia, can adversely affect microvascular function; in turn, microvascular disease can enhance the risk of CVD.
- Recent data suggest that insulin resistance per se may be associated with dysfunction in the skeletal microvasculature while nonglucose intermediary metabolites may contribute to renovascular hypertension.

- A multi-factorial therapeutic strategy is advocated for high-risk patients with the metabolic syndrome.
- The potential for synergy between drugs with cardioprotective properties merits further investigation.

INTRODUCTION

The metabolic syndrome (International Classification of Disease ninth revision code 277.7) has come to be regarded as a major global threat to cardiovascular health (1). The syndrome is a precursor both of Type 2 diabetes and atherosclerotic CVD (2). Through this link, the concept of the metabolic syndrome has helped to bring together diabetologists and cardiologists pursuing better outcomes for their patients (3). It has also led clinicians and scientists to reevaluate traditional concepts about pathogenesis and management of vascular disease. Inconsistencies in definitions and competing hypotheses concerning the pathogenesis of the metabolic syndrome have contributed to some recent tensions between clinical specialties (3–8).

In this chapter we extend the view of metabolic syndrome to incorporate recent evidence implicating the syndrome in the development and progression of microvascular as well as macrovascular disease. We suggest that interactions between disease of large and small blood vessels are more important than is often realized. We also explore new evidence that may help illuminate the underlying causes of the metabolic syndrome. We conclude that a broader view of vasculopathy in the context of the metabolic syndrome\diabetes spectrum may be advantageous in pursuit of strategies to prevent or attenuate the clinical sequelae associated with these disorders.

CLASSIFICATION OF VASCULOPATHY: TIME FOR A REAPPRAISAL?

The metabolic syndrome confers approximately a fivefold increase in the risk of developing Type 2 diabetes (9). The cardiovascular consequences of diabetes are well-recognized by cardiologists (10–12). In some populations a middle-aged adult with established Type 2 diabetes has a risk of myocardial infarction (MI) as high as an age-matched non-diabetic individual with a history of prior MI (13). The high prevalence of other risk factors such as dyslipidemia and high blood pressure contribute to the coronary risk equivalence of diabetes (3). Using data from the Third National Health and Nutrition Examination Survey Alexander et al. reported that nearly 90% of patients with diabetes over the age of 50 years have the metabolic syndrome by National Cholesterol Education Program (NCEP) Adult Treatment Panel III criteria (14). The highest prevalence of coronary heart disease (CHD) was observed among those with both metabolic syndrome and diabetes but the small proportion of individuals with diabetes without metabolic syndrome had similar prevalence of CHD to people with neither diabetes nor the metabolic syndrome (14). Outcomes for patients with diabetes who develop CVD remain worse to those for non-diabetics (15). People with both CVD and diabetes are regarded as being at particularly high risk that merits consideration of more aggressive risk factor modification (16).

There is an increasing realization that defects in the function of other major organs, e.g., the kidney (17), have important implications for CVD. Endocrinologists have conventionally divided diabetes-related vascular disease into two main subtypes (18). First are the purportedly disease-specific microvascular complications of retinopathy, nephropathy, and arguably polyneuropathy (19). The microvasculature comprises small arterioles which branch into the capillary circulation, the latter being organized into units of 15 to 20 capillaries which coalesce to form post-capillary venules. The surface area of the microvasculature greatly exceeds that of medium- and large-diameter arteries. Diabetic microangiopathy is the result of multiple defects affecting the structure and reactivity of the vessel wall and of blood cells and their interactions with the vasculature (20). Second are the non-specific macrovascular complications of large vessels that result in CHD, stroke, and peripheral arterial disease (PAD). Among these clinical manifestations, CHD is the principal cause of mortality in patients with diabetes and is also responsible for much morbidity and incapacity (21). It should also be recalled that diabetes is a risk factor for sudden cardiac death (15,22). Both the updated NCEP (23) and International Diabetes Federation (IDF) guidelines (8) allow for a diagnosis of the metabolic syndrome to be made in patients with diabetes who exhibit clustering of other risk factors. We endorse this view since the available evidence indicates that the combination of diabetes and the metabolic syndrome is associated with a higher incidence and prevalence of CVD and other adverse outcomes.

The dramatic increase observed in the incidence and prevalence of the metabolic syndrome (1,24,25) prompted us to reconsider this widely-accepted paradigm of vascular disease. It is becoming increasingly apparent that microvascular and macrovascular complications show similarities in pathogenesis and often share common risk factors (Table 1). Accordingly, we believe that there may be merit in protecting the microvasculature and macrovasculature simultaneously wherever possible. At present such an approach requires a multi-factorial assault on modifiable shared risk factors using lifestyle and pharmacologic interventions. Theoretically, interventions that target endothelial dysfunction or other putative fundamental defects such as insulin resistance might be particularly advantageous (26).

INSULIN RESISTANCE: A FUNDAMENTAL DEFECT IN THE METABOLIC SYNDROME?

Insulin resistance, defined generically as a reduced biological action of the hormone, is widely regarded as a key, possibly initiating biochemical, underpinning the metabolic syndrome (27,28). At present, management of the syndrome hinges on efforts directed at ameliorating the characteristic defects in glucose and lipid

Table 1 Potential Pathogenic Links Between Microvascular
and Macrovascular Disease

Microvascular and macrovascular disease often co-exist with the potential for negative
  clinical interactions
Lesser degrees of hyperglycemia, i.e., impaired glucose tolerance, may be associated
  with microvascular disease traditionally ascribed to diabetes
There is considerable overlap of modifiable risk factors for microvascular and
  macrovascular disease
Animal models and clinical studies suggest that insulin resistance per se may be associated may be associated with microvascular dysfunction as well as macrovascular disease

metabolism that in the long-term result in vascular damage. Defective cellular
insulin action may have direct implications for the vasculature (29). It has been
suggested that endothelial dysfunction, an early vascular defect associated with
insulin resistance, might leads to progression from the metabolic syndrome to
overt Type 2 diabetes (29).

Obesity, Insulin Resistance, and Cardiovascular Risk

As outlined in more detail in Chapter 1, a new definition of the metabolic syndrome has recently been proposed by the IDF (8). Central obesity is placed at the
core of the definition with sex- and ethnicity-specific thresholds proposed for
waist circumference. This recognizes the wealth of data implicating central
obesity with adverse clinical outcomes. It is well-established that obesity, a
highly prevalent cause of acquired insulin resistance, is a potent risk factor for the
development of Type 2 diabetes and atherothrombotic CVD (30,31). Calorie
consumption that outweighs expenditure will, over time, inevitable lead to the
accumulation of body fat. Excessive weight may serve to accentuate cardiovascular risk by further reducing levels of aerobic capacity that are already sub-optimal
and impairing insulin sensitivity (32). Adiposity, with a central, abdominal or
upper-body distribution, is associated with the other major components of the
metabolic syndrome, i.e., dyslipidemia, high blood pressure, a prothrombotic
state and chronic inflammation (1,25).

It remains uncertain whether the metabolic syndrome reflects a single
underlying pathological process, e.g., insulin resistance (6). Much evidence
gleaned from experimental and epidemiologic studies support this hypothesis
(27). Several groups of investigators have addressed this issue by applying the
multivariate correlation technique known as factor analysis. This is a means for
reducing a large number of variables to a lower number of so-called factors that
may represent underlying domains that cannot be directly observed. Studies using
this approach have consistently reported that the metabolic syndrome can be
reduced to between two and four factors (6). Critics have argued that these studies provide evidence for the presence of more than one distinct pathophysiologic

process (6). Attempts at confirmatory factor analysis, a complementary statistical technique, have produced mixed results. Shen et al. proposed a four-factor model (insulin resistance, obesity, lipids and blood pressure) (33) whereas a more recent report using three separate datasets accords with the current definition of the syndrome and is consistent with the existence of a single factor that links the core components (34).

THE METABOLIC SYNDROME AND VASCULAR DISEASE

In recent years, the collusion of cardiovascular risk factors in subjects at increased risk of diabetes has been increasingly appreciated. However, acceptance of the concept of the metabolic syndrome has not been universal. Recent papers from the diabetes community have questioned the existence and clinical relevance of the syndrome (5,6). We believe that current evidence provides a convincing case for cardiovascular risk factor clusters united by one or more underlying biochemical defects. First, risk factors tend to congregate in affected individuals more commonly that expected by chance and second, global CVD risk, rather than the magnitude of single risk factors, is usually more relevant in deciding when to intervene therapeutically (23). Strategies for estimating CVD risk are discussed in more detail in Chapter 2.

Coronary Heart Disease

Evidence from cross-sectional and prospective demonstrates that the metabolic syndrome, as currently defined by NCEP (10) or World Health Organization criteria (35,36), is associated with an increased risk of atherosclerosis, predominantly CHD (1,6,23). It should be acknowledged that the data are not unanimous on this issue (6) although given the impact of different definitions and the characteristics of populations studied some inconsistencies are perhaps to be expected. This increase in CVD risk is predictable since diagnosis of the syndrome hinges on identification of traditional and emerging risk factors for CVD (37). Current estimates derived from prospective population studies suggest a two- to fivefold increase in the relative risk of atherosclerotic CVD, and, as already mentioned, an even higher risk of developing Type 2 diabetes (23). In a joint paper from the American Diabetes Association (ADA) and European Association for the Study of Diabetes (EASD), Kahn et al. questioned whether diagnosing the metabolic syndrome adds to the prediction of CVD obtained using the Framingham equation (6). A recent prospective study of 5128 British men aged 40 to 59 years followed for more than 20 years confirmed that the presence of the metabolic syndrome was a significant predictor of both CVD and Type 2 diabetes (38). There was evidence of a dose-effect association between the risk of developing CVD or diabetes and an increasing number of metabolic syndrome components (38). However, the metabolic syndrome did not predict CHD as well as the Framingham risk score (0.68 vs. 0.59 for area under the receiver-operating characteristic curves, $p < 0.001$) (38). Other investigators have found evidence of a similar association between the number of risk factors and subsequent cardiovascular morbidity and mortality (39). Malik et al. analysed data on 6255 subjects 30 to 75 years of age (54% female) (representative of 64 million adults in the United States) derived from the Second National Health and Nutrition Examination Survey who were followed for a mean of 13.3 years (40). In those with metabolic syndrome but without diabetes, risks of CHD and CVD mortality were elevated compared with those without the syndrome. Diabetes predicted all mortality end points. Subjects with even 1 to 2 metabolic syndrome risk factors, as defined by the NCEP, were at increased risk for mortality from CHD and CVD. Moreover, the metabolic syndrome predicted CHD, CVD, and total mortality more strongly than its individual components (40). In another recent British study the prognostic value of the Framingham equation and the United Kingdom Prospective Diabetes Study (UKPDS) risk engine were compared in patients with newly diagnosed Type 2 diabetes in Poole, southern England. The Framingham equation underestimated the overall number of cardiovascular events by 33% and coronary events by 32%; the overall underestimate was lower and not statistically significant using the UKPDS risk engine for CHD (13%). The inclusion of patients with Type 2 diabetes in the definition of the metabolic syndrome was also called into question in the ADA-EASD statement (6). The impact of the metabolic syndrome and the implication of individual components of the metabolic syndrome on CVD and CHD were also examined prospectively in the Poole cohort. Among 428 participants, metabolic syndrome at baseline was associated with an increased risk of incident CVD in the five years following diagnosis of Type 2 diabetes (hazard ratio 2.05; $p = 0.019$ compared with patients with Type 2 diabetes in the absence of the metabolic syndrome). CVD-free survival rates declined incrementally as the number of metabolic syndrome features increased (41). Thus, identifying the features of metabolic syndrome at diagnosis of Type 2 diabetes may be a useful prognostic tool for identifying individuals at increased risk of CVD. However, it remains uncertain which components of the metabolic syndrome have the greatest predictive value for CVD (6). This is a rapidly moving area of research and it may be anticipated that as more data accrue some of these issues will be resolved.

   Whether the metabolic syndrome is predictive of vascular events beyond that conferred by the sum of its component parts has been debated (42,43). In the view of some authorities, accumulated evidence of multiplicative risk with multiple risk factors, i.e., increases in risk that are more than the sum of each, argues strongly in favor of this notion (3). Even critics of the current construct of the metabolic syndrome have acknowledged that it provides a useful reminder of risk factor clustering (6). Another important clinical point encompassed by the syndrome is the frequency of conditions including non-alcoholic fatty liver disease, gout and sleep apnea, that often complicate management (3). Recent data from a community-based study in Sweden suggests that the metabolic syndrome, defined according to NCEP criteria, is predictive of total as well as cardiovascular mortality (44). Subjects at age 50 years with the metabolic syndrome continued to have an increased risk of total and cardiovascular mortality when established risk factors for CVD were taken into account (44).

Impact of the Metabolic Syndrome on Outcomes After Myocardial Infarction

In addition to increasing the risk of CHD the metabolic syndrome may also have prognostic implications for subjects who present with MI. A U.S. case-control study concluded that the presence of the metabolic syndrome increased infarct size and the risk of in-patient complications notably acute renal failure (45). In a recent analysis of post-MI patients in the Gruppo Italiano per lo Studio della Sopravvivenza nell'Infarto miocardico-Prevenzione Trial, both the metabolic syndrome and diabetes were associated with increased risk of mortality and major cardiovascular events during follow-up (46). These risks tended to be more pronounced in women. Of note, weight reduction of 6% to 10% or greater decreased the risk of developing diabetes among patients with the metabolic syndrome at baseline, whereas weight gain significantly increased the risk of developing diabetes (46). In a study from France among 633 patients hospitalized with MI 46% fulfilled the NCEP Adult Treatment Panel (ATP) III criteria for diagnosis of the metabolic syndrome. Affected patients tended to be older and were more likely to be female. In multivariate analyses, the metabolic syndrome was a significant independent predictor of severe heart failure (47). These studies suggest that identification of patients with metabolic syndrome may be helpful in stratifying risk of adverse clinical outcomes after acute MI.

Stroke

The metabolic syndrome is also independently associated with ischemic stroke (37,38,48). In an analysis of the Framingham Offspring Study, the combination of metabolic syndrome and diabetes carried a higher risk (relative risk 3.28, 95% confidence interval 1.82–5.92) than either condition in isolation (metabolic syndrome alone: relative risk 2.01, 95% confidence interval 1.37–3.22; diabetes alone: relative risk 2.47, 95% confidence interval 1.31–4.65). Since the prevalence of metabolic syndrome is greater than that of diabetes, the population-attributable risk was higher for the former (19% vs. 7%) with more marked differences for women than men (48).

Peripheral Arterial Disease

There is a paucity of studies concerning the association between the metabolic syndrome and PAD (49). In a recent analysis of the population-based Edinburgh Artery Study 25% of the study population (1538 men and women aged 55–74 years) had the metabolic syndrome, defined using a modification of the NCEP ATP III criteria (50). Low (<0.9) ankle-brachial pressure index was more prevalent among people with the metabolic syndrome compared to those without the syndrome (24% vs. 15%, $p < 0.001$) and was associated with an increased risk of

CVD independent of the metabolic syndrome and other major cardiovascular risk factors (50).

MICROVASCULAR AND MACROVASCULAR FUNCTION

While the molecular basis of the metabolic syndrome remains to be delineated it is becoming increasingly apparent that shared mechanisms initiate and promote dysfunction in both the microvasculature and larger arteries. Generalized endothelial dysfunction can result from disparate insults that include hyperglycemia (51), hyperinsulinemia (52), elevated circulating levels of non-esterified (free) fatty acids (53), reactive oxygen species (54), hyperleptinemia (55), enhanced cytokine-mediated inflammation (56,57), activation of the sympathoadrenal system (58), and the induction of a pro-thrombotic diathesis (59). These insults are often present in combination thereby serving to magnify the potential for vascular damage. Current evidence supports links between the inflammatory response induced by hypercholesterolemia and other risk factors and events in the microcirculation as well as in larger vessels, e.g., coronary arteries (60). Early pathological events are very similar within small and larger vessels and it has been hypothesised that changes within the microcirculation may drive the development and progression of large vessel disease (60).

As already mentioned, the metabolic syndrome, which is highly prevalent (~85%) among patients with Type 2 diabetes, contributes to elevated rates of atherothrombotic CVD events (1). In addition, some observational studies have suggested that diabetic patients with the metabolic syndrome, as defined according to the criteria of the aforementioned expert groups, may also have a higher prevalence of diabetes-specific microvascular complications (61,62). While plausible mechanisms exist (Table 2) the effects of confounders such as differences in

Table 2   Recent Evidence and Hypotheses Supporting an Expanded Role for the Metabolic Syndrome in the Pathogenesis of Microvascular as well as Macrovascular Disease

---

Renal dysfunction in relation to the metabolic syndrome
Obesity-associated glomerulonephropathy is an increasingly important cause of chronic renal impairment; microalbuminuria and renal impairment are important predictors of atherosclerosis and cardiovascular outcomes after myocardial infarction
Microvascular disease in association with the metabolic syndrome
Inconsistent reports of increased prevalence of microvascular complications in patients with Type 2 diabetes who also have the metabolic syndrome
Microvascular complications of impaired glucose tolerance
Postulated to be a risk factor for microvascular as well as macrovascular disease: supportive epidemiological and experimental evidence, although inconclusive data at present
Disordered regulation of intermediary metabolism
Intermediates of citric acid cycle may interact with specific cellular receptors to promote renovascular hypertension

---

long-term glycemic control between those with and those without the metabolic syndrome leave this issue in some doubt at present. A recent analysis of UKPDS data showed no association between the presence of the metabolic syndrome and microvascular complications (63)

Microvascular and Macrovascular Disease: Potential for Interaction

The literature contains numerous examples of inter-relationships between microvascular complications and atherosclerosis in patients with diabetes. In the World Health Organization Multinational Study of Vascular Disease in Diabetes retinopathy was related to the incidence of MI and death from CVD (64). The Atherosclerosis Risk in Communities study showed that retinal arteriolar narrowing was related to risk of CHD in women (65). This study has also shown that microvascular abnormalities are associated with the metabolic syndrome even in the absence of diabetes or hypertension (66). In the European Diabetes study of Type 1 diabetes, retinopathy, again in women, was associated with increased risk of CHD (67). Microvascular and macrovascular disease frequently co-exist in patients with diabetes (68). These complications often conspire to the detriment of the patient (Fig. 1). Organ dysfunction resulting from microvascular disease may also promote atherosclerosis, through direct and indirect mechanisms, thereby further increasing CVD risk; the impact of nephropathy on CVD events and mortality is perhaps the most pertinent example of this interaction (69–72). It is noteworthy that progressive glomerulosclerosis has similarities to atherosclerosis, both in terms of shared risk factors and histopathology (73). It is well-established that the presence of nephropathy greatly accentuates the risk of macrovascular disease (74). The burden of cardiac disease in chronic kidney disease (CKD) patients is high with left ventricular hypertrophy, dilated cardiomyopathy and CHD frequently encountered. In turn, these factors predispose to congestive heart failure, angina, MI, and premature death. Multiple risk factors for cardiac disease often co-exist and include hypertension, diabetes, smoking, anemia, defective calcium and phosphate metabolism, and inflammation (71). As a consequence, many patients with diabetic nephropathy succumb to fatal CHD before they reach the late stages of established renal failure (ERF) (69). Not only is CKD a risk factor for atherothrombotic CVD, but the components of the metabolic syndrome predispose to renal damage in a vicious cycle (75,76). Accordingly, there are concerns that obesity (77) and the metabolic syndrome (78) may be adding to the population burden of ERF.

It has been argued that the close links between albuminuria progression, insulin resistance and Type 2 diabetes should lead to consideration of renal dysfunction being included as a component of the metabolic syndrome (17).

Nephropathy-associated hypertension has major adverse consequences for the microvasculature by promoting loss of glomerular function and progression of retinopathy (79) and neuropathy (80). The Joint National Committee for Detection and Treatment of Hypertension recognizes CKD as a major independent

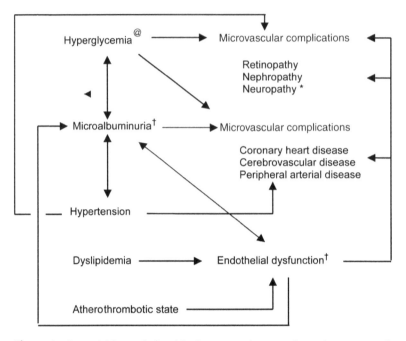

Figure 1 Potential interrelationships between microvascular and macrovascular complications in patients with the metabolic syndrome.

Note: # denotes impaired glucose tolerance is a risk marker for macrovascular disease; recent data, which require confirmation, suggest a possible role in microvascular complications.

* denotes includes impaired cardiovascular autonomic reflexes.

† denotes the relationship between microalbuminuria and macrovascular disease is not presented as being causal; rather, microalbuminuria is regarded as a marker of generalized endothelial dysfunction and is a predictor of macrovascular disease.

@ denotes in addition to hyperglycemia, hyperinsulinemia, elevated circulating non-esterified fatty acid concentrations, reactive oxygen species, cytokine-mediated inflammation, activation of the sympathoadrenal system, vasoconstriction and a prothrombotic diathesis may all contribute to endothelial dysfunction.

risk factor for CVD. Recent evidence, e.g., from the Valsartan in Acute Myocardial Infarction Trial (VALIANT) (81) and the Antihypertensive and Lipid-Lowering Treatment to prevent Heart Attack (ALLHAT) trial (82), has highlighted the importance of even minor degrees of renal impairment on cardiovascular outcomes. The term microalbuminuria has come to denote a urinary albumin excretion of 30 to 300 mg\day. Not only is microalbuminuria an early indicator of CKD but it also serves as an important risk marker for atherosclerotic disease (Fig. 1); greater degrees of clinical proteinuria, i.e., more than 300 mg\day, are associated with further increases in the risk of atherothrombosis (83). The adverse prognostic value of persistent microalbuminuria and albuminuria in patients with patients with diabetes is well-recognised, predicting not only progressive renal failure but premature cardiovascular mortality (84,85).

Microvascular dysfunction is held to contribute to cardiac disease in subjects with diabetes with women being particularly disadvantaged (86). Non-diabetic women with non-obstructive coronary disease, as judged by angiography, may nonetheless have early stage atherosclerosis and endothelial dysfunction that signal an adverse prognosis in the presence of symptoms (87). The heart is an insulin-responsive organ and evidence for cardiac insulin resistance has been found in association with obesity and Type 2 diabetes (88). Retinopathy in patients with Type 2 diabetes is reportedly associated with greater mortality after percutaneous coronary intervention, an association perhaps reflecting the presence of serious co-morbidites (89). Microvascular defects within the myocardium may contribute to the high risk of cardiac failure among patients with diabetes (90) while obesity may exacerbate cardiac failure independently of other major risk factors (91). In diabetic and non-diabetic women microvascular spasm has been implicated in the syndrome of acute myocardial stunning associated with emotional stress (92). A further manifestation of the diverse interactions between macrovascular disease and the microvasculature comes in the form of a recently described acute retinopathy following percutaneous coronary intervention (93).

HYPERTENSION

Moreover, the microvascular function of tissues such as skeletal muscle may be affected by disease of conduit arteries. Thus, proximal PAD leads to secondary impairment of microvascular function, partial denervation, and reduced metabolic capacity of downstream skeletal muscle (94,95). Such inter-relationships may also operate to initiate or sustain threats to the vasculature via more general mechanisms. For example, reduced retinal vessel diameter has been implicated in the pathogenesis of hypertension, perhaps reflecting widespread small vessel abnormalities (96). The early stages of essential hypertension are associated with tissue capillary rarefaction (97) and ultrastructural changes (98) that may be only partially reversible with attainment of good blood pressure control. When hypertension becomes established the adverse consequences for small and large blood vessels are well-recognized in the diabetic patient (99). The adverse lipid profile (52) commonly co-exists in subjects with essential hypertension has at least an additive effect on cardiovascular risk. Other mechanisms, e.g., deleterious cardiac effects of diabetic autonomic dysfunction (100) may also contribute to premature death. The relationship between autonomic dysfunction and cardiovascular complications is complex and incompletely delineated. Relative sympathetic overactivity may contribute to the development of hypertension and has also been implicated in the high rates of sudden death among patients with diabetes (15). Similar mechanisms may operate in obesity, it has been proposed, even in the absence of diabetes (101,102). High blood pressure is a highly prevalent modifiable cardiovascular risk factor in patients with Type 2 diabetes. Hypertension is also a major component of the metabolic syndrome, an association in which obesity is thought to play a pivotal role (103). The renin-angiotensin system is activated in the metabolic syndrome (17), a defect that is amenable to pharmacological intervention (see below). Evidence is also accumulating that arterial stiffness is associated with whole-body insulin resistance and may contribute to systolic hypertension in subjects with obesity and diabetes (104). Hypertension exacerbates diabetic retinopathy and nephropathy and is undisputedly an important modifiable risk factor for atherosclerosis. In contrast to the disparities observed in relation to glucose control in the UKPDS tight control of hypertension produced unequivocal benefits for microvascular and macrovascular complications (105). Based on this evidence and the results from other major trials that have included diabetic patients effective treatment of hypertension is regarded as an important strategy of protection against vascular complications in patients with Type 2 diabetes (106). As discussed in more detail below, targeting treatment to pre-diabetic subjects with hypertension may diminish the risk of diabetes, CVD, and renal complications (107).

A Pathogenic Role for Nonglucose Intermediary Metabolites?

In his Banting Lecture to the British Diabetic Association in 1973, Sir George Alberti proposed that derangements of circulating intermediary metabolites other than glucose might contribute to vascular damage (108). A recent report suggests that certain citric acid (Kreb's) cycle intermediates may promote renovascular hypertension through novel cellular mechanisms (109). GPR91, a previously orphan G-protein–coupled receptor (GPCR), functions as a receptor for succinate while GPR99, a relative of GPR91, responds to α-ketoglutarate. Acting as ligands for GPCRs, succinate and α-ketoglutarate have unexpected signaling functions. In the same paper, the investigators showed that succinate can increase blood pressure in animals, an effect that involves activation of the renin-angiotensin system. Thus, a potential role has emerged for GPR91 in renovascular hypertension, which in turn is closely linked to atherosclerosis, diabetes, and CKD. The role of mitochondrial dysfunction, the site of citric acid cycle activity, in the pathogenesis of Type 2 diabetes requires further clarification (110,111).

Quantifying the potential for vascular damage induced by non-glucose metabolites is problematic and its impact may have been underestimated. The discovery of interactions between adipocytes and other metabolically active tissues suggests that this might be a fertile area for further research (112). Leptin, for example, is an adipocytokine secreted by adipocytes, is present at high circulating concentrations in obese subjects and which stimulates glucose and fatty acid metabolism in skeletal muscle (113). Adiponectin, circulating concentrations of which are reduced in states of insulin resistance, also influences hepatic and skeletal muscle metabolism (114,115). Thus, cross-talk between these tissues and the vasculature might ultimately contribute to vascular damage in subjects with obesity-related insulin resistance.

Caveolae: A Novel Link Between Metabolism and Vascular Disease?

Other common defects at the cellular level may be relevant to the association between metabolism and vascular disease. For example, the vesicular organelles known as caveolae, and their structural proteins, caveolins, play prominent roles in disorders with overlapping clinical phenotypes including atherosclerosis and diabetes (116). A relationship between caveolin-1 and insulin signaling has been demonstrated which involves tyrosine phosphorylation of the caveolins protein (117). The facilitative glucose transporter GLUT-4 localizes to caveolae where it is modulated by insulin (118).

Role of Hyperglycemia in Microvascular and Macrovascular Disease

Tight control of hyperglycemia has traditionally been the principal therapeutic goal in preventing microvascular complications in subjects with diabetes. However, it has proved more difficult to demonstrate the impact of glycemic control on atherosclerotic disease. Pari passu, evidence of pathogenic roles for non-glucose factors has been steadily accumulating.

Evidence from Clinical Trials

Among the young and relatively healthy patients with Type 1 diabetes who participated in the Diabetes Control and Complications Trial (DCCT) better glycemic control was associated with significant reductions in the development and progression of retinopathy, early nephropathy, and measures of neural function (119). Whilst unequivocally demonstrating benefits on microvascular complications, the DCCT was neither designed nor powered to demonstrate the impact of intensified therapy on macrovascular disease. Nonetheless, a non-significant trend towards a reduction in macrovascular events was observed in subjects randomised to intensified insulin therapy. A clearer picture has emerged with further follow-up of the DDCT cohort. In the Epidemiology of Diabetes Interventions and Complications (EDICs) follow-up study carotid intima media thickness (IMT) progressed less rapidly in those patients assigned to intensive treatment during the randomized phase of the DCCT (120). It has been proposed that a "legacy effect" of earlier improved metabolic control provides durable protection for the macrovasculature. Further follow-up of the EDIC cohort has subsequently demonstrated that cardiovascular events were reduced in the intensive therapy group (121). Persuasive evidence for benefits of near-normalization of blood glucose on macrovascular disease comes from studies of pancreatic transplantation (122). Carotid IMT improves after transplantation possibly even without changes in non-glucose cardiovascular risk factors. Extending these observations are intriguing data showing better survival in patients with impaired autonomic cardiovascular reflexes who receive successful pancreatic grafts (123,124).

Compelling evidence from observational studies and interventional clinical trials also links the degree and duration of hyperglycemia with the development and progression of microvascular disease in patients with Type 2 diabetes (125). In the UKPDS, a reduction in microvascular complications was evident with better long-term glycemic control, although this required a decade of intensified treatment with sulfonylureas or insulin to become apparent. However, the benefits of better long-term glycemic control for reducing risk of macrovascular disease were less clear cut. Thus, a 16% reduction in MI was observed with sulphonylurea or insulin therapy that did not reach conventional statistical significance ($p = 0.052$). However, median HbA_{1c} measurements of the so-called intensified and conventional treatment arms were 7.0% and 7.9%, respectively, and it seems plausible that more rigorous reductions of glucose concentrations might have produced a further reduction in MI in the intensive treatment arm of the UKPDS. In practice, the limited efficacy of oral anti-diabetic agents and the risk of hypoglycemia with insulin therapy constrain the improvements in glycemia that can be safely achieved. A smaller group of overweight patients who were randomized to metformin as monotherapy in the UKPDS enjoyed significant reductions in microvascular complications and MI (126); this contrasts with the aforementioned borderline results for MI with sulfonylureas and insulin—agents that increase insulin levels. This dichotomy between the drug classes points to the potential of a drug-specific effect, a possibility that is supported by other evidence from other studies (127). While this issue remains to be clarified experimental evidence points to effects on vasomotor function, rheology vascular permeability through which metformin may improve microvascular function (128).

GLUCOSE INTOLERANCE: A RISK FACTOR FOR VASCULAR DISEASE

As noted earlier, current diagnostic criteria for diabetes comprise of thresholds for chronic hyperglycemia above which the risk of classic microvascular complications increases dramatically (129,130). However, while diabetes confers an increased risk of macrovascular disease of approximately two- to fourfold (15,131), no clear glycemic threshold for atherosclerosis can be identified (132,133). Lesser degrees of glucose intolerance, referred to as states of "pre-diabetes," i.e., impaired glucose tolerance (IGT) and impaired fasting glucose, are also associated with an increased risk of macrovascular disease (134). Recent data, notably from the large Diabetes Epidemiology: Collaborative analysis of diagnostic criteria in Europe study (135), have demonstrated that an elevated two-hour plasma glucose concentration following oral glucose challenge predicts cardiovascular mortality better than fasting hyperglycaemia. Postulated mechanisms of post-challenge vascular damage include acute oxidative stress (136,137), activation of protein kinase-C activity and non-enzymatic glycation of structural proteins (15,21).

The Common Soil Hypothesis

Such is the intimacy of the relationship between Type 2 diabetes and atherosclerosis that it has been suggested that they might result from a common, shared antecedent or "common soil" (138). It is clear that, after excluding patients with known diabetes, undiagnosed hyperglycemia is highly prevalent among patients with acute MI (139). Elevation of post-prandial glucose levels during the long pre-clinical phase of Type 2 diabetes may explain why macrovascular complications are often present when diabetes is diagnosed (138). An alternative hypothesis is the so-called "ticking clock" wherein aggregations of cardiovascular risk factors conspire to promote atherogenesis (140). The latter possibility is supported by epidemiological data showing that major risk factors such as dyslipidemia, hypertension and hyperinsulinemia worsen in line with deteriorating glucose tolerance (141). However, it can be argued that the relationship between glycated hemoglobin concentrations and the chronic vascular complications of diabetes is not as clear cut as is often assumed (142). Interventional studies have provided some interesting data. In the recently reported Study to Prevent Non-Insulin Dependent Diabetes Mellitus (STOP-NIDDM) trial (143), the α-glucosidase inhibitor acarbose, which lowers post-prandial hyperglycemia (without increasing plasma insulin concentrations), reduced the incidence of new cases of Type 2 diabetes in high-risk subjects with IGT. Acarbose therapy was also associated with a reduction in incident cases of MI and of new cases of hypertension. An attenuated progression of carotid IMT among the acarbose treated group compared to control group lends support to a cause-and-effect relationship between post-prandial hyperglycemia and CVD risk (144) but at present, the STOP-NIDDM results must be regarded as hypothesis-generating.

Does Impaired Glucose Tolerance Increase the Risk of Microvascular Complications?

The effect of lesser degrees of chronic hyperglycemia on microvascular function is an area of controversy. It has long been recognized that glucose intolerance, as well as being a predictor of future Type 2 diabetes, confers some of the increased risk of atherosclerosis associated with diabetes (134). Recently, Singleton et al. suggested that chronic glucose intolerance may also have clinically-relevant adverse effects on microvascular function (145). Epidemiological and experimental evidence has been advanced in support of this assertion (145). Mechanistically, the link between glucose intolerance and microvascular disease might plausibly lie in superoxide formation by mitochondria during acute hyperglycemia resulting in endothelial dysfunction (146). Rapid increases in circulating glucose and lipid levels also trigger carbonyl stress; the latter, whether through independent pathways or by potentiating oxidative stress, may contribute to vasculopathy within the microvascular and macrovascular arterial networks (147). In our view, additional data from animal and human studies are required before the thesis that IGT directly causes microvascular disease can be considered to be proven. It is uncertain, for instance, whether chronic polyneuropathy (148) can be regarded as a reliable indicator of diabetic microvascular disease (149,150). Imprecision in defining the clinical phenotype may also be relevant when considering erectile dysfunction as a complication of diabetes since neuropathic and vascular disease may both contribute. The erectile vasculature is vulnerable to the effects of impaired endothelial function (151); erectile dysfunction is associated with risk factors for macrovascular disease (152).

MICROVASCULAR AND MACROVASCULAR DISEASE SHARE COMMON RISK FACTORS

Occlusive disease within the vasa nervorum is regarded as an important contributor to diabetic polyneuropathy (153) and acute mononeuropathies (154). The case for overlap between small vessel disease and atherosclerosis was strengthened by a recent report from the European Diabetes (EURODIAB) Prospective Complications Study. This report, confined to patients with Type 1 diabetes, suggested that the incidence of distal neuropathy is associated with classic risk factors for atherosclerosis. The latter included raised serum triglycerides, together with elevated body mass index, smoking and hypertension (155). Expanding on this theme, the overlap in risk factors shared by conditions as diverse as CVD, Type 2 diabetes, dementia and some forms of cancer points to the potential for a plurality of clinical benefits from a combined therapeutic approach (156).

Dyslipidemia and Microvascular Disease

Risk factors for atherosclerosis may also have implications for the development of the microvascular complications of diabetes. In addition to the aforementioned impact of hyperglycemia and hypertension on diabetic retinopathy there is evidence that disturbed lipoprotein metabolism may contribute to damage of the ocular microvasculature (157,158). In the aforementioned DCCT\EDIC cohort the technique of nuclear magnetic resonance lipoprotein subclass profiling revealed associations between serum lipoproteins and severity of retinopathy in Type 1 diabetes (159). Taken together these data are consistent with a role for dyslipoproteinemia involving lipoprotein subclasses in the pathogenesis of diabetic retinopathy. Dyslipidemia may also be of relevance to the progression of diabetic nephropathy (see below).

INSULIN RESISTANCE—A DIRECT LINK WITH MICROVASCULAR FUNCTION?

In addition to the well-accepted association between insulin resistance-hyperinsulinemia complex and macrovascular disease (160,161) recent human studies provide support for a direct link between impaired insulin action and microvascular dysfunction. These observations build on the proposal that functional microangiopathy might be integral to the metabolic syndrome (128,162). In a group of obese insulin-resistant women, de Jongh et al. examined microvascular responses finding impaired skin capillary recruitment and endothelium-independent vasodilatation (163). A correlation was observed between capillary recruitment and whole-body insulin sensitivity, measured using the glucose clamp technique. Using an invasive approach, these investigators have also shown impairment of intramuscular microvascular function during exogenous insulin infusion in healthy volunteers (164). These results raise the possibility that capillary dysfunction in a key insulin-responsive tissue, namely skeletal muscle, might contribute to whole-body insulin resistance. This defect could have secondary implications for macrovascular disease through the myriad mechanisms discussed above.

A role for a heritable component of insulin resistance on microvascular complication of diabetes has been proposed. In a recent report from the Genesis France-Belgium Study composite insulin resistance scores, which included vascular risk factors such as high blood pressure and diabetes, were higher in relatives of probands with Type 1 diabetes who had diabetic retinopathy or nephropathy compared to those without these complications (165).

A Combined Therapeutic Approach to Vascular Disease in the Metabolic Syndrome

Health economic analyses show that the highest costs incurred by diabetic patients are in those with a combination of microvascular and macrovascular complications (166). Targeting classic cardiovascular risk factors would be expected to decrease the incidence of vascular events in subjects with the metabolic syndrome, many of whom at intermediate or high risk, as determined using the Framingham equation (167). In our view, the increasing threat from the metabolic syndrome strengthens the case for using therapies proven to reduce atherosclerotic events and microvascular disease in parallel wherever feasible. Given the high mortality among patients with hyperglycemia after MI (168) primary prevention of the metabolic syndrome seems a logical and worthwhile aspiration. Recently published data from the VALIANT trial, confirms the continuing poor prognosis of patients with diabetes after MI (169). Such data serve as a reminder of the high toll that often accompanies known, or even newly-diagnosed, diabetes. In high-risk patients with diabetes, a multi-factorial, target-driven approach to management, such as that adopted in the Steno-2 study in patients with Type 2 diabetes and microalbuminura, has been shown to be highly effective in preventing microvascular and macrovascular events (170). Data from the Munich registry also support a multipronged approach to the high-risk diabetic patient after MI with greater use of insulin treatment along with other cardioprotective measures (171)

Lifestyle and Societal Issues

Since adverse western lifestyles have fuelled the epidemic of obesity countering measures have enormous potential to prevent the metabolic syndrome (172). However, it is so often the case that such approaches are underutilized or poorly adhered to by those in most need (172,173). For example, recent evidence indicates that a Mediterranean-style diet reduces the prevalence of the metabolic syndrome while improving endothelial function (174). Moreover, a Mediterranean diet is associated with increasing longevity (175) and improved survival after MI (176). Minimising the development of cardiovascular risk factors by middle age is the key to avoidance of occlusive events in later life (177).

The impact of social status on cardiovascular risk may operate, at least in part, through development of the metabolic syndrome. Data from the prospective Whitehall II study of British civil servants indicates that occupational psychological stressors are associated with the metabolic syndrome in a dose-response relationship (178). The suggestion that passive exposure to tobacco smoke is associated with the metabolic syndrome in adolescents (179), while requiring confirmation, underscores the potential importance of changes in lifestyle at societal level on the accrual of risk factors over decades of adult life. At the population level, measures such as improved maternal and infant nutrition may have a role in reducing the risk of the metabolic syndrome in future generations (180); this may be particularly relevant to the developing countries that face the greatest increases in Type 2 diabetes in coming years (181).

Insulin Therapy

The issue of insulin therapy in patients with Type 2 diabetes has been a topic of much debate and merits a brief discussion in the context of the metabolic syndrome and vascular risk (182). The much debated Diabetes Mellitus, Insulin Glucose Infusion in Acute Myocardial Infarction (DIGAMI) study reported a significant and impressive reduction in mortality after MI in patients with elevated plasma glucose concentrations treated with an insulin-based regimen (183). The effects of insulin on atherothrombosis have been clouded by studies with limited relevance to human pathophysiology (184). Failure to distinguish between hyperinsulinemia on one hand and impaired cellular tissue action on the other has not helped bring a clear view the risks and benefits of timely insulin therapy (185). In between publication of the DCCT and the UKPDS came the Kumamoto study. This randomized trial showed a trend towards a reduction in CVD events in middle-aged Japanese patients with Type 2 diabetes treated with an intensified insulin regimen, in concert with a reduced risk of onset and progression of microvascular complications (186). There are theoretical reasons on which to base a case for insulin therapy in patients in whom insulin—or insulin action—is deficient. Insulin has vasodilatory properties, which, by augmenting muscle blood flow, may reduce insulin resistance through enhanced glucose uptake (162). Recent evidence supports an early direct effect of insulin on microvascular function in muscle, mediated through a nitric oxide-dependent mechanism, that regulates glucose disposal in vivo (187). Insulin therapy might also have favourable effects of local expression of plasminogen activator inhibitor-1 which retards fibrinolysis in the coronary vasculature of patients with diabetes (188). In addition, an anti-inflammatory effect of insulin may mediate some of the vascular protective effects of the hormone: C-reactive protein, circulating levels of which are reduced by insulin therapy (189), reportedly has detrimental effects on endothelial progenitor cells (190). When excessive, endothelial activation is associated with compromise of the microcirculation. Insulin exerts protective effects on the endothelium in patients with critical illness, an action that may help to prevent organ failure and so improve prognosis (191).

While the DIGAMI 2 trial failed to clarify the relative benefits of acute versus chronic insulin therapy hyperglycemia was independently associated with higher mortality after MI (192). Recent results from animal studies support a cardioprotective effect of normalizing glucose levels, a reduction in reactive oxygen species being a postulated mechanism of benefit (193). Animal (194) and other human studies suggest beneficial effects of timely insulin treatment on aspects of vascular function ands clinical outcomes in patients with Type 2 diabetes. Recent clinical trials show improvements in surrogate markers of atherosclerosis, i.e., endothelial function (195) and measures of aortic waveforms (196) in patients with Type 2 diabetes treated with modern insulin preparations. The failure of insulin therapy to provide unequivocal evidence of protection against macrovascular disease in the UKPDS should not necessarily detract from more enthusiastic use of insulin by clinicians: several aspects of insulin therapy, e.g., the enhanced pharmacokinetics of novel insulin analogues and strategies for effective implementation, have improved considerably since the 1980s when the UKPDS was conducted (182). While there have been calls for more extensive use of insulin in crically ill hospitalized patients (197) issues concerning optimal levels of glycemia, the selection of patients, i.e., medical versus post-surgical patients, (198) and the practicalities of safe implementation of such treatment in busy clinical settings require further study (199,200).

New Drugs for the Metabolic Syndrome and Type 2 Diabetes

Clearly, insulin treatment is suitable only for subjects who have developed diabetes. This represents the end-point of a long and complex journey from normal glucose tolerance, through a state of glucose intolerance, culminating in clinical diabetes. In the future, the antihyperglycemic and cardioprotective actions of metformin and acarbose, discussed earlier, may find application in the treatment of subjects prior to the development of diabetes. If the aforementioned "legacy effect" or "metabolic memory" operates at this stage of the natural history of the metabolic syndrome early attainment of strict glucose control might alter the course of chronic tissue complications (201).

Antidiabetic Agents: Cost-Effective Treatment of Prediabetes?

An analysis of the Diabetes Prevention Program has suggested that intervention with metformin in obese pre-diabetic subjects might retard the development of microvascular and cardiovascular complications in the longer term; it is estimated that this would be cost-effective (202). It is noteworthy that, unlike sulfonylureas, metformin has favorable effects on insulin action and vascular risk factors. Since the results of UKPDS were published in 1998, considerable interest has focused on the thiazolidinedione class of insulin-sensitising agents, synthetic ligands for the peroxisome proliferator-activated receptor-γ (PPAR-γ). These drugs, which have multiple effects on the metabolic syndrome and cellular events that lead to atherogenesis (203), are currently being assessed in large clinical trials with hard cardiovascular endpoints (204). Thiazolidinediones may also prevent, or at least defer, the development of Type 2 diabetes through effects on insulin action and preservation of β-cell function (205,206). In obese glucose-intolerant subjects, intensive lifestyle interventions (207), metformin and troglitazone have each been shown to retard progression to Type 2 diabetes (208). The potential benefits of early treatment of hyperglycemia are considered in more detail in Chapter 6. Note, however, that no drugs are currently approved for treating hyperglycemia in states of pre-diabetes.

Statins and Other Lipid-Modifying Drugs

Of the other classes of vasculoprotective agents currently available statins reduce inflammation and low-density lipoprotein-cholesterol levels and have been shown to dramatically reduce cardiovascular events in patients with or without diabetes in the settings of primary and secondary prevention (209–212). Reports of renoprotective benefits of lipid-lowering (74,213) and suggestions of favourable effects of statins on microalbuminuria require confirmation (214,215). A report suggesting a significant protective effect of pravastatin against the development of diabetes in the West of Scotland study (216) has not been confirmed in studies of other statins (217). Of note, in the Fenofibrate Intervention and Event Lowering in Diabetes study, fenofibrate therapy was associated with less ocular laser treatment (5.2% vs. 3.6%, $p = 0.0003$) and reduced the progression of microalbuminuria($p = 0.002$) in patients with Type 2 diabetes compared with placebo (218). A reduction in total CVD events, mainly attributable to a lower incidence of non-fatal MI and fewer revascularizations, was also observed in this relatively low-risk population (hazard ratio 0.89, 95% confidence interval 0.80–0.99, $p = 0.035$) (218).

Drugs Acting on the Renin-Angiotensin System

The high cardiovascular risk associated with established diabetic nephropathy warrants intensive pharmacotherapy, including use of drugs that block the renin-angiotensin system, i.e., angiotensin converting enzyme inhibitors (ACEIs) and angiotensin receptor blockers (ARBs), wherever it is safe to do so (219–222). Effective reduction of blood pressure will simultaneously attenuate microvascular and macrovascular disease thereby disrupting the proposed vicious cycle of tissue injury. Endothelial dysfunction resulting from activation of the renin-angiotensin system is a subclinical precursor of atheroma that facilitates continuing damage from hypertension and dyslipidemia (17). Theoretically, effective intervention at this early stage might avoid the advance to vascular remodelling and irreversible tissue damage (223).

A recently recognized bonus of ACE inhibitors and ARBs is a consistent reduction in the incidence of new-onset diabetes among patients with essential hypertension (224). Thus, pharmacological blockade of the renin-angiotensin system, in addition to having proven benefits in reducing cardiovascular events, may also be able to prevent the development of diabetes. Elucidation of the mechanism(s) by which these drugs prevent or delay diabetes (225) might open the door to new therapeutic strategies. The results of recently reported DREAM study "Diabetes REduction with ramipril and rosiglitazone medication" were negative for ramipril, i.e., the combined endpoint of new cases of diabetes and deaths was not significantly reduced in glucose-intolerant subjects initially free of CVD (Yusuf S. Data presented at the European Association for the Study of Diabetes, Copenhagen, September 2006). Another factorial study using valsartan and nateglinide in prediabetic subjects is still in progress (230). Another aspect of the different metabolic-hemodynamic profiles of older and newer antihypertensive agents is the demonstration that some classes of drugs—notably those with disadvantageous metabolic effects—do not they impair glucose tolerance?, i.e., β–blockers and diuretics—may be more effective at reducing central blood pressure (227). This effect may contribute to more effective prevention of left ventricular hypertrophy and may be associated with better protection of renal function (227).

Insulin-Sensitizing Drugs

At a more fundamental level, directly improving defective insulin action, ideally through non-pharmacological modifications by increasing levels of physical activity and weight loss, or through the use of insulin-sensitizing drugs offers a logical and attractive means of improving a multiplicity of risk factors. Lifestyle changes which are effective, cheap, have multiple benefits and few side-effects are difficult to achieve and several clinical trials of thiazolidinediones are currently in progress. To date, the only placebo-controlled study to measure clinical end-points, the Prospective Pioglitazone Clinical Trial In Macrovascular Events (PROactive) study has generated a degree of controversy (228). While the primary composite endpoint of cardiovascular events, including leg revascularization, did not attain statistical significance ($p = 0.095$) the main secondary endpoint (all-cause mortality, non-fatal MI, and stroke was significant (hazard ratio 0.84, 95% confidence interval 0.72–0.98, $p = 0.027$). Concerns about the validity of the secondary endpoint analysis (229) allied to concerns about hospital admissions for heart failure (a non-adjudicated adverse event) and weight gain have led to some uncertainties about the clinical implications of this trial (230).

As mentioned above, the results of the DREAM study have recently been reported. The effects of rosiglitazone and ramipril were assessed in subjects with impaired glucose tolerance or fasting hyperglycaemia using a 2×2 factorial design. Rosiglitazone 8 mg daily was associated with a hazard ratio of 0.4 for progression to Type 2 diabetes or death compared to placebo over a median follow up of 3 years ($p < 0.0001$). Overall cardiovascular event rates were similar in both treatment arms but there was a significantly higher incidence of heart failure in the rosiglitazone-treated subjects (0.5% vs. 0.1%, $p = 0.01$) (230).

Reducing the need for polypharmacy is becoming an important part of the therapeutic challenge (173). Whether therapies based on new approaches, e.g., targeting PPAR-δ, will prove safe and effective remains to be determined (232). Recent doubts about the safety of the new class of combined PPAR-α and -γ agonists (glitazars) cautions against over-optimistic expectations (233). More data are required on the potential benefits of existing PPAR-?α agonists, i.e., fibrates, in the light of data suggesting a protective role for these agents in secondary prevention after MI in patients with the metabolic syndrome (234).

CONCLUSIONS

There are fears that the current global explosion of obesity-related insulin resistance (235) will create a tidal wave of diabetes and CVD (172,236–238). From a practical point of view, prevention of the metabolic syndrome, diabetes and CVD requires a combination of therapeutic lifestyle interventions, i.e., a prudent diet and adequate physical activity, allied to the judicious use of safe and effective drugs including ACEIs, statins, and possibly insulin-sensitizers (239, 240). The possibility of synergy between agents from these different classes merits further study (239). Selecting drugs that have proven efficacy in preventing CVD and that may reduce the risk of Type 2 diabetes is to be preferred in high-risk prediabetic subjects.

It is estimated that 65% of U.S. adults are currently overweight or obese (241). The metabolic consequences of obesity are set to affect huge numbers of ever younger subjects. Affected individuals are destined to face decades of exposure to a multiplicity of cardiovascular risk factors—optimization of current and emerging therapeutic interventions may improve the chances of preventing or at least retarding vascular complications. Carefully designed clinical trials will be required to assess the risk-benefit and economic implications of these approaches. We suggest that the potential to influence the progression of microvascular and macrovascular disease simultaneously should be considered in the design of future studies. Efforts to elucidate the molecular basis of the metabolic syndrome must continue if attempts to change lifestyles at a population level continue to fail and more specific therapeutic interventions are to be developed.

REFERENCES

1. Eckel RH, Grundy SM, Zimmet PZ. The metabolic syndrome. Lancet 2005; 365(9468):1415–1428.
2. Grundy SM, Cleeman JI, Daniels SR, et al. Diagnosis and management of the metabolic syndrome: an American Heart Association\National Heart, Lung, and Blood Institute scientific statement. Curr Opin Cardiol 2006; 21(1):1–6.

3. Grundy SM. Metabolic syndrome: connecting and reconciling cardiovascular and diabetes worlds. J Am Coll Cardiol 2006; 47(6):1093–1100.

4. Leslie BR. Metabolic syndrome: historical perspectives. Am J Med Sci 2005; 330(6):264–268.

5. Gale EA. The myth of the metabolic syndrome. Diabetologia 2005; 48(9):1679–1683.

6. Kahn R, Buse J, Ferrannini E, Stern M. The metabolic syndrome: time for a critical appraisal. Joint statement from the American Diabetes Association and the European Association for the Study of Diabetes. Diabetologia 2005; 48(9):1684–1699.

7. Kim SH, Reaven GM. The metabolic syndrome: one step forward, two steps back. Diab Vasc Dis Res 2004; 1(2):68–75.

8. Alberti KG, Zimmet P, Shaw J. The metabolic syndrome—a new worldwide definition. Lancet 2005; 366(9491):1059–1062.

9. Wild S, Byrne CD. The global burden of the metabolic syndrome and its consequences for diabetes and cardiovascular disease. In: Wild S, Byrne CD, eds. The Metabolic Syndrome. Chichester: John Wiley & Sons, 2005:1–41.

10. Executive Summary of The Third Report of The National Cholesterol Education Program (NCEP) Expert Panel on Detection, Evaluation, And Treatment of High Blood Cholesterol In Adults (Adult Treatment Panel III). JAMA 2001; 285(19):2486–2497.

11. De Backer G, Ambrosioni E, Borch-Johnsen K, et al. European guidelines on cardiovascular disease prevention in clinical practice. Third Joint Task Force of European and Other Societies on Cardiovascular Disease Prevention in Clinical Practice. Eur Heart J 2003; 24(17):1601–1610.

12. Williams B, Poulter NR, Brown MJ, et al. British Hypertension Society guidelines for hypertension management 2004 (BHS-IV): summary. BMJ 2004; 328(7440):634–640.

13. Haffner SM, Lehto S, Ronnemaa T, Pyorala K, Laakso M. Mortality from coronary heart disease in subjects with Type 2 diabetes and in nondiabetic subjects with and without prior myocardial infarction. N Engl J Med 1998; 339(4):229–234.

14. Alexander CM, Landsman PB, Teutsch SM, Haffner SM. NCEP-defined metabolic syndrome, diabetes, and prevalence of coronary heart disease among NHANES III participants age 50 years and older. Diabetes 2003; 52(5):1210–1214.

15. Nesto RW. Correlation between cardiovascular disease and diabetes mellitus: current concepts. Am J Med 2004; 116(Suppl 5A):11S–22S.

16. Grundy SM, Cleeman JI, Merz CN, et al. Implications of recent clinical trials for the National Cholesterol Education Program Adult Treatment Panel III guidelines. Circulation 2004; 110(2):227–239.

17. Ritz E. Heart and kidney: fatal twins? Am J Med 2006; 119(5 Suppl 1):S31–S39.

18. Nathan DM. Long-term complications of diabetes mellitus. N Engl J Med 1993; 328(23):1676–1685.

19. He Z, King GL. Microvascular complications of diabetes. Endocrinol Metab Clin North Am 2004; 33(1):215–238, xi–xii.

20. Kollros PR, Konkle BA. Microvascular disease in diabetes mellitus. J Cardiovasc Risk 1997; 4(2):70–75.

21. Creager MA, Luscher TF, Cosentino F, Beckman JA. Diabetes and vascular disease: pathophysiology, clinical consequences, and medical therapy: part I. Circulation 2003; 108(12):1527–1532.

22. Jouven X, Lemaitre RN, Rea TD, Sotoodehnia N, Empana JP, Siscovick DS. Diabetes, glucose level, and risk of sudden cardiac death. Eur Heart J 2005; 26(20):2142–2147.

23. Grundy SM, Cleeman JI, Daniels SR, et al. Diagnosis and management of the metabolic syndrome: an American Heart Association\National Heart, Lung, and Blood Institute Scientific Statement. Circulation 2005; 112(17):2735–2752.

24. Kereiakes DJ, Willerson JT. Metabolic syndrome epidemic. Circulation 2003; 108(13):1552–1553.

25. Grundy SM. Obesity, metabolic syndrome, and cardiovascular disease. J Clin Endocrinol Metab 2004; 89(6):2595–2600.

26. Quinones MJ, Nicholas SB, Lyon CJ. Insulin resistance and the endothelium. Curr Diab Rep 2005; 5(4):246–253.

27. Reaven GM. Banting lecture 1988. Role of insulin resistance in human disease. Diabetes 1988; 37(12):1595–1607.

28. Krentz A. Insulin Resistance. Oxford: Blackwell Science, 2002.

29. Hsueh WA, Quinones MJ. Role of endothelial dysfunction in insulin resistance. Am J Cardiol 2003; 92(4A):10J–17J.

30. Sowers JR. Obesity as a cardiovascular risk factor. Am J Med 2003; 115(Suppl 8A): 37S–41S.

31. Reaven G, Abbasi F, McLaughlin T. Obesity, insulin resistance, and cardiovascular disease. Recent Prog Horm Res 2004; 59:207–223.

32. LaMonte MJ, Blair SN, Church TS. Physical activity and diabetes prevention. J Appl Physiol 2005; 99(3):1205–1213.

33. Shen BJ, Todaro JF, Niaura R, et al. Are metabolic risk factors one unified syndrome? Modeling the structure of the metabolic syndrome X. Am J Epidemiol 2003; 157(8):701–711.

34. Pladevall M, Singal B, Williams LK, et al. A single factor underlies the metabolic syndrome: a confirmatory factor analysis. Diabetes Care 2006; 29(1):113–122.

35. Alberti KG, Zimmet PZ. Definition, diagnosis and classification of diabetes mellitus and its complications. Part 1: diagnosis and classification of diabetes mellitus provisional report of a WHO consultation. Diabet Med 1998; 15(7):539–553.

36. Organization WH. Definition, diagnosis and classification of diabetes mellitus and its complications: reports of a WHO consultation. Part 1: diagnosis and classification of diabetes mellitus. Geneva: World Health Organization.

37. Ninomiya JK, L'Italien G, Criqui MH, Whyte JL, Gamst A, Chen RS. Association of the metabolic syndrome with history of myocardial infarction and stroke in the Third National Health and Nutrition Examination Survey. Circulation 2004; 109(1):42–46.

38. Wannamethee SG, Shaper AG, Lennon L, Morris RW. Metabolic syndrome vs. Framingham Risk Score for prediction of coronary heart disease, stroke, and Type 2 diabetes mellitus. Arch Intern Med 2005; 165(22):2644–2650.

39. Dekker JM, Girman C, Rhodes T, et al. Metabolic syndrome and 10-year cardiovascular disease risk in the Hoorn Study. Circulation 2005; 112(5):666–673.

40. Malik S, Wong ND, Franklin SS, et al. Impact of the metabolic syndrome on mortality from coronary heart disease, cardiovascular disease, and all causes in United States adults. Circulation 2004; 110(10):1245–1250.

41. Guzder RN, Gatling W, Mullee MA, Byrne CD. Impact of metabolic syndrome criteria on cardiovascular disease risk in people with newly diagnosed Type 2 diabetes. Diabetologia 2006; 49(1):49–55.

42. Reilly MP, Rader DJ. The metabolic syndrome: more than the sum of its parts? Circulation 2003; 108(13):1546–1551.
43. Farmer A. Metabolic syndrome and mortality. BMJ 2006; 332(7546):882.
44. Sundstrom J, Riserus U, Byberg L, Zethelius B, Lithell H, Lind L. Clinical value of the metabolic syndrome for long term prediction of total and cardiovascular mortality: prospective, population based cohort study. BMJ 2006; 332(7546):878–882.
45. Clavijo LC, Pinto TL, Kuchulakanti PK, et al. Metabolic syndrome in patients with acute myocardial infarction is associated with increased infarct size and in-hospital complications. Cardiovasc Revasc Med 2006; 7(1):7–11.
46. Levantesi G, Macchia A, Marfisi R, et al. Metabolic syndrome and risk of cardiovascular events after myocardial infarction. J Am Coll Cardiol 2005; 46(2):277–283.
47. Zeller M, Steg PG, Ravisy J, et al. Prevalence and impact of metabolic syndrome on hospital outcomes in acute myocardial infarction. Arch Intern Med 2005; 165(10):1192–1198.
48. Najarian RM, Sullivan LM, Kannel WB, Wilson PW, D'Agostino RB, Wolf PA. Metabolic syndrome compared with Type 2 diabetes mellitus as a risk factor for stroke: the Framingham Offspring Study. Arch Intern Med 2006; 166(1):106–111.
49. Watson G, Fowkes G. Peripheral arterial disease. In: Wild S, Byrne CD, eds. The Metabolic Syndrome. Chichester: John Wiley & Sons, 2005:263–277.
50. Wild SH, Byrne CD, Smith FB, Lee AJ, Fowkes FG. Low ankle-brachial pressure index predicts increased risk of cardiovascular disease independent of the metabolic syndrome and conventional cardiovascular risk factors in the Edinburgh artery study. Diabetes Care 2006; 29(3):637–642.
51. Cipollone F, Iezzi A, Fazia M, et al. The receptor RAGE as a progression factor amplifying arachidonate-dependent inflammatory and proteolytic response in human atherosclerotic plaques: role of glycemic control. Circulation 2003; 108(9):1070–1077.
52. Beckman JA, Creager MA, Libby P. Diabetes and atherosclerosis: epidemiology, pathophysiology, and management. JAMA 2002; 287(19):2570–2581.
53. Steinberg HO, Baron AD. Vascular function, insulin resistance and fatty acids. Diabetologia 2002; 45(5):623–634.
54. Evans JL, Goldfine ID, Maddux BA, Grodsky GM. Oxidative stress and stress-activated signaling pathways: a unifying hypothesis of Type 2 diabetes. Endocr Rev 2002; 23(5):599–622.
55. Rahmouni K, Haynes WG. Leptin and the cardiovascular system. Recent Prog Horm Res 2004; 59:225–244.
56. Biondi-Zoccai GG, Abbate A, Liuzzo G, Biasucci LM. Atherothrombosis, inflammation, and diabetes. J Am Coll Cardiol 2003; 41(7):1071–1077.
57. Plutzky J. The vascular biology of atherosclerosis. Am J Med 2003; 115(Suppl 8A): 55S–61S.
58. Saruta T, Kumagai H. The sympathetic nervous system in hypertension and renal disease. Curr Opin Nephrol Hypertens 1996; 5(1):72–79.
59. Faxon DP, Fuster V, Libby P, et al. Atherosclerotic vascular disease conference: Writing Group III: pathophysiology. Circulation 2004; 109(21):2617–2625.
60. Stokes KY, Granger DN. The microcirculation: a motor for the systemic inflammatory response and large vessel disease induced by hypercholesterolaemia? J Physiol 2005; 562(Pt 3):647–653.

61. Isomaa B, Henricsson M, Almgren P, Tuomi T, Taskinen MR, Groop L. The metabolic syndrome influences the risk of chronic complications in patients with Type II diabetes. Diabetologia 2001; 44(9):1148–1154.

62. Costa LA, Canani LH, Lisboa HR, Tres GS, Gross JL. Aggregation of features of the metabolic syndrome is associated with increased prevalence of chronic complications in Type 2 diabetes. Diabet Med 2004; 21(3):252–255.

63. Cull CA JC, Holman RR. Metabolic syndrome is associated with an increased risk of microvascular but not macrovascular complications in Type 2 diabetes. Diabetes 2004; 53(Suppl 2):A28.

64. Fuller JH, Stevens LK, Wang SL. Risk factors for cardiovascular mortality and morbidity: the WHO Multinational Study of Vascular Disease in Diabetes. Diabetologia 2001; 44(Suppl 2):S54–S64.

65. Wong TY, Klein R, Sharrett AR, et al. Retinal arteriolar narrowing and risk of coronary heart disease in men and women. The Atherosclerosis Risk in Communities Study. JAMA 2002; 287(9):1153–1159.

66. Wong TY, Duncan BB, Golden SH, et al. Associations between the metabolic syndrome and retinal microvascular signs: the atherosclerosis risk in communities study. Invest Ophthalmol Vis Sci 2004; 45(9):2949–2954.

67. Soedamah-Muthu SS, Chaturvedi N, Toeller M, et al. Risk factors for coronary heart disease in Type 1 diabetic patients in Europe: the EURODIAB Prospective Complications Study. Diabetes Care 2004; 27(2):530–537.

68. Bailey CC, Sparrow JM. Co-morbidity in patients with sight-threatening diabetic retinopathy. Eye 2001; 15(Pt 6):719–722.

69. Molitch ME, DeFronzo RA, Franz MJ, et al. Nephropathy in diabetes. Diabetes Care 2004; 27(Suppl 1):S79–S83.

70. Wali RK, Henrich WL. Chronic kidney disease: a risk factor for cardiovascular disease. Cardiol Clin 2005; 23(3):343–362.

71. Curtis BM, Levin A, Parfrey PS. Multiple risk factor intervention in chronic kidney disease: management of cardiac disease in chronic kidney disease patients. Med Clin North Am 2005; 89(3):511–523.

72. Krentz AJ. Diabetes, the kidney and vascular disease: a complex relationship. Prac Diab Int 2006; 23:1–3.

73. Meguid El Nahas A, Bello AK. Chronic kidney disease: the global challenge. Lancet 2005; 365(9456):331–340.

74. Mogensen CE, Cooper ME. Diabetic renal disease: from recent studies to improved clinical practice. Diabet Med 2004; 21(1):4–17.

75. Zhang R, Liao J, Morse S, Donelon S, Reisin E. Kidney disease and the metabolic syndrome. Am J Med Sci 2005; 330(6):319–325.

76. Govindarajan G, Whaley-Connell A, Mugo M, Stump C, Sowers JR. The cardiometabolic syndrome as a cardiovascular risk factor. Am J Med Sci 2005; 330(6):311–318.

77. Kambham N, Markowitz GS, Valeri AM, Lin J, D'Agati VD. Obesity-related glomerulopathy: an emerging epidemic. Kidney Int 2001; 59(4):1498–1509.

78. Chen J, Muntner P, Hamm LL, et al. The metabolic syndrome and chronic kidney disease in U.S. adults. Ann Intern Med 2004; 140(3):167–174.

79. Jawa A, Kcomt J, Fonseca VA. Diabetic nephropathy and retinopathy. Med Clin North Am 2004; 88(4):1001–1036, xi.

80. McGowan T, McCue P, Sharma K. Diabetic nephropathy. Clin Lab Med 2001; 21(1):111–146.

81. Anavekar NS, McMurray JJ, Velazquez EJ, et al. Relation between renal dysfunction and cardiovascular outcomes after myocardial infarction. N Engl J Med 2004; 351(13):1285–1295.

82. Rahman M, Pressel S, Davis BR, et al. Cardiovascular outcomes in high-risk hypertensive patients stratified by baseline glomerular filtration rate. Ann Intern Med 2006; 144(3):172–180.

83. Yuyun MF, Khaw KT, Luben R, et al. A prospective study of microalbuminuria and incident coronary heart disease and its prognostic significance in a British population: the EPIC-Norfolk study. Am J Epidemiol 2004; 159(3):284–293.

84. Mogensen CE. Microalbuminuria and hypertension with focus on Type 1 and Type 2 diabetes. J Intern Med 2003; 254(1):45–66.

85. Donnelly R, Yeung JM, Manning G. Microalbuminuria: a common, independent cardiovascular risk factor, especially but not exclusively in Type 2 diabetes. J Hypertens Suppl 2003; 21(Suppl 1):S7–S12.

86. Blendea MC, McFarlane SI, Isenovic ER, Gick G, Sowers JR. Heart disease in diabetic patients. Curr Diab Rep 2003; 3(3):223–229.

87. Bugiardini R, Bairey Merz CN. Angina with "normal" coronary arteries: a changing philosophy. JAMA 2005; 293(4):477–484.

88. Abel ED. Myocardial insulin resistance and cardiac complications of diabetes. Curr Drug Targets Immune Endocr Metabol Disord 2005; 5(2):219–226.

89. Kim YH, Hong MK, Song JM, et al. Diabetic retinopathy as a predictor of late clinical events following percutaneous coronary intervention. J Invasive Cardiol 2002; 14(10):599–602.

90. Bell DS. Heart failure: the frequent, forgotten, and often fatal complication of diabetes. Diabetes Care 2003; 26(8):2433–2441.

91. Kenchaiah S, Evans JC, Levy D, et al. Obesity and the risk of heart failure. N Engl J Med 2002; 347(5):305–313.

92. Wittstein IS, Thiemann DR, Lima JA, et al. Neurohumoral features of myocardial stunning due to sudden emotional stress. N Engl J Med 2005; 352(6):539–548.

93. Kinoshita N, Kakehashi A, Yasu T, et al. A new form of retinopathy associated with myocardial infarction treated with percutaneous coronary intervention. Br J Ophthalmol 2004; 88(4):494–496.

94. Regensteiner JG, Wolfel EE, Brass EP, et al. Chronic changes in skeletal muscle histology and function in peripheral arterial disease. Circulation 1993; 87(2):413–421.

95. Brass EP, Hiatt WR, Gardner AW, Hoppel CL. Decreased NADH dehydrogenase and ubiquinol-cytochrome c oxidoreductase in peripheral arterial disease. Am J Physiol Heart Circ Physiol 2001; 280(2):H603–H609.

96. Wong TY, Shankar A, Klein R, Klein BE, Hubbard LD. Prospective cohort study of retinal vessel diameters and risk of hypertension. BMJ 2004; 329(7457):79.

97. Sowers JR, Stump CS. Insights into the biology of diabetic vascular disease: what's new? Am J Hypertens 2004; 17(11 Pt 2):2S–6S; quiz A2–A4.

98. Thom S. Arterial structural modifications in hypertension. Effects of treatment. Eur Heart J 1997; 18(Suppl E):E2–E4.

99. Landsberg L, Molitch M. Diabetes and hypertension: pathogenesis, prevention and treatment. Clin Exp Hypertens 2004; 26(7–8):621–628.

100. Veglio M, Chinaglia A, Cavallo-Perin P. QT interval, cardiovascular risk factors and risk of death in diabetes. J Endocrinol Invest 2004; 27(2):175–181.

101. Liatis S, Tentolouris N, Katsilambros N. Cardiac autonomic nervous system activity in obesity. Pediatr Endocrinol Rev 2004; 1(Suppl 3):476–483.

102. Dandona P, Aljada A, Chaudhuri A, Mohanty P, Garg R. Metabolic syndrome: a comprehensive perspective based on interactions between obesity, diabetes, and inflammation. Circulation 2005; 111(11):1448–1454.

103. Morse SA, Zhang R, Thakur V, Reisin E. Hypertension and the metabolic syndrome. Am J Med Sci 2005; 330(6):303–310.

104. Westerbacka J, Yki-Jarvinen H. Arterial stiffness and insulin resistance. Semin Vasc Med 2002; 2(2):157–164.

105. Tight blood pressure control and risk of macrovascular and microvascular complications in Type 2 diabetes: UKPDS 38. UK Prospective Diabetes Study Group. BMJ 1998; 317(7160):703–713.

106. Sowers JR, Frohlich ED. Insulin and insulin resistance: impact on blood pressure and cardiovascular disease. Med Clin North Am 2004; 88(1):63–82.

107. Segura J, Campo C, Ruilope LM, Rodicio JL. Do we need to target "prediabetic" hypertensive patients? J Hypertens 2005; 23(12):2119–2125.

108. Alberti KG. Blood metabolites in the diagnosis and treatment of diabetes mellitus. Postgrad Med J 1973; 49(Suppl 7):955–963.

109. He W, Miao FJ, Lin DC, et al. Citric acid cycle intermediates as ligands for orphan G-protein-coupled receptors. Nature 2004; 429(6988):188–193.

110. Lowell BB, Shulman GI. Mitochondrial dysfunction and Type 2 diabetes. Science 2005; 307(5708):384–387.

111. Stumvoll M, Goldstein BJ, van Haeften TW. Type 2 diabetes: principles of pathogenesis and therapy. Lancet 2005; 365(9467):1333–1346.

112. Bergman RN, Mittelman SD. Central role of the adipocyte in insulin resistance. J Basic Clin Physiol Pharmacol 1998; 9(2–4):205–221.

113. Ceddia RB, William WN Jr, Curi R. The response of skeletal muscle to leptin. Front Biosci 2001; 6:D90–D97.

114. Rajala MW, Scherer PE. Minireview: the adipocyte—at the crossroads of energy homeostasis, inflammation, and atherosclerosis. Endocrinology 2003; 144(9):3765–3773.

115. Bouskila M, Pajvani UB, Scherer PE. Adiponectin: a relevant player in PPARgamma-agonist-mediated improvements in hepatic insulin sensitivity? Int J Obes (Lond) 2005; 29(Suppl 1):S17–S23.

116. Williams TM, Lisanti MP. The Caveolin genes: from cell biology to medicine. Ann Med 2004; 36(8):584–595.

117. Kimura A, Mora S, Shigematsu S, Pessin JE, Saltiel AR. The insulin receptor catalyzes the tyrosine phosphorylation of caveolin-1. J Biol Chem 2002; 277(33):30153–30158.

118. Karlsson M, Thorn H, Parpal S, Stralfors P, Gustavsson J. Insulin induces translocation of glucose transporter GLUT4 to plasma membrane caveolae in adipocytes. Faseb J 2002; 16(2):249–251.

119. The effect of intensive treatment of diabetes on the development and progression of long-term complications in insulin-dependent diabetes mellitus. The Diabetes Control and Complications Trial Research Group. N Engl J Med 1993; 329(14):977–986.

120. Nathan DM, Lachin J, Cleary P, et al. Intensive diabetes therapy and carotid intima-media thickness in Type 1 diabetes mellitus. N Engl J Med 2003; 348(23):2294–2303.

121. Nathan DM, Cleary PA, Backlund JY, et al. Intensive diabetes treatment and cardiovascular disease in patients with Type 1 diabetes. N Engl J Med 2005; 353(25):2643–2653.

122. Larsen JL, Colling CW, Ratanasuwan T, et al. Pancreas transplantation improves vascular disease in patients with Type 1 diabetes. Diabetes Care 2004; 27(7):1706–1711.

123. Navarro X, Kennedy WR, Sutherland DE. Autonomic neuropathy and survival in diabetes mellitus: effects of pancreas transplantation. Diabetologia 1991; 34(Suppl 1):S108–S112.

124. Tyden G, Bolinder J, Solders G, Brattstrom C, Tibell A, Groth CG. Improved survival in patients with insulin-dependent diabetes mellitus and end-stage diabetic nephropathy 10 years after combined pancreas and kidney transplantation. Transplantation 1999; 67(5):645–648.

125. Intensive blood-glucose control with sulphonylureas or insulin compared with conventional treatment and risk of complications in patients with Type 2 diabetes (UKPDS 33). UK Prospective Diabetes Study (UKPDS) Group. Lancet 1998; 352(9131):837–853.

126. Effect of intensive blood-glucose control with metformin on complications in overweight patients with Type 2 diabetes (UKPDS 34). UK Prospective Diabetes Study (UKPDS) Group. Lancet 1998; 352(9131):854–865.

127. Simpson SH, Majumdar SR, Tsuyuki RT, Eurich DT, Johnson JA. Dose-response relation between sulfonylurea drugs and mortality in Type 2 diabetes mellitus: a population-based cohort study. CMAJ 2006; 174(2):169–174.

128. Wiernsperger NF, Bouskela E. Microcirculation in insulin resistance and diabetes: more than just a complication. Diabetes Metab 2003; 29(4 Pt 2):6S77–6S87.

129. Gabir MM, Hanson RL, Dabelea D, et al. Plasma glucose and prediction of microvascular disease and mortality: evaluation of 1997 American Diabetes Association and 1999 World Health Organization criteria for diagnosis of diabetes. Diabetes Care 2000; 23(8):1113–1118.

130. Report of the Expert Committee on the Diagnosis and Classification of Diabetes Mellitus. Diabetes Care 2002; 25(90001):5S–20S.

131. Haffner SJ, Cassells H. Hyperglycemia as a cardiovascular risk factor. Am J Med 2003; 115(Suppl 8A):6S–11S.

132. Gerstein HC, Yusuf S. Dysglycaemia and risk of cardiovascular disease. Lancet 1996; 347(9006):949–950.

133. Khaw KT, Wareham N, Luben R, et al. Glycated haemoglobin, diabetes, and mortality in men in Norfolk cohort of European prospective investigation of cancer and nutrition (EPIC-Norfolk). BMJ 2001; 322(7277):15–18.

134. Alberti KG. Impaired glucose tolerance: what are the clinical implications? Diabetes Res Clin Pract 1998; 40(Suppl):S3–S8.

135. Glucose tolerance and mortality: comparison of WHO and American Diabetes Association diagnostic criteria. The DECODE study group. European Diabetes Epidemiology Group. Diabetes Epidemiology: Collaborative analysis of diagnostic criteria in Europe. Lancet 1999; 354(9179):617–621.

136. Ceriello A. The emerging role of post-prandial hyperglycaemic spikes in the pathogenesis of diabetic complications. Diabet Med 1998; 15(3):188–193.

137. Abrahamson MJ. Optimal glycemic control in Type 2 diabetes mellitus: fasting and postprandial glucose in context. Arch Intern Med 2004; 164(5):486–491.

138. Stern MP. Diabetes and cardiovascular disease. The "common soil" hypothesis. Diabetes 1995; 44(4):369–374.

139. Norhammar A, Tenerz A, Nilsson G, et al. Glucose metabolism in patients with acute myocardial infarction and no previous diagnosis of diabetes mellitus: a prospective study. Lancet 2002; 359(9324):2140–2144.

140. affner SM, Stern MP, Hazuda HP, Mitchell BD, Patterson JK. Cardiovascular risk factors in confirmed prediabetic individuals. Does the clock for coronary heart disease start ticking before the onset of clinical diabetes? JAMA 1990; 263(21): 2893–2898.

141. Meigs JB, Nathan DM, Wilson PW, Cupples LA, Singer DE. Metabolic risk factors worsen continuously across the spectrum of nondiabetic glucose tolerance. The Framingham Offspring Study. Ann Intern Med 1998; 128(7):524–533.

142. Jeffcoate SL. Diabetes control and complications: the role of glycated haemoglobin, 25 years on. Diabet Med 2004; 21(7):657–665.

143. Chiasson JL, Josse RG, Gomis R, Hanefeld M, Karasik A, Laakso M. Acarbose treatment and the risk of cardiovascular disease and hypertension in patients with impaired glucose tolerance: the STOP-NIDDM trial. JAMA 2003; 290(4):486–494.

144. Hanefeld M, Chiasson JL, Koehler C, Henkel E, Schaper F, Temelkova-Kurktschiev T. Acarbose slows progression of intima-media thickness of the carotid arteries in subjects with impaired glucose tolerance. Stroke 2004; 35(5):1073–1078.

145. Singleton JR, Smith AG, Russell JW, Feldman EL. Microvascular complications of impaired glucose tolerance. Diabetes 2003; 52(12):2867–2873.

146. Garcia Soriano F, Virag L, Jagtap P, et al. Diabetic endothelial dysfunction: the role of poly(ADP-ribose) polymerase activation. Nat Med 2001; 7(1):108–113.

147. Heine RJ, Balkau B, Ceriello A, Del Prato S, Horton ES, Taskinen MR. What does postprandial hyperglycaemia mean? Diabet Med 2004; 21(3):208–213.

148. Lee RH, Dellon AL. Insulin resistance. Does it play a role in peripheral neuropathy? Diabetes Care 1999; 22(11):1914–1915.

149. Perkins BA, Bril V. Early vascular risk modification in Type 1 diabetes. N Engl J Med 2005; 352:408–409.

150. Krentz AJ, Honigsberger L, Nattrass M. Selection of patients with symptomatic diabetic neuropathy for clinical trials. Diabetes Metab 1989; 15(6):416–419.

151. Solomon H, Man JW, Jackson G. Erectile dysfunction and the cardiovascular patient: endothelial dysfunction is the common denominator. Heart 2003; 89(3):251–253.

152. Fung MM, Bettencourt R, Barrett-Connor E. Heart disease risk factors predict erectile dysfunction 25 years later: the Rancho Bernardo Study. J Am Coll Cardiol 2004; 43(8):1405–1411.

153. Cameron NE, Cotter MA. Metabolic and vascular factors in the pathogenesis of diabetic neuropathy. Diabetes 1997; 46(Suppl 2):S31–S37.

154. Vinik AI. Diabetic neuropathy: pathogenesis and therapy. Am J Med 1999; 107(2B):17S–26S.

155. Tesfaye S, Chatuvedi N, Eaton SEM, et al. Vascular risk factors and diabetic neuropathy. N Engl J Med 2005; 352:592–597.

156. Tuomilehto J. Primary prevention of Type 2 diabetes: lifestyle intervention works and saves money, but what should be done with smokers? Ann Intern Med 2005; 142(5):381–383.

157. Jenkins AJ, Rowley KG, Lyons TJ, Best JD, Hill MA, Klein RL. Lipoproteins and diabetic microvascular complications. Curr Pharm Des 2004; 10(27):3395–3418.

158. Leiter LA. The prevention of diabetic microvascular complications of diabetes: is there a role for lipid lowering? Diabetes Res Clin Pract 2005; 68(Suppl 2):S3–S14.

159. Lyons TJ, Jenkins AJ, Zheng D, et al. Diabetic retinopathy and serum lipoprotein subclasses in the DCCT\EDIC cohort. Invest Ophthalmol Vis Sci 2004; 45(3):910–918.

160. Hu G, Qiao Q, Tuomilehto J, Eliasson M, Feskens EJ, Pyorala K. Plasma insulin and cardiovascular mortality in non-diabetic European men and women: a meta-analysis of data from eleven prospective studies. Diabetologia 2004; 47(7):1245–1256.

161. Zethelius B, Lithell H, Hales CN, Berne C. Insulin sensitivity, proinsulin and insulin as predictors of coronary heart disease. A population-based 10-year, follow-up study in 70-year old men using the euglycaemic insulin clamp. Diabetologia 2005; 48(5):862–867.

162. Baron AD. Insulin resistance and vascular function. J Diabetes Complications 2002; 16(1):92–102.

163. De Jongh RT, Serne EH, RG IJ, de Vries G, Stehouwer CD. Impaired microvascular function in obesity: implications for obesity-associated microangiopathy, hypertension, and insulin resistance. Circulation 2004; 109(21):2529–2535.

164. De Jongh RT, Clark AD, RG IJ, Serne EH, De Vries G, Stehouwer CD. Physiological hyperinsulinaemia increases intramuscular microvascular reactive hyperaemia and vasomotion in healthy volunteers. Diabetologia 2004; 47(6):978–986.

165. Hadjadj S, Pean F, Gallois Y, et al. Different patterns of insulin resistance in relatives of Type 1 diabetic patients with retinopathy or nephropathy: the Genesis France-Belgium Study. Diabetes Care 2004; 27(11):2661–2668.

166. Williams R, Van Gaal L, Lucioni C. Assessing the impact of complications on the costs of Type II diabetes. Diabetologia 2002; 45(7):S13–S17.

167. Wong ND, Pio JR, Franklin SS, L'Italien GJ, Kamath TV, Williams GR. Preventing coronary events by optimal control of blood pressure and lipids in patients with the metabolic syndrome. Am J Cardiol 2003; 91(12):1421–1426.

168. Capes SE, Hunt D, Malmberg K, Gerstein HC. Stress hyperglycaemia and increased risk of death after myocardial infarction in patients with and without diabetes: a systematic overview. Lancet 2000; 355(9206):773–778.

169. Aguilar D, Solomon SD, Kober L, et al. Newly diagnosed and previously known diabetes mellitus and 1-year outcomes of acute myocardial infarction: the VALsartan In Acute myocardial iNfarcTion (VALIANT) trial. Circulation 2004; 110(12):1572–1578.

170. Gaede P, Vedel P, Larsen N, Jensen GV, Parving HH, Pedersen O. Multifactorial intervention and cardiovascular disease in patients with Type 2 diabetes. N Engl J Med 2003; 348(5):383–393.

171. Schnell O, Schafer O, Kleybrink S, Doering W, Standl E, Otter W. Intensification of therapeutic approaches reduces mortality in diabetic patients with acute myocardial infarction: the Munich registry. Diabetes Care 2004; 27(2):455–460.

172. Libby P. The forgotten majority: unfinished business in cardiovascular risk reduction. J Am Coll Cardiol 2005; 46(7):1225–1228.

173. Grundy SM. Drug therapy of the metabolic syndrome: minimizing the emerging crisis in polypharmacy. Nat Rev Drug Discov 2006; 5(4):295–309.

174. Esposito K, Marfella R, Ciotola M, et al. Effect of a Mediterranean-style diet on endothelial dysfunction and markers of vascular inflammation in the metabolic syndrome: a randomized trial. JAMA 2004; 292(12):1440–1446.

175. Trichopoulou A, Orfanos P, Norat T, et al. Modified Mediterranean diet and survival: EPIC-elderly prospective cohort study. BMJ 2005; 330(7498):991.

176. Trichopoulou A, Bamia C, Trichopoulos D. Mediterranean diet and survival among patients with coronary heart disease in Greece. Arch Intern Med 2005; 165(8):929–935.

177. Lloyd-Jones DM, Leip EP, Larson MG, et al. Prediction of lifetime risk for cardiovascular disease by risk factor burden at 50 years of age. Circulation 2006; 113(6):791–798.

178. Chandola T, Brunner E, Marmot M. Chronic stress at work and the metabolic syndrome: prospective study. BMJ 2006; 332(7540):521–525.

179. Weitzman M, Cook S, Auinger P, et al. Tobacco smoke exposure is associated with the metabolic syndrome in adolescents. Circulation 2005; 112(6):862–869.

180. Byrne CD, Phillips DI. Fetal origins of adult disease: epidemiology and mechanisms. J Clin Pathol 2000; 53(11):822–828.

181. Wild S, Roglic G, Green A, Sicree R, King H. Global prevalence of diabetes: estimates for the year 2000 and projections for 2030. Diabetes Care 2004; 27(5):1047–1053.

182. Evans A, Krentz AJ. Benefits and risks of transfer from oral agents to insulin in Type 2 diabetes mellitus. Drug Saf 1999; 21(1):7–22.

183. Malmberg K. Prospective randomised study of intensive insulin treatment on long term survival after acute myocardial infarction in patients with diabetes mellitus. DIGAMI (Diabetes Mellitus, Insulin Glucose Infusion in Acute Myocardial Infarction) Study Group. BMJ 1997; 314(7093):1512–1515.

184. Stout RW. The impact of insulin upon atherosclerosis. Horm Metab Res 1994; 26(3):125–128.

185. Sjoholm A, Nystrom T. Endothelial inflammation in insulin resistance. Lancet 2005; 365(9459):610–612.

186. Ohkubo Y, Kishikawa H, Araki E, et al. Intensive insulin therapy prevents the progression of diabetic microvascular complications in Japanese patients with non-insulin-dependent diabetes mellitus: a randomized prospective 6-year study. Diabetes Res Clin Pract 1995; 28(2):103–117.

187. Vincent MA, Clerk LH, Lindner JR, et al. Microvascular recruitment is an early insulin effect that regulates skeletal muscle glucose uptake in vivo. Diabetes 2004; 53(6):1418–1423.

188. Sobel BE, Woodcock-Mitchell J, Schneider DJ, Holt RE, Marutsuka K, Gold H. Increased plasminogen activator inhibitor Type 1 in coronary artery atherectomy specimens from Type 2 diabetic compared with nondiabetic patients: a potential factor predisposing to thrombosis and its persistence. Circulation 1998; 97(22):2213–2221.

189. Takebayashi K, Aso Y, Inukai T. Initiation of insulin therapy reduces serum concentrations of high-sensitivity C-reactive protein in patients with Type 2 diabetes. Metabolism 2004; 53(6):693–699.

190. Verma S, Kuliszewski MA, Li SH, et al. C-reactive protein attenuates endothelial progenitor cell survival, differentiation, and function: further evidence of a mechanistic link between C-reactive protein and cardiovascular disease. Circulation 2004; 109(17):2058–2067.

191. Langouche L, Vanhorebeek I, Vlasselaers D, et al. Intensive insulin therapy protects the endothelium of critically ill patients. J Clin Invest 2005; 115(8):2277–2286.
192. Malmberg K, Ryden L, Wedel H, et al. Intense metabolic control by means of insulin in patients with diabetes mellitus and acute myocardial infarction (DIGAMI 2): effects on mortality and morbidity. Eur Heart J 2005; 26(7):650–661.
193. Marfella R, D'Amico M, Di Filippo C, et al. Myocardial infarction in diabetic rats: role of hyperglycaemia on infarct size and early expression of hypoxia-inducible factor 1. Diabetologia 2002; 45(8):1172–1181.
194. Nordestgaard BG, Agerholm-Larsen B, Stender S. Effect of exogenous hyperinsulinaemia on atherogenesis in cholesterol-fed rabbits. Diabetologia 1997; 40(5):512–520.
195. Vehkavaara S, Yki-Jarvinen H. 3.5 years of insulin therapy with insulin glargine improves in vivo endothelial function in Type 2 diabetes. Arterioscler Thromb Vasc Biol 2004; 24(2):325–330.
196. Tamminen MK, Westerbacka J, Vehkavaara S, Yki-Jarvinen H. Insulin therapy improves insulin actions on glucose metabolism and aortic wave reflection in Type 2 diabetic patients. Eur J Clin Invest 2003; 33(10):855–860.
197. Bryer-Ash M, Garber AJ. Point: inpatient glucose management: the emperor finally has clothes. Diabetes Care 2005; 28(4):973–975.
198. Watkinson P, Barber VS, Young JD. Strict glucose control in the critically ill. BMJ 2006; 332(7546):865–866.
199. Mesotten D, Van den Berghe G. Clinical potential of insulin therapy in critically ill patients. Drugs 2003; 63(7):625–636.
200. Van den Berghe G, Wilmer A, Hermans G, et al. Intensive insulin therapy in the medical ICU. N Engl J Med 2006; 354(5):449–461.
201. LeRoith D, Fonseca V, Vinik A. Metabolic memory in diabetes—focus on insulin. Diabetes Metab Res Rev 2005; 21(2):85–90.
202. Herman WH, Hoerger TJ, Brandle M, et al. The cost-effectiveness of lifestyle modification or metformin in preventing Type 2 diabetes in adults with impaired glucose tolerance. Ann Intern Med 2005; 142(5):323–332.
203. Glass CK. Antiatherogenic effects of thiazolidinediones? Arterioscler Thromb Vasc Biol 2001; 21(3):295–296.
204. Martens FM, Visseren FL, Lemay J, de Koning EJ, Rabelink TJ. Metabolic and additional vascular effects of thiazolidinediones. Drugs 2002; 62(10):1463–1480.
205. Buchanan TA, Xiang AH, Peters RK, et al. Preservation of pancreatic beta-cell function and prevention of Type 2 diabetes by pharmacological treatment of insulin resistance in high-risk Hispanic women. Diabetes 2002; 51(9):2796–2803.
206. Bell DS. Beta-cell rejuvenation with thiazolidinediones. Am J Med 2003; 115(Suppl 8A):20S–23S.
207. Tuomilehto J, Lindstrom J, Eriksson JG, et al. Prevention of Type 2 diabetes mellitus by changes in lifestyle among subjects with impaired glucose tolerance. N Engl J Med 2001; 344(18):1343–1350.
208. Knowler WC, Barrett-Connor E, Fowler SE, et al. Reduction in the incidence of Type 2 diabetes with lifestyle intervention or metformin. N Engl J Med 2002; 346(6):393–403.
209. Collins R, Armitage J, Parish S, Sleigh P, Peto R. MRC\BHF Heart Protection Study of cholesterol-lowering with simvastatin in 5963 people with diabetes: a randomised placebo-controlled trial. Lancet 2003; 361(9374):2005–2016.

210. Krentz AJ. Lipoprotein abnormalities and their consequences for patients with Type 2 diabetes. Diabetes Obes Metab 2003; 5(Suppl 1):S19–S27.

211. Armitage J, Bowman L. Cardiovascular outcomes among participants with diabetes in the recent large statin trials. Curr Opin Lipidol 2004; 15(4):439–446.

212. Colhoun HM, Betteridge DJ, Durrington PN, et al. Primary prevention of cardiovascular disease with atorvastatin in Type 2 diabetes in the Collaborative Atorvastatin Diabetes Study (CARDS): multicentre randomised placebo-controlled trial. Lancet 2004; 364(9435):685–696.

213. Fried LF, Forrest KY, Ellis D, Chang Y, Silvers N, Orchard TJ. Lipid modulation in insulin-dependent diabetes mellitus: effect on microvascular outcomes. J Diabetes Complications 2001; 15(3):113–119.

214. Fried LF, Orchard TJ, Kasiske BL. Effect of lipid reduction on the progression of renal disease: a meta-analysis. Kidney Int 2001; 59(1):260–269.

215. Athyros VG, Papageorgiou AA, Elisaf M, Mikhailidis DP. Statins and renal function in patients with diabetes mellitus. Curr Med Res Opin 2003; 19(7):615–617.

216. Freeman DJ, Norrie J, Sattar N, et al. Pravastatin and the development of diabetes mellitus: evidence for a protective treatment effect in the West of Scotland Coronary Prevention Study. Circulation 2001; 103(3):357–362.

217. Padwal R, Majumdar SR, Johnson JA, Varney J, McAlister FA. A systematic review of drug therapy to delay or prevent Type 2 diabetes. Diabetes Care 2005; 28(3):736–744.

218. Keech A, Simes RJ, Barter P, et al. Effects of long-term fenofibrate therapy on cardiovascular events in 9795 people with Type 2 diabetes mellitus (the FIELD study): randomised controlled trial. Lancet 2005; 366(9500):1849–1861.

219. McLaughlin K, Jardine AG. Clinical management of diabetic nephropathy. Diabetes Obes Metab 1999; 1(6):307–315.

220. Opie LH, Parving HH. Diabetic nephropathy: can renoprotection be extrapolated to cardiovascular protection? Circulation 2002; 106(6):643–645.

221. Marshall SM. Inhibition of the renin-angiotensin system: added value in reducing cardiovascular and renal risk? Diabet Med 2004; 21(1):1–3.

222. Viberti G. Regression of albuminuria: latest evidence for a new approach. J Hypertens Suppl 2003; 21(Suppl 3):S24–S28.

223. McVeigh GE, Plumb R, Hughes S. Vascular abnormalities in hypertension: cause, effect, or therapeutic target? Curr Hypertens Rep 2004; 6(3):171–176.

224. McFarlane SI, Kumar A, Sowers JR. Mechanisms by which angiotensin-converting enzyme inhibitors prevent diabetes and cardiovascular disease. Am J Cardiol 2003; 91(12A):30H–37H.

225. Scheen AJ. Prevention of Type 2 diabetes mellitus through inhibition of the Renin-Angiotensin system. Drugs 2004; 64(22):2537–2565.

226. Williams B, Lacy PS, Thom SM, et al. Differential impact of blood pressure-lowering drugs on central aortic pressure and clinical outcomes: principal results of the Conduit Artery Function Evaluation (CAFE) study. Circulation 2006; 113(9):1213–1225.

227. Dormandy JA, Charbonnel B, Eckland DJ, et al. Secondary prevention of macrovascular events in patients with Type 2 diabetes in the PROactive Study (PROspective pioglitAzone Clinical Trial In macroVascular Events): a randomised controlled trial. Lancet 2005; 366(9493):1279–1289.

228. Freemantle N. How well does the evidence on pioglitazone back up researchers' claims for a reduction in macrovascular events? BMJ 2005; 331(7520):836–838.

229. Yki-Jarvinen H. The PROactive study: some answers, many questions. Lancet 2005; 366(9493):1241–1242.

230. The DREAM (Diabetes REduction Assessment with ramipril and rosiglitazone Medication) investigators. Effect of rosiglitazone on the frequency of diabetes in patients with impaired glucose tolerance or impaired fasting glucose: a randomised controlled trial. Lancet 2006; 368:1096–1105.

231. Barish GD, Narkar VA, Evans RM. PPAR delta: a dagger in the heart of the metabolic syndrome. J Clin Invest 2006; 116(3):590–597.

232. Nissen SE, Wolski K, Topol EJ. Effect of muraglitazar on death and major adverse cardiovascular events in patients with Type 2 diabetes mellitus. JAMA 2005; 294(20):2581–2586.

233. Tenenbaum A, Motro M, Fisman EZ, Tanne D, Boyko V, Behar S. Bezafibrate for the secondary prevention of myocardial infarction in patients with metabolic syndrome. Arch Intern Med 2005; 165(10):1154–1160.

234. Weiss R, Dziura J, Burgert TS, et al. Obesity and the metabolic syndrome in children and adolescents. N Engl J Med 2004; 350(23):2362–2374.

235. Ten S, Maclaren N. Insulin resistance syndrome in children. J Clin Endocrinol Metab 2004; 89(6):2526–2539.

236. Tounian P, Aggoun Y, Dubern B, et al. Presence of increased stiffness of the common carotid artery and endothelial dysfunction in severely obese children: a prospective study. Lancet 2001; 358(9291):1400–1404.

237. Lorenzo C, Williams K, Hunt KJ, Haffner SM. Trend in the prevalence of the metabolic syndrome and its impact on cardiovascular disease incidence: the San Antonio Heart Study. Diabetes Care 2006; 29(3):625–630.

238. Caglayan E, Blaschke F, Takata Y, Hsueh WA. Metabolic syndrome-interdependence of the cardiovascular and metabolic pathways. Curr Opin Pharmacol 2005; 5(2):135–142.

239. Rosenson RS. New approaches in the intensive management of cardiovascular risk in the metabolic syndrome. Curr Probl Cardiol 2005; 30(5):241–279.

240. Hedley AA, Ogden CL, Johnson CL, Carroll MD, Curtin LR, Flegal KM. Prevalence of overweight and obesity among US children, adolescents, and adults, 1999–2002. JAMA 2004; 291(23):2847–2850.

6

Glycemic Control and the Metabolic Syndrome

John E. Gerich and Regina Dodis

*Department of Medicine, University of Rochester School of Medicine,
Rochester, New York, U.S.A.*

SUMMARY

■ The metabolic syndrome represents a cluster of factors that increase the risk for atherothrombotic cardiovascular disease (CVD).

■ An imbalance between caloric intake and caloric expenditure leads to an accumulation of visceral fat, leading to insulin resistance with a reduction in the beneficial effects of insulin on (i) carbohydrate and lipid metabolism, (ii) vascular health, and (iii) inflammatory mechanisms.

■ Numerous epidemiologic surveys indicate that hyperglycemia is an independent risk factor for CVD with no apparent threshold so that even isolated postprandial hyperglycemia not severe enough to lead to the diagnosis of Type 2 diabetes increases the risk for CVD.

■ Lifestyle interventions form the foundation of treatment of Type 2 diabetes and its prevention; weight reduction in obese individuals and increased physical activity reduce insulin resistance, decrease cardiovascular risk factors, and improve β-cell function.

■ In people with impaired glucose tolerance and Type 2 diabetes, pharmacologic therapy will probably be necessary for most patients. In theory, the ideal pharmacologic agent to treat the hyperglycemia of the metabolic syndrome should be safe, effective, and, rather than adversely affect other cardiovascular risk factors, improve them.

INTRODUCTION

The metabolic syndrome represents a cluster of cardiovascular risk factors that occur together more commonly than expected from the prevalence of their individual rates (1–5). The definition and diagnostic criteria of the metabolic syndrome are extensively discussed in Chapter 1. Currently there is considerable controversy and confusion about the metabolic syndrome, because its definition includes diagnostic criteria, potential causes, mediators, and consequences, because it is uncertain whether having the syndrome conveys no additional cardiovascular risk than the sum of its components, and because at the present time, having the syndrome does not alter treatment (6–10).

Insulin resistance is widely believed to be the common denominator causing, in susceptible individuals, the development of various cardiovascular risk factor components of the syndrome (e.g., hyperlipidemia, hypertension, and hyperglycemia) (11). The major cause of this insulin resistance appears to be obesity, especially the accumulation of visceral fat (12–14). This obesity is due to the combination of excessive caloric intake and inadequate physical activity rather than alterations in energy utilization (15). Psychosocial factors rather than genetic factors appear to be primarily involved. However, not all obese individuals have visceral obesity and conversely some nonobese individuals [i.e., with normal body mass index (BMI)] can have excessive visceral fat (13,16). It has been estimated that about 50% of the variation in body fat deposition is genetic (17). Theoretically, other causes of insulin resistance [e.g., high saturated fat diets, physical inactivity, aging, drugs (e.g., corticosteroids), and concomitant conditions (e.g., polycystic ovary syndrome, uremia, and liver disease)] could also produce the same sequelae. At the present time, there is no convincing evidence that the molecular defects associated with the insulin resistance of the metabolic syndrome differ from those due to other common causes of insulin resistance.

It also should be pointed out that just as not all insulin-resistant individuals are hyperlipidemic, hypertensive, and hyperglycemic, not all hyperlipidemic, hypertensive, and hyperglycemic individuals are insulin resistant (16,18–20). Nevertheless, as indicated earlier, hyperlipidemia, hypertension, and hyperglycemia occur more often in insulin-resistant individuals than would be expected from their relative prevalence rates. This suggests that insulin resistance may not in itself be sufficient to cause these cardiovascular risk factors except in genetically predisposed individuals [e.g., people with a genetically impaired capacity to secrete insulin, as in the case of diabetes mellitus (DM)]. Alternatively and/or additionally, it is possible that insulin resistance exacerbates the consequences of environmental factors (e.g., high-salt diet as in the case of hypertension).

Approximately 60% of people with the metabolic syndrome have obesity. Only 10% to 20% of patients with the metabolic syndrome actually have impaired glucose tolerance (IGT). Conversely, many studies have shown that only a minority of nondiabetics with insulin resistance [but who may have impaired fasting glucose (IFG) or IGT] will have the metabolic syndrome (21).

The 20-year results from the Epidemiology of Diabetes Interventions and Complications (EDIC) trial, presented at the American Diabetes Association's (ADA's) 65th Annual Scientific Sessions, showed evidence that early, aggressive glycemic control in Type 1 diabetes significantly decreases the long-term risk of cardiovascular disease (CVD). EDIC is a long-term follow-up to the Diabetes Control and Complications Trial (DCCT), which started in 1983 with a cohort of 1441 patients. At the end of DCCT, 93% of participants joined EDIC. The 20-year cumulative incidence of any CVD event was 11% in the former conventional therapy group, compared to 6% in the former intensive therapy group. This translated into a 42% CVD risk reduction. Furthermore, formerly intensively treated patients experienced a 57% risk reduction for severe CVD events. This provides evidence that achieving and sustaining a hemoglobin (Hb) A_{1c} level of approximately 7% in Type 1 DM provides definitive cardiovascular benefits.

The Prospective Pioglitazone Clinical Trial in Macrovascular Events (PROactive) is a prospective, randomized controlled trial involving 5238 patients with Type 2 diabetes who had evidence of macrovascular disease. Patients were assigned to oral pioglitazone (titrated from 15–45 mg) or matching placebo in addition to their other medications. After three years of therapy, the pioglitazone group showed an absolute risk reduction of approximately 2% in all-cause mortality, nonfatal myocardial infarction (MI), and stroke. Various metabolic effects could contribute to this cardiovascular protection; i.e., an absolute reduction of 0.5% in HbA_{1c}, a 13% reduction in triglycerides, a 3 mmHg reduction in systolic blood pressure, a 9% increase in high-density lipoprotein (HDL) cholesterol in the pioglitazone group compared to placebo. It is not possible to extrapolate these results to patients with the metabolic syndrome without diabetes, and additional studies are required (22–25).

Recently released by the European Association for the Study of Diabetes (Copenhagen, September 2006) were the results of the Diabetes REduction Assessment with Ramipril and Rosiglitazone Medication (DREAM) study. 5,269 presons with prediabetes randomized to rosiglitazone (8 mg daily) versus placebo and ramipril versus placebo for an average of 3 years. 10.6% of those on rosiglitazone progressed to Type 2 diabetes versus 25% on placebo, representing a 62% risk reduction ($p < 0.0001$), and there was a 60% reduction in the primary endpoint of development of diabetes or death from any cause. Moreover, 51% of those on rosiglitazone versus 30% on placebo returned to normal blood sugar. There was a higher rate of heart failure in the rosiglitazone (0.5%) versus placebo (0.1%) arm, however. This study provides significant evidence for the efficacy of thiazolidinediones for the prevention of new diabetes onset in those with prediabetes or the metabolic syndrome (26).

A key question is whether the overall metabolic syndrome should be a target of therapy or should the individual components of the syndrome be treated specifically. At the present time, there are no drugs approved with an indication to treat the metabolic syndrome. However, there are effective pharmacologic treatments available to treat its individual components such as fibrates, which reduce plasma triglycerides and increase plasma HDL. Moreover, there are several weight-loss agents available that could be expected to improve all components of the syndrome (27,28).

This chapter deals specifically with the treatment of hyperglycemia associated with the syndrome. The goals of such treatment are to prevent the complications of chronic hyperglycemia—micro- and macrovascular disease. For people with IGT or Type 2 diabetes, the major problem is CVD (29).

EPIDEMIOLOGY AND MECHANISMS OF HYPERGLYCEMIA AND CVD

Numerous epidemiologic surveys indicate that hyperglycemia is an independent risk factor for CVD with no apparent threshold (30–32), so that even isolated postprandial hyperglycemia not severe enough to lead to the diagnosis of Type 2 diabetes increases the risk for CVD (30,31).

The Funagata Study (33), for example, demonstrated that individuals with IGT have seven-year cardiovascular mortality rates that are nearly as increased as those of patients with Type 2 diabetes. The European Prospective Investigation into Cancer Study found that individuals with HbA_{1c} levels between 5.0% and 5.5% had a roughly twofold increased risk of dying from CVD than those with HbA_{1c} values less than 5.0% (34). People with HbA_{1c} values between 5.0% and 5.5% generally have fasting and two-hour postprandial plasma glucose levels averaging 92 mg/dL (5.1 mmol/L) and 124 mg/dL (6.9 mmol/L), respectively (35). The implications of these observations are that the ideal therapeutic target of treatment of glycemia should be an HbA_{1c} of 5.0% or less and that people with CVD should be treated just as vigorously as people with Type 2 diabetes.

Currently no drugs have been approved for the treatment of IGT. However, controlled clinical trials have shown that several drugs [e.g., metformin, acarbose, orlistat, and thiazolidinediones (TZDs)] are safe and effective in improving glucose tolerance and preventing progression to overt diabetes in such individuals (23,36–39) (see Chapter 3). Two drugs used in these studies have been shown to reduce cardiovascular events (23,38). Perhaps when the results of several ongoing clinical trials with cardiovascular outcomes become available, this situation may change. At present, major organizations such as the ADA, the American College of Endocrinology, and the International Diabetes Federation recommend target HbA_{1c} levels no lower than 6.5% (40–42). Such a high target would still leave many individuals at increased risk for CVD. To some extent, this situation is the result of a lack of large-scale clinical trials demonstrating that reduction in HbA_{1c} levels to values less than 5.5% can reduce cardiovascular mortality and can do so without unacceptable side effects (i.e., hypoglycemia). Again, this may change when the results of clinical trials underway become known.

Another issue is the lack of early and aggressive treatment. For example, according to the latest National Health and Nutrition Examination Study (NHANES) data, glycemic control of diabetes has not improved over the past 10 years, and nearly 40% of diabetic patients have HbA_{1c} levels above 7% (43). This is probably not simply the result of the absence of safe and effective treatments, but rather the lack of sufficient follow-up by health-care providers, the lack of understanding and complimentary resources of caregivers, and the lack of patient motivation and cooperation (44). Theoretically, these barriers could be overcome by improved education of caregivers and patients and by increasing caregiver compensation, allowing them more time with patients.

The epidemiologic data suggesting that glycemia is an independent risk factor for CVD is supported by studies demonstrating biochemical mechanisms by which hyperglycemia may cause CVD (Fig. 1). Hyperglycemia by its mass action increases tissue glucose uptake and metabolism by ordinarily minor pathways such as the polyol and glucosamine pathways. In addition, hyperglycemia will lead to glycosylation of extracellular proteins [such as low-density lipoprotein (LDL), which renders it more oxidizable and more atherogenic] and to generation of free radicals (increased oxidative stress) and advanced glycation endproducts. Binding of advanced glycation endproducts to receptors on endothelial, smooth muscle, and fibroblast cells can lead to increased vascular permeability, increased coagulability, decreased thrombolysis, cell proliferation, and increased production of extracellular matrix proteins such as fibronectin, type IV collagen, laminin, and proteoglycans (45). Generation of free radicals by hyperglycemia may promote atherogenesis (i) through peroxidation of LDL, leading to a more atherogenic molecule, (ii) by oxidation of fibrinogen, leading to products that enhance coagulation, (iii) by increasing platelet activation by collagen (46,47), and (iv) by decreasing production of nitric oxide (NO) (48).

Endothelium-derived NO causes vasodilation and also inhibits platelet aggregation and adhesion of inflammatory cells to endothelium (49). Endothelium-dependent vasodilatation is reduced in healthy volunteers after six hours of a hyperglycemic clamp (50). A similar impairment in endothelium-dependent

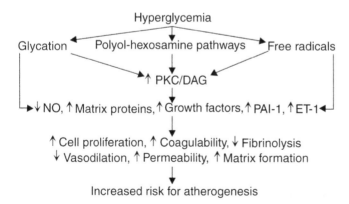

Figure 1 Mechanisms by which hyperglycemia may cause macrovascular disease. *Abbreviations*: NO, nitric oxide; PAI-1, plasminogen activator inhibitor-1; ET-1, endothelium-1; PKC, protein kinase-C; DAG, diacylgycerol. *Source*: From Ref. 31; courtesy of American Medical Association.

vasodilatation is seen in healthy individuals after oral glucose intake (51). Endothelium-dependent vasodilatation is impaired in people with diabetes and is improved by vitamin C intake, thus implicating inactivation of NO by oxygen-derived free radicals (52,53).

Many of the above processes are thought to be mediated to a large extent by the activation of protein kinase-C (PKC) and generation of diacylgycerol (DAG) (54–56). Hyperglycemia itself can directly increase PKC and DAG, because tissues incubated with high glucose concentrations have increased levels of DAG and PKC (47,56). Activation of PKC and increased DAG promotes expression, formation, and enhanced activity of transforming growth factor B, Type IV collagen, fibronectin, vascular endothelial growth factor, endothelin-1, caldesmon, plasminogen activator inhibitor-1, phospholipase A_2, prostaglandin E_2, and intercellular adhesion molecules. These have been identified to play a role in basement membrane thickness, extracellular matrix formation, angiogenesis, increased vascular permeability, smooth muscle cell proliferation, increased inflammatory cell adhesion, and decreased fibrinolysis (54). In summary, there are now several plausible mechanisms by which hyperglycemia occurring post-prandially may directly or indirectly promote atherogenesis and thus predispose both nondiabetic and diabetic individuals to CVD.

Finally, there have been several controlled clinical trials demonstrating that improved glycemic control can reduce cardiovascular events or surrogates there-fore. These include the following: (i) the U.K. Prospective Diabetes Study (UKPDS) in which an approximately 1% decrease in HbA_{1c} was shown to reduce the risk of MI by 16% in people with Type 2 diabetes (57); (ii) the 10-year fol-low-up of the DCCT—the EDIC Study—in which intensive insulin therapy (HbA_{1c} 7.0% vs. 9.0%) reduced cardiovascular events by 57% in patients with Type 1 diabetes (58); (iii) the Study to Prevent Noninsulin Dependent Diabetes Mellitus (STOP-NIDDM) in which specific treatment of postprandial hyper-glycemia reduced cardiovascular events by about 50% in patients with IGT (38), and (iv) the Proactive Study, whose results were consistent with the UKPDS (23).

PATHOPHYSIOLOGY OF HYPERGLYCEMIA

Normal Glucose Homeostasis

Plasma glucose levels increase because the amount of glucose entering the circu-lation exceeds the amount of glucose leaving the circulation. In people with IGT or Type 2 diabetes, excessive release of glucose into the circulation rather than a reduction in removal of glucose is the primary problem (59). As glucose tolerance deteriorates, postprandial plasma glucose levels increase earlier and at a faster rate than fasting plasma glucose levels (Fig. 2) (35). Normally after meal inges-tion, release of glucose into plasma due to glycogenolysis and gluconeogenesis is markedly suppressed (60). Glycogenolysis is virtually completely suppressed, thereby permitting hepatic glycogen repletion. The gluconeogenic pathway

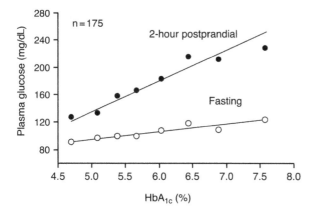

Figure 2 Changes in fasting and two-hour postprandial plasma glucose levels as hemoglobin. A_{lc} (HBA_{1c}) levels increase. *Source*: From Ref. 31; courtesy of American Medical Association.

remains operative, but in the postprandial state, more of the three-carbon precursors (lactate, alanine, pyruvate, and glycerol) are diverted into glycogen (indirect pathway) rather than into plasma glucose. As a consequence, most of the glucose entering the systemic circulation represents carbohydrate from the meal that has escaped initial splanchnic (mainly liver) sequestration (glycogen) or utilization (glycolysis), and to renal gluconeogenesis, which actually increases after meal ingestion (61).

Regulation of postprandial glucose release is largely a function of changes in insulin and glucagon secretion, alterations in sympathetic nervous system activity, and the sensitivity of the liver and kidney to these factors. Preeminent among these is the insulin:glucagon molar ratio (62).

The major tissues taking up glucose after meal ingestion are, in order of importance (Table 1): liver, muscle, brain, adipose tissue, and kidney.

The metabolic pathways for postprandial glucose disposal have recently been delineated (Fig. 3) (61). About two-thirds of glucose taken up by tissues

Table 1 Tissues Responsible for Postprandial Glucose Uptake

	Normal	Type 2 diabetes
Liver	~30%	~20%
Muscle	~25%	~20%
Brain	~15%	~15%
Kidney	~10%	~15%
Other	~20%	~30%

Source: From Ref. 62.

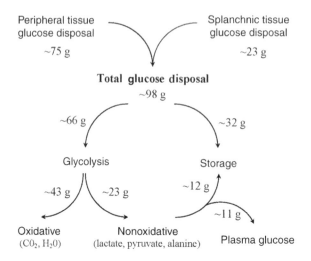

Figure 3 Metabolic pathways during postprandial glucose disposal. *Source*: From Ref. 64; courtesy of The American Physiological Society.

undergo glycolysis, and the remainder is stored mainly as glycogen, but also, to a lesser extent, as the glyceride backbone of adipose tissue triglycerides. Of the glucose undergoing glycolysis, about two-thirds are oxidized, and the remainder is converted to three-carbon compounds that enter the gluconeogenic pathway, half of which end up in plasma glucose and half of which end up being incorporated into hepatic glycogen (indirect pathway) (64).

Abnormalities in Type 2 Diabetes

Most people progress to Type 2 diabetes by first developing isolated postprandial hyperglycemia (i.e., IGT). A smaller percentage (~10%) first develop IFG (i.e., fasting plasma glucose > 100 mg/dL), but less than 126 mg/dL and a two-hour plasma glucose level during an oral glucose tolerance test less than 140 mg/dL. Both of these prediabetic states are associated with insulin resistance and impaired (-cell function. Limited data are available on IFG.

In people with IGT or Type 2 diabetes, various abnormalities have been identified (60). First of all, suppression of glycogenolysis and gluconeogenesis is reduced, and there is increased hepatic glycogen cycling, so that early on more of the ingested glucose escapes splanchnic sequestration and enters the systemic circulation. As a consequence, the overall release of glucose into the systemic circulation is increased, and net hepatic glycogen repletion is reduced. This can largely be explained by abnormalities in insulin and glucagon secretion and, to a lesser extent, by hepatic insulin resistance: Early insulin release is reduced, and glucagon secretion is not suppressed and may even increase, resulting in a markedly reduced plasma insulin:glucagon molar ratio (60). Overall tissue glucose uptake in people with IGT and Type 2 diabetes is not different from that of people with normal glucose tolerance (60). This can be most readily explained by the mass action effects of hyperglycemia "forcing" glucose into cells. The discrepancy between the rate of entry of glucose into the systemic circulation (increased) and its rate of removal (normal) explains the exaggerated and prolonged increases in postprandial glucose levels in these individuals.

Despite "normal" rates of tissue glucose uptake, the intracellular fates of glucose and the tissue distribution of its uptake are abnormal in Type 2 diabetes (Table 1). Although overall tissue uptake and glycolysis are quantitatively normal, less of the glucose undergoing glycolysis is oxidized, so that nonoxidative glycolysis is increased in people with Type 2 diabetes and presumably also those with IGT (60). As a result, more three-carbon precursors are available to enter the gluconeogenic pathway. In people with normal glucose tolerance, half of these are converted into plasma glucose and the other half is converted into hepatic glycogen (Fig. 2). In contrast, in people with Type 2 diabetes, more is released back into the circulation as glucose.

Regarding the tissues taking up glucose, in people with Type 2 diabetes, muscle glucose uptake and net hepatic glucose storage are reduced, whereas renal glucose uptake and uptake by other tissues are increased (Table 1). The exact mechanisms for this abnormal disposal have not been delineated, but reduced insulin secretion and insulin resistance and secondary effects thereof, e.g., increased free (nonesterified) fatty acid (FFA) levels, no doubt are involved.

Roles and Causes of β-Cell Dysfunction and Insulin Resistance

Normal glucose tolerance is maintained by a balance between insulin availability and the sensitivity of tissues to insulin. There exists a hyperbolic relationship between these factors such that their normal product (β-cell function x tissue insulin sensitivity) is a constant (Fig. 4).

This is commonly referred to as the Disposition Index (66). Thus, in people who are very insulin sensitive, less insulin is secreted in response to a standard stimulus than in insulin-resistant individuals. In other words, there is an adjustment in the amount of insulin secreted, depending on the body's need for insulin. As glucose tolerance deteriorates, the Disposition Index decreases. Both β-cell function and insulin sensitivity may decrease, but it is primarily the failure of β-cell function to compensate for insulin resistance that leads to a deterioration of glucose tolerance (67). A clear illustration of this is the changes that take place during pregnancy. All women become insulin resistant during the third trimester of pregnancy (68). Some of these women develop diabetes (gestational diabetes). The degree of insulin resistance is similar in women who do and do not develop diabetes (69,70). What distinguishes them is that those who develop diabetes have lower plasma insulin levels (70–73). In other words, the women who develop diabetes have β-cells, which cannot compensate for their insulin resistance. A similar process may explain why some people develop diabetes with

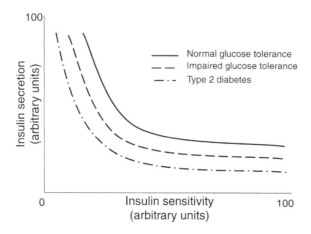

Figure 4   Relationship between β-cell function and insulin sensitivity. *Source*: From Ref. 65.

stress or steroid therapy and others do not. Both environmental and genetic factors influence β-cell function and insulin sensitivity. It has long been controversial whether an alteration in β-cell function or insulin sensitivity is the underlying genetic defect ultimately leading to the development of Type 2 diabetes. Recent evidence indicates that abnormalities in β-cell function are the main genetic factor, whereas changes in insulin sensitivity are largely acquired (environmental) (74).

It was once widely thought that insulin resistance preceded the impairment of β-cell function (75–77). This discredited view was largely based on the failure to recognize the relationship between β-cell function and insulin sensitivity, the failure to distinguish between insulin secretion (as reflected in plasma insulin levels) and β-cell function, and the failure to take into consideration the dynamics of insulin release. Thus early studies compared nonobese insulin-sensitive individuals with obese insulin-resistant persons. The findings of higher plasma insulin levels in the latter led to the erroneous conclusion that insulin resistance preceded β-cell dysfunction (75). Similarly, the findings that plasma insulin levels in fasting and in those two hours after glucose ingestion were often higher in people with IGT or mild diabetes led to the conclusion that insulin resistance preceded β-cell dysfunction. This interpretation did not take into consideration that the plasma insulin levels were inappropriate for the prevailing plasma glucose levels. This fallacy persisted for many years, despite the fact that Perley and Kipnis had demonstrated that individuals with normal glucose tolerance made comparably hyperglycemic as diabetic individuals by infusion of glucose secreted much more insulin than the diabetic individuals (78). Finally, insulin secretion is biphasic, consisting of first and second phases (Fig. 5).

When insulin secretion is stimulated by a square wave of hyperglycemia such as during a hyperglycemic clamp experiment, plasma insulin levels increase to a peak at 5 to 10 minutes and then decrease over the next 5 to 10 minutes. This

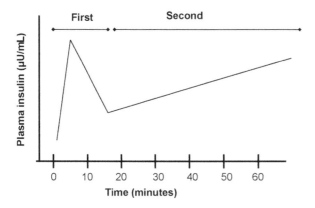

Figure 5   Phases of insulin secretion.

is referred to as first-phase insulin release. Thereafter plasma insulin levels gradually increase to a stable plateau. This is referred to as second-phase insulin release (79). The first phase of insulin release is thought to reflect early (e.g., 30 minutes) insulin release after meal or glucose ingestion and to be a very important determinant of glucose tolerance. Observations that two-hour plasma insulin levels initially increased as two-hour plasma glucose level increased but then decreased when two-hour plasma glucose levels exceeded 200 mg/dL (11 mmol/L) decreased were interpreted to indicate that β-cell dysfunction was a late event (75). However, examination of early- and first-phase insulin release has clearly demonstrated that they progressively decreased as glucose tolerance deteriorated even when fasting plasma glucose levels are in the normal range (Fig. 6) (31,62). It is now well established that (i) β-cell dysfunction occurs in people with IGT (62,80); (ii) early insulin release decreases as glucose tolerance deteriorates over the normal range (65); and (iii) impaired early insulin release is detectable in individuals with normal glucose tolerance who have first-degree relatives with Type 2 diabetes at a time when their insulin sensitivity is normal (81). The most convincing data come from studies of monozygotic twins who are discordant for Type 2 diabetes. The twins who have not yet developed diabetes have been shown to have reduced first-phase insulin release and normal insulin sensitivity (82). Finally, recent studies in adolescents who have developed diabetes have found that when compared to comparably obese adolescents with normal glucose tolerance, the adolescents who developed diabetes have comparable insulin sensitivity but reduced β-cell function (83).

Taken together, the above experimental data indicate that β-cell abnormalities can be demonstrated before individuals become insulin resistant or glucose intolerant and are therefore likely to be genetically determined. In contrast, the insulin resistance seen in the general population and in people with abnormal glucose tolerance appears to be largely acquired and to be due to obesity, especially visceral obesity, physical inactivity, high-fat diets, and other factors. A clear

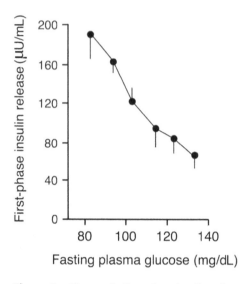

Figure 6   Changes in first-phase insulin release as a function of fasting plasma glucose. *Source*: From Ref. 31; courtesy of American Medical Association.

example comes from studies of the Pima Indians who have one of the highest incidences of diabetes (84). Several hundred years ago, the population split— some members remaining in the United States and others traveling south to Mexico. Those who remained in the United States were settled on reservations, led sedentary lives, became obese, and developed diabetes. Those who went to Mexico became free-living farmers, were physically active, did not become obese, and did not develop diabetes despite having the same genetic background as their brethren in the United States. This is not to say that environmental factors are not important for β-cell function or conversely that genetic factors are not involved in insulin resistance. For example, visceral fat accumulation is a more important determinant of insulin sensitivity than mere weight as reflected by BMI. The distribution of body fat is, at least in part, genetically determined. Having a genetic predisposition to accumulate visceral fat may explain why individuals with comparable degrees of obesity as reflected by BMI may differ in their insulin sensitivity. Conversely, environmental factors can have an important influence on β-cell function. Chronic hyperglycemia (glucose toxicity) adversely affects β-cell function (e.g., high glucose levels can induce β-cell apoptosis in vitro), and improvements in glycemic control improve β-cell function. Adipocytes release FFAs (lipotoxicity) and cytokines [e.g., resistin, leptin, tumor necrosis factor-α (TNF-α), and interleukin-6, which can impair β-cell function (85)].

It is beyond the scope of this chapter to go into specific molecular mechanisms that may be involved in impaired insulin release and insulin resistance, but it is important to point out that the impaired insulin release involves reductions in β-cell mass as well as abnormal function (86), and that the decrease in β-cell insulin release is progressive. In the UKPDS, β-cell function was reduced by about 50% at the time of diagnosis and decreased further at a rate of approximately 6% per year (87). With normal aging, β-cell function decreases annually at a rate of only about 0.6% (88). As a consequence of this progressive deterioration in β-cell function, patients progressively need additional drugs to maintain satisfactory control and many, if not most, will need insulin therapy.

TREATMENT AND PREVENTION

Role of Hyperinsulinemia

Before discussing specific therapeutic agents, it is important to consider the role of hyperinsulinemia in the manifestations of the metabolic syndrome and its link to CVD. Originally, it was proposed that insulin resistance, not simply due to environmental factors such as obesity, physical inactivity, etc., was the fundamental lesion of the metabolic syndrome. According to this hypothesis the resultant hyperinsulinemia further exacerbated the insulin resistance leading to hyperlipidemia and hypertension, damaging the vasculature and, as a consequence of all these effects, promoted CVD (1,89). This view became widespread, and led to a reduction in the use of insulin secretagogues and the withholding, delay or inadequate use of insulin in patients who needed it. We now know the above formulation to be wrong.

Hyperinsulinemia appears to be an innocent bystander, a marker for insulin resistance—the real culprit (90). Insulin is a vasodilator (91); diminution of this action in a susceptible individual can increase blood pressure. Insulin suppresses lipolysis and the release of triglycerides from the liver (92). Diminution of these actions can raise plasma triglycerides and lower plasma levels of HDL-cholesterol in susceptible individuals. Insulin may also have many beneficial effects on endothelial and platelet function and inflammatory cytokines (Table 2).

Table 2 Effects of Insulin and Potential Consequences of Insulin Resistance

Effect	Potential consequence of insulin resistance
Vasodilation	Hypertension
Suppression of lipolysis and hepatic triglyceride release	Hyperlipidemia
Suppression of glucose production and stimulation of tissue glucose uptake	Impaired glucose tolerance and Type 2 diabetes
Maintenance of endothelial health and inhibition of inflammatory cytokine production	Atherosclerosis
Stimulation of satiety; inhibition of appetite	Obesity

Diminution of these actions would tend to promote occlusive CVD. Finally, as demonstrated in the EDIC study (58), intensive treatment with insulin decreases cardiovascular events, and studies such as DIGAMI (Diabetes Insulin Glucose Infusion in Acute Myocardial Infarction) 1 and DIGAMI 2 failed to demonstrate any adverse effect of intensive insulin therapy (93). Therefore, whether an antidiabetic drug increases or decreases circulating insulin levels should not be a consideration of its appropriateness for treating dysglycemia associated with the metabolic syndrome.

Prevention

Variations in both physical activity and body composition predict cardiovascular mortality (94,95). Moreover, the main causes of the metabolic syndrome and its associated dysglycemia seem to be largely explained by obesity, especially visceral obesity (12,13), which results from a combination of increased caloric consumption and reduced physical activity. It would seem logical, therefore, that institution of a healthy lifestyle would prevent development of the metabolic syndrome. Virtually all lifestyle intervention studies have been conducted in people who have already become obese and acquired various elements of the metabolic syndrome. The results of such studies have demonstrated that hypocaloric diets with or without increased physical activity can prevent deterioration in glucose tolerance, lower blood pressure, and improve plasma lipids (96). The main problem is that compliance with such programs is poor, and participation is not maintained in the longer term (97,98). For those failing to follow lifestyle interventions, pharmacologic therapy is available, although no drugs are approved for this purpose. In controlled clinical trials, metformin, TZDs, orlistat, and acarbose have all been shown to be safe and effective in improving glucose tolerance and preventing or delaying the onset of Type 2 diabetes—sometimes with success rates approaching or superior to lifestyle interventions (36–39,99). The problem with pharmacologic approaches is one of cost-effectiveness and the fact that they do not treat the underlying etiologic factors.

Obesity is a public health issue, and a public health approach is needed to address the medical problems that ensue (97). Early on, children should be instructed in healthy nutritional habits. Schools should serve healthy foods and limit access to junk food (e.g., fried foods and caloric soft drinks). In addition, schools should have serious physical education programs in which there is substantial preplanned energy expenditure and individualized documentable end points for students [attainment of a certain aerobic capacity (VO_2 max), weight loss, time to run a certain distance, etc.]. These healthy habits should be reinforced by providing the public with safe facilities for exercise. Companies could subsidize healthy foods in their cafeterias, and governments could tax unhealthy foods (e.g., fast foods). Insurance companies could support weight loss programs and offer incentives in terms of premium reductions for achievement and maintenance of weight targets. Government could limit the use of polyunsaturated fat in prepared food and subsidize use of monounsaturated fats. These are only a few examples of what could be done.

Therapeutic Goals

As indicated earlier, there is evidence that glycemia is an independent risk factor for CVD, with no apparent threshold (30). Moreover, like blood pressure and plasma lipids, glycemia is a continuous variable. The criteria of diabetes [e.g., fasting or two-hour postchallenge plasma glucose = 126 (7.0 mmol/L) and 200 mg/dL (11.1 mmol/L), respectively] were originally based on epidemiologic data concerning the risk of developing microvascular complications. The criteria for prediabetes, i.e., IFG 100 to 125 mg/dL (5.56–6.90 mmol/L) and IGT postchallenge glucose levels between 140 and 199 mg/dL (7.8–11.1 mmol/L), respectively, are arbitrary. It would be better to consider glycemia in terms of relative risk for CVD, taking into consideration the presence or absence of other risk factors as illustrated in Table 2 (100–102). In the Interheart Study, which compared over 10,000 subjects in 52 countries (100), having diabetes was a greater risk for a MI than having hypertension. Because this study did not examine the effect of degree of glycemic control, the risk attributable to diabetes was probably underestimated (Table 3).

The goal of glycemic control for individuals with the metabolic syndrome should be to prevent the HbA_{1c} from exceeding a value, which increases cardiovascular risk. The American Heart Association and the National Heart, Lung, and Blood Institute Scientific Statement recommend a target HbA_{1c} of less than 7% to minimize the risk of CVD (103).

Lifestyle and/or pharmacologic intervention should be initiated if the desirable HbA_{1c} is exceeded (Table 4).

This aggressive approach would no doubt increase the costs of healthcare, especially if not accompanied by preventative public health measures. But one would not be surprised if in the long run, it would not be cost-effective in terms of reducing morbidity, mortality, days lost from work, and in improving quality of life indicators. Such an approach as outlined above is far off and will require a paradigm change in the way we view dysglycemia and at least initially an infusion of considerable monies and resources into the health-care system and substantial education of industry and the public. Therefore, one must deal with present time realities and changes expected in the near future. It can be anticipated

Table 3 Risk of Acute Myocardial Infarction from the Interheart Study

Risk factor	Odds ratio
Smoking	~3.0
Diabetes	~2.5
Hypertension	~2.0
Hyperlipidemia	~3.8

Source: From Ref. 100.

Table 4 Hemoglobin A_{1c} Target Depending on Presence
or Absence of Cardiovascular Risk Factors

Desirable hemoglobin A_{1c}	Other risk factors (family history, obesity, hypertension, hyperlipidemia)
<6.0%	0
<5.8%	1
<5.6%	2
<5.4%	3
<5.2%	4

that, if some of the ongoing clinical trials demonstrate cardiovascular benefit from treating people with glucose intolerance, the Food and Drug Administration (FDA) will give drugs an indication to treat IGT, and insurance companies will reimburse such treatment. Should this happen, one would expect more routine screening for IGT. Currently, no organization endorses this approach, and screening is recommended only for those over a certain age or those with risk factors for developing diabetes. Currently, the ADA recommends screening based on fasting plasma glucose levels. Such an approach is relatively insensitive compared to the two-hour plasma glucose following a 75 goral glucose load. Identification of individuals with IGT will increase the frequency of postprandial self-glucose testing, because many of these newly identified individuals will have fasting plasma glucose and HbA_{1c} levels within what is considered the normal range. For example, most people with IGT have HbA_{1c} values between 5.4% and 5.9%. Finally, therapeutic glycemic goals will be reduced, and postprandial plasma glucose levels will be taken into consideration along with HbA_{1c} values.

Let us assume, therefore, that new targets for glycemic control include two-hour postprandial plasma glucose levels less than 140 mg/dL (7.8 mmol/L) and/or HbA_{1c} values less than 5% when they can be safely achieved without unacceptable side effects. These should be viewed as upper limits, so that once exceeded initiation of or additional treatment should be introduced. In other words, emphasis should be placed on preventing these goals from being exceeded rather than waiting for them to be exceeded. Such an approach will probably lead to earlier pharmacologic intervention and use of agents that may be less effective in the maximum reduction in HbA_{1c} they can achieve and in the use of lower doses of more powerful agents with a reduction in their dose-related side effects (e.g., hypoglycemia with insulin secretagogues). Most clinical trials of safety and efficacy of agents used to treat dysglycemia have been performed in patients with diabetes, whose HbA_{1c} levels have ranged between 7.5% and 10.5%. Except for the intervention trials in people with IGT, there are no data in treating people with much lower HbA_{1c} levels. However, all of the drugs used in these trials have been shown to be reasonably safe and effective.

New Treatment Paradigm

In the past, a step-wise approach has been used to treat diabetes. Initially, one drug is commenced (monotherapy); a titration period is then followed by addition of a second drug (dual therapy) if monotherapy failed to achieve or maintain the desired HbA_{1c}. In turn, this is followed by titration and addition of a third oral agent or insulin if dual therapy is unsuccessful. The Kaiser Permanente Study indicated that such an approach exposed the majority of patients to unacceptable glycemia (e.g., HbA_{1c} > 8%) for an average of five years before insulin therapy was initiated (104). Unfortunately, NHANES data indicate 60% of patients treated with insulin have HbA_{1c} levels above 7% (105). Thus insulin therapy is being initiated late and is not being used aggressively enough. What is needed is a new paradigm.

Initial therapy should be based on the HbA_{1c} level at presentation. Table 5 gives the reductions in HbA_{1c} levels expected to be achieved with monotherapy based on a patient's initial presenting (drug-naive) HbA_{1c} level.

In general, the greater the pretreatment HbA_{1c}, the greater the decrease in HbA_{1c} with intervention. Nevertheless, despite these greater decrements in HbA_{1c} levels, a greater proportion of patients fail to reach their goal. Thus, assuming a target HbA_{1c} level of less than 6.5%, monotherapy with various agents can be expected to be successful in attaining that goal if the HbA_{1c} is less than 7.0% to 7.5%. Presenting HbA_{1c} levels between 7.5% and 8.5% will probably require initial dual therapy, and most patients with present HbA_{1c} levels above 8.5% will probably need some form of insulin therapy alone or in conjunction with oral agents.

Table 5 Expected Reductions in Hemoglobin A_{1c} Levels in Drug Naive-Patients with Initial Hemoglobin A_{1c} Approximately 8%

Class—drug	Hemoglobin A_1 reduction	References
Insulin sensitizers		
Biguanide–metformin	1.5–2.0%	(106,107)
Thiazolidinediones (pioglitazone/rosiglitazone)	1.0–1.2%	(106,108)
Insulin secretagogues		
Sulfonylureas (glyburide, glipizide, and glimepiride)	1.5–2.0%	(107)
Meglitinides		
Nateglinide	0.5–1.0%	(107,109)
Repaglinide	1.5–2.0%	(107,109)
α-glucosidase inhibitors		
Acarbose, miglitol	0.5–1.0%	(107,110)
Glucagon-like peptide-1 agonists/dipeptidyl peptidase-IV Inhibitors		
Exenatide	1.0–1.5%	(111–113)
Vildagliptin	0.5–1.0%	(114)

Lifestyle Interventions

Many of those diagnosed with the metabolic syndrome will be obese individuals with IGT rather than Type 2 diabetes. Therefore, emphasis needs to be placed on treatment regimens for people with IGT. We have data from several clinical trials looking at interventions to prevent (and therefore treat) progression of IGT to Type 2 diabetes. These studies can be divided into lifestyle changes and pharmacologic intervention trials.

Lifestyle interventions form the foundation of treatment of Type 2 diabetes and its prevention and should be part of any comprehensive treatment regimen (115). The basis for this concept are studies showing that weight reduction in obese individuals and increased physical activity reduce insulin resistance, decrease cardiovascular risk factors, and improve β-cell function (96,98,116–119). It should be emphasized that the weight loss to achieve these effects need only be modest, i.e., approximately 10% (120). Such decreases are more achievable in clinical practice than attempt to attain ideal body weight.

Patient Education

A key to the successful lifestyle intervention is the ability and willingness of the patient to comply with the therapeutic goals established collaboratively by the patient and the primary health-care provider. This requires that the patient understands his condition, actively assumes the necessary self-management skills, and initiates lifestyle changes. This process can be facilitated by a support system (e.g., dietitian, diabetes educator, exercise physiologist, and family) and an awareness of additional resources (e.g., mental health provider, foot specialist, and endocrinologist). As part of a comprehensive program, patients should be evaluated for risk factors and the presence of complications (coronary artery disease, nephropathy, retinopathy, and neuropathy) on a regular basis.

After completing an initial evaluation, the treatment team and the patient should construct a management plan that establishes the following:

- Treatment goals (before- and after-meal blood glucose levels and A_{1C} targets)
  Short term
  Long term
- Self-management education
- Lifestyle modification guidelines
  Diet
  Exercise

In the Diabetes Prevention Program (DPP) (37,121) that followed more than 3000 nondiabetic individuals with IGT for a mean of 2.8 years, the cumulative incidence of diabetes was approximately 30% of untreated patients. Intervention with a lifestyle-modification program (diet and exercise) reduced the incidence by 58%. Furthermore, in obese patients with established Type 2 diabetes weight loss is associated with a reversal of insulin resistance (120,122) and reduces the risk of CVD (99,123,124). Thus, it is not surprising that diet or medical nutrition therapy (MNT) and physical activity are considered essential (i.e., first line) components of the standard of care recommended by all organizations that provide guidelines for the management of diabetes; and this applies to people with IGT (125).

Diet

Patients with IGT or Type 2 diabetes should receive individualized MNT in accordance with achieving treatment goals. A registered dietitian familiar with the goals and treatment of diabetes should assist the patient in developing and implementing MNT (40). An initial assessment of the patient's eating habits, lifestyle, cultural preferences, and level of physical activity should be conducted prior to developing an MNT program.

Following are the goals of MNT as outlined by the ADA for people with Type 2 diabetes (40):

- Attain and maintain metabolic goals, including blood glucose and A_{1C} levels, cholesterol, triglycerides, blood pressure, and bodyweight
- Prevent and address complications and associations of diabetes, including obesity, dyslipidemia, hypertension, and nephropathy
- Improve health via nutrition and exercise programs
- Consider individual needs (i.e., lifestyle, personal, and cultural preferences)

The most recent ADA guidance on MNT stresses the importance of dietary carbohydrates, including sugars, starch, and fiber (40). The total amount of carbohydrate, type of sugar or starch, method of processing, and additional food components have an impact on glycemic response to a given food. However, it is recommended that total carbohydrate intake, rather than type of carbohydrate intake, be monitored in order to maintain glycemic control. As with the general population, fiber-containing foods are recommended for patients with Type 2 diabetes. Nevertheless, a recent randomized controlled trial found no difference in weight loss and reduction of cardiovascular risk factors with the Atkins, Ornish, Weight Watchers, and Zone diets that differ substantially in their carbohydrate and fat content (126). Nutrition recommendations from the ADA include (40,127) the following:

- Carbohydrates and monounsaturated fats should provide 60% to 70% of daily energy intake; fat intake should be individualized with regard to weight loss and metabolic profile.
- Carbohydrate intake influences blood glucose levels; the recommended range of carbohydrates is 45% to 65% of total calorie intake; low carbohydrate diets are not recommended.
- Polysaturated fat intake should be less than 10% of total energy intake.

■ Protein intake can be similar to recommendations for the general population (15–20% of daily energy) if renal function is normal.

The 2005 ADA recommendations now indicate that the use of the glycemic index (GI)/glycemic load can provide an additional benefit when considering carbohydrate intake. The GI ranks carbohydrates based on their postprandial glucose excursion rate into bloodstream as compared to reference food (pure glucose). Studies suggest that ingestion of high-GI meals increases hunger and promotes overeating in a subsequent meal relative to low-GI meals. Quickly digested high-GI carbohydrates produce a greater and more rapid rise in blood glucose than the more slowly digested low-GI ones. GI values can be found on an online database (128). Incorporation of low-GI carbohydrates into daily meals is an effective behavioral lifestyle change that improves glycemic control and weight management.

Several epidemiologic studies showed that whole-grain cereals and diets with a low GI protect against the development of Type 2 DM and heart disease. The major mechanism is thought to be through decreased insulin resistance and improved β-cell function (improved first-phase insulin response and acute insulin response). Controlled feeding studies have generally shown a benefit of whole compared with refined grain intake on insulin sensitivity and glucose metabolism. Beneficial effects were also shown by increasing fiber content.

In conclusion, it appears that whole grain foods low GI/glycemic load foods, and fiber-rich foods such as fruits and vegetables should be preferred and over refined foods (129,130).

Other diet plans proven to be successful in reducing cardiovascular risk include the Dietary Approach to Stop Hypertension Eating Plan (DASH) and the Mediterranean diet. The DASH Eating Plan is very appropriate for hypertensive patients. It causes significant lowering of blood pressure in hypertensive individuals, particularly African Americans and other minority population groups. DASH is rich in fruits, vegetables, and low-fat dairy foods and reduced in total and saturated fat. Compared with the usual American diet, it also is reduced in red meat, sweets, and sugar-containing drinks. It is rich in potassium, calcium, magnesium, fiber, and protein. A DASH Eating Plan with lower sodium content (DASH-II) reduces blood pressure levels beyond what the DASH-I diet can produce. Studies have shown that the DASH Eating Plan lowers blood pressure, LDL-cholesterol, and plasma homocysteine levels (131–133) and reduces insulin resistance among diabetic patients. Information concerning the DASH Eating Plan is available at National Institute of Health website (134). The Mediterranean Diet also reduces markers of vascular inflammation in the metabolic syndrome patients (135). This diet has been associated with a significant reduction in CVD and is a worthy alternative to the DASH Eating Plan (135).

Short-term studies in obese patients with Type 2 DM showed that during the low-carbohydrate diet, 24-hour glucose profiles improved dramatically and mean HbA_{1c} decreased approximately 0.5% to 1.5%. Insulin sensitivity also improved (136,137). Long-term effects still remain uncertain, particularly because long-term adherence to these diets has been poor. Daily incorporation of low-GI carbohydrates in meal planning can be an effective self-management strategy for glycemic control and weight management (129).

Exercise

Increased physical activity is paramount to long-term maintenance of weight loss and is associated with lowering blood glucose, improving insulin sensitivity, and reducing CVD risk (138,139). Physical activity has also been demonstrated to decrease the risk of developing Type 2 diabetes in patients with IGT (140,141). An exercise program should be initiated gradually after a complete medical evaluation, including assessment of microvascular and macrovascular complications that may be negatively impacted by increased physical activity (142), e.g., peripheral neuropathy predisposing to foot ulceration or undiagnosed myocardial ischemia. The ADA recommends that patients gradually increase their activity to 30 to 45 minutes of moderate aerobic activity three to five times per week (40). More rigorous exercise programs may be needed to maintain long-term weight loss.

Daily, low-impact aerobic activity should be encouraged. Reduced physical activity promotes obesity. Low levels of daily activity are particularly common among African American women, a group with a higher rate of cardiovascular mortality than white women (143). Daily physical activity of 60 minutes will assist in weight loss, hypertension, and dyslipidemia control and reduction of insulin resistance to help prevent the onset of, and to assist in glycemic control of, Type 2 diabetes (144,145). A formal exercise program is not necessary, but it can be very beneficial. Daily walking or any daily activity that maintains the pulse rate at 70% of 220 minus one's age for 30 to 60 minutes should be undertaken to increase aerobic capacity and to assist with weight loss. Less-intense exercise for a shorter time can also reduce cardiovascular risk among patients with Type 2 diabetes. Cardiovascular mortality correlates inversely with the distance of walking (145). Supervised low-intensity resistance exercise for 30 minutes, three to four times a week, can improve lean muscle mass (thereby helping to offset any reduction in resting energy expenditure during weight loss), reduce insulin resistance, and improve glycemic control in patients with Type 2 diabetes (146).

Regular exercise has a positive effect on HbA_{1c} and blood glucose, as well as on cholesterol. In studies with diabetic subjects, blood glucose significantly declines during exercise in comparison with the controls. Clinical benefits of acute exercise on glycemic control can be seen during and up to 24 hours following exercise (147).

In the Da Qing Trial, 597 subjects with IGT were treated with exercise, diet, combined diet, and exercise or neither (control group). There was a significant decrease in the development of Type 2 DM in the intervention groups compared with the control group after a six-year follow-up (DM was reduced by 31%, 46%, and 42% in the diet, exercise, and diet plus exercise interventions, respectively) (148).

The Finnish Diabetes Prevention Trial studied 522 middle-aged, overweight subjects with IGT for a mean of 3.2 years. Subjects were assigned to two groups: intervention group, which comprises a diet high in fiber and low in saturated and trans fats, and regular moderate exercise or control group. The risk of Type 2 DM decreased in the intervention group by 58% compared to controls. There also was a significantly greater weight loss in the intervention group than in the control group (140).

The Oslo Diet and Exercise study reported beneficial effects of exercise on glycemic control, but noted better results with diet and exercise than with exercise alone (149). Similar positive effects of aerobic (vs. stretching) exercise were reported by Liao et al. in a two-year study of Japanese American men (150).

In the DPP, 3234 obese subjects with IGT were treated with lifestyle changes (aim for a weight loss of at least 7% of initial body weight through a low-calorie, low-fat diet and participation in moderate intensity exercise for at least 150 minutes per week), metformin, or placebo. There was 58% decrease in the development of Type 2 DM in the lifestyle modification group compared to controls (37).

Pharmacotherapy

Introduction

Lifestyle changes are difficult to initiate in the primary-care setting and patient adherence to such programs is notoriously poor (97,98,119). Considering this and the fact that β-cell function deteriorates with time in people with IGT and Type 2 diabetes, pharmacologic therapy will probably be necessary for most patients. In theory, the ideal pharmacologic agent to treat the hyperglycemia of the metabolic syndrome should be safe and effective, and, rather than adversely affect other cardiovascular risk factors, improve them. There are several up-to-date detailed reviews of antidiabetic agents currently in use, which delineate their pharmacology, pharmacokinetics, mechanism of action, side effects, relative efficacy, and contraindications (151–153). In this section, therefore, emphasis will be placed on characteristics of these agents relative to individuals with the metabolic syndrome and on newer agents which have recently become available or which may soon reach the market. Besterman et al. (154) have recently summarized the optimal actions of drugs for treating the metabolic syndrome (Table 6). Unfortunately, no single drug provides all these benefits. However, metformin has many.

Weight Loss–Promoting Drugs

A number of weight loss agents are available. These include agents that decrease appetite, e.g., sibutramine and the glucagon-like peptide-1 (GLP-1) agonist exenatide, an agent that reduces absorption of ingested fat, e.g., orlistat, and a new class of agents—endocannabanoid-1 receptor blockers, e.g., rimonabant, which decrease the positive feedback of food ingestion. Most data are available for

Table 6 Optimal Drug Effects in the Metabolic Syndrome

Improve endothelial function and arterial compliance
Improve insulin resistance
Cause no adverse effect on weight
Improve dyslipidemia
Control hypertension
Reduce vascular inflammation and the surrogate markers such as C-reactive protein or
  microalbuminuria
Reduce prothrombotic activity
Prevent or reverse atherosclerosis
Have minimal side effects
Provide best efficacy at the lowest price

Source: From Ref. 154.

orlistat and sibutramine whose clinical trials have recently been reviewed (155–157). Padwal et al. (155) compared year-long results of 10 studies of orlistat and three studies of sibutramine. Compared to placebo, orlistat resulted in an average weight loss of 2.7 kg (2.9%), whereas sibutramine resulted in an average weight loss compared to placebo of 4.3 kg (4.6%). About 12% of orlistat-treated patients and 15% of sibutramine patients lost more than 10% of their initial weight. The major side effects with orlistat were fatty/oily stools, fecal urgency, and oily spotting, which occurred in 15% to 30% of patients. Seven percent of patients reported fecal incontinence. These side effects were related to the fat content of diets and could be minimized by prudent reductions in dietary fat. Levels of fat-soluble vitamins (A, D, and E) were reduced. Although no clinically evident consequences were observed, supplementation of these vitamins is recommended. Side effects of sibutramine included increases in blood pressure, pulse rate, insomnia, nausea, dry mouth, and constipation, occurring in 7% to 20% of patients. DeRosa et al. (156) performed a head to head yearlong comparison of orlistat and sibutramine in a randomized controlled study of obese Type 2 diabetes patients (Table 7).

After 12 months' therapy, orlistat resulted in more weight loss, a reduction in blood pressure versus no change in sibutramine patients. Regarding side

Table 7 Comparison of Orlistat and Sibutramine in Obese Type 2 Diabetes

	Orlistat	Sibutramine
Body mass index (kg/m^2)	-3.9	-3.6
Hemoglobin A$_{1c}$ (%)	-0.8	-0.9
Systolic blood pressure (mmHg)	-3.0	+2.0
Diastolic blood pressure (mmHg)	-3.0	0
Heart rate (bpm)	0	+2

Source: From Refs. 155–157.

effects, about a third of patients treated with orlistat experienced abdominal pain, fatty/oily stools, flatulence, and increased defecation or fecal urgency, whereas about 15% of patients treated with sibutramine experienced headache, insomnia, dry mouth, and increased blood pressure. The overall conclusions of reviews of antiobesity drugs are that orlistat produces somewhat more weight loss than sibutramine, but is associated with more gastrointestinal side effects, whereas sibutramine is associated with more central nervous system and blood pressure side effects. Thus, because the side effects of orlistat are not related to cardiovascular risk and can be controlled by diet alterations, it would be preferable to sibutramine. Moreover, there is evidence that orlistat may have actions unrelated to its weight loss effects. It has been reported to augment postprandial GLP-1 levels (158) and, compared to comparable weight loss with diet and exercise, to produce greater reductions in plasma FFAs and greater increases in insulin sensitivity (120).

Rimonabant is an agent that blocks cannabinoid-1 (CB-1) receptors and thus blocks the positive feedback with pleasure and food ingestion. Although there have been no head-to-head comparisons of the weight loss efficacy of this agent with others, recent studies (27,141) indicate that, compared to placebo, its weight loss efficacy may be superior to those of orlistat and sibutramine. At a dose of 20 mg, rimonabant after one year, relative to placebo, caused weight loss of 4.8 kg (~4%) in one study (28) and 5.4 kg (~6%) in another (27). As expected, plasma LDL-cholesterol, triglycerides, insulin resistance (homeostasis model assessment), leptin, and C-reactive decreased, while plasma HDL-cholesterol and adiponectin increased. Both systolic and diastolic blood pressure decreased. In terms of side effects, the most common, which occurred with greater frequency, with rimonabant compared to placebo were dizziness, nausea, diarrhea, anxiety, and depression (27,28). However, these were generally mild. Like orlistat, there is evidence that rimonabant may have actions in addition to those causing a decrease in food consumption. CB-1 receptors have been identified in various peripheral tissues such as adipocytes, gastrointestinal tract, liver, adrenal glands, and sympathetic ganglia (159). Regression analysis indicated that changes in weight could not account for all of the beneficial changes in plasma lipids (28). Moreover, in pair-fed animals, the rimonabant-treated group lost more weight, suggesting an effect on caloric expenditure (160).

When compared with placebo, exenatide showed the decrease in HbA_{1c} of 0.8% to 1% depending on baseline (111–113). Patients taking orlistat can expect to decrease HbA_{1c} levels by 0.7% to 0.9% (161,162). Patients taking sibutramine experienced a 0.3% decrease in HbA_{1c} (155–157,163). Rimonabant In Obesity Diabetes Trial followed 1045 patients with Type 2 DM taking rimonabant 20 mg/day for over one year. It showed a 0.7% reduction in HbA_{1c}, with 43% of subjects achieving HbA_{1c} levels less than 6.5% (27,28).

Metformin

Metformin is a biguanide that has been used to treat Type 2 diabetes for over 50 years (151,164). It is at least as effective in lowering HbA_{1c} levels as any other class of oral agent (e.g., sulfonylureas and TZDs). It is classified as an insulin sensitizer (164) and has its major effect on the liver to reduce hepatic glucose output (165) by suppressing gluconeogenesis and possibly glycogenolysis (165–167). It also improves muscle glucose uptake in skeletal muscle (168) and systemic glucose clearance (165), although these may be indirect actions through alleviation of glucose toxicity (164). It has no direct effects on insulin secretion or lipolysis (165). Current evidence indicates that the metaboliceffects of metformin are mediated by stimulating adenosine monophosphate–activated PK (164).

In contrast to most other oral antidiabetic agents, metformin use is generally associated with weight loss rather than weight gain (164), an action attributable to appetite reduction because the drug does not alter energy expenditure (165). Although metformin is generally neutral in terms of blood pressure and lipids (106,169), various nonglycemic actions have been reported (Table 8) (124), which suggest that metformin may reduce cardiovascular risk independent of its effect on glycemic control. In the multicenter UKPDS (182), metformin as part of an intensive treatment regimen in obese patients reduced diabetes-related death and all-cause mortality by 42% and 36%, respectively, compared to the conventional treatment regimen. Moreover, despite comparable reductions in HbA_{1c} levels, metformin showed greater reductions in all-cause mortality and stroke than did sulfonylurea-treated groups (182). These beneficial results with metformin appear to be superior to those of a TZD reported in the Proactive Study (23).

As monotherapy, metformin does not cause hypoglycemia and thus can be safely used in people without diabetes as demonstrated in various clinical trials to

Table 8 Potential Beneficial Cardiovascular Effects of Metformin Therapy

Decreases oxidative stress (170)
Improves vascular relaxation (170)
Reduces hypercoagulation state (170)
Decreases plasminogen activator inhibitor-1 levels (170)
Increases tissue plasminogen activator activity (170)
Decreases von Willebrand factor levels (170)
Decreases platelet aggregation and adhesion (170)
Reduction of C-reactive protein (171)
Improves diastolic dysfunction (170)
Inhibition of protein glycation (172)
Improvement of vascular wall structure (173)
Improves vascular redox balance (174,175)
Increases functional capillary density (176,177)
Reduces cross-linkage of fibrin (178)
Reduces neovascularization (178)
Improves postischemic arterial flow (179,180)
Improves endothelial function (181)

Source: From Ref. 154.

prevent diabetes in people with glucose intolerance (183). In addition to monotherapy, metformin can be used in combination with insulin, secretagogues (sulfonylureas and meglitinides), GLP-1 analogs, and insulin. Its most common side effects are diarrhea and nausea—dose-dependent effects that necessitate its discontinuation in 10% to 15% of patients (184). The most serious adverse event associated with metformin use is lactic acidosis. Its incidence has been estimated as 1 in 30,000 (185,186). Most cases have occurred in individuals who had contraindications to its use, which include renal insufficiency (serum creatinine > 1.4 mg/dL), liver disease, heart failure requiring pharmacologic treatment, hypoxia, acute hemodynamic compromise, dehydration, and iodinated contrast studies (164)—conditions that can increase anaerobic glycolysis and raise metformin concentrations. When used judiciously, the use of metformin is probably not associated with an increased risk of lactic acidosis (185). For example, in the UKPDS (182) and the Cosmic Study (184), a one-year trial of over 7000 patients treated with metformin, not a single case was reported. Because of its relative safety and proven efficacy in controlling glycemia and preventing progression of IGT to Type 2 diabetes, beneficial effects on cardiovascular risk factors including weight loss, reduction in mortality demonstrated in controlled clinical trials, and low cost, metformin should be considered the initial drug of choice to treat hyperglycemia associated with the metabolic syndrome.

The degree of expected HbA_{1c} reduction ranges from 1.5% to 2% depending on baseline (106,107). In the DPP, the incidence of Type 2 DM was reduced by 31% with metformin as compared with placebo in 3234 subjects with IGT or IFG. Metformin reduced the incidence of the metabolic syndrome by 17% during a follow-up of 3.2 years compared with placebo in those participants who did not have the metabolic syndrome at baseline. For those subjects who had the metabolic syndrome at baseline, and received metformin, 23% no longer had the syndrome after three years (37,187,188).

Thiazolidinediones

TZDs are insulin sensitizers, which are synthetic ligands for the nuclear transcription peroxisome proliferator–activated receptor-γ (PPAR-γ) (189). After ligand binding, the PPAR-γ undergoes conformational changes that result in binding a numerous coactivators and corepressors. As a general principle, ligands can vary in their ability to recruit different activators. This may explain differences in biologic responses between individual drugs within a class. PPAR-γ regulates gene transcription by two mechanisms: (i) transactivation, a deoxyribonucleic acid (DNA)-dependent process involves binding to DNA response elements of target genes and heterodimerization with the retinoid X receptor and (ii) transrepression, a DNA-independent mechanism that involves interference with other transcription-factor pathways. PPAR-γ is expressed mostly in adipose tissue, but is also present in pancreatic β-cells, the vascular endothelium, and macrophages. Very low levels are found in liver, heart, and skeletal muscle. Other PPAR subtypes—α and δ—also exist. PPAR-α is expressed in liver, heart, and muscle.

Fibrates (such as fenofibrate and gemfibrozil) are full or partial agonists for these receptors that regulate lipoprotein and FFA metabolism and have anti-inflammatory effects. PPAR-δ is expressed in many tissues, mainly skin, brain, and adipose tissue. Their physiologic role is unclear at present. PPAR-γ activation leads to changes in more than 100 different genes, and responses vary with the ligand (189). Many of these genes regulate aspects of fatty acid and glucose metabolism, e.g., via fatty acid–binding protein and glut-4-transporters. PPAR-γ is essential for adipose tissue differentiation and, therefore, production of various adipocytokines, e.g., adiponectin, resistin, and TNF-α.

There are therefore two current theories of how TZDs improve insulin sensitivity. One proposes that the main action is via changes in lipid redistribution and alteration of adipocyte release of FFAs and adipocytokines. According to this theory, expansion of subcutaneous adipose tissue mass leads to a transfer of triglyceride from visceral tissues to subcutaneous tissue, resulting in improved insulin sensitivity in tissues from which the lipid has been removed. TZD treatment of patients with Type 2 diabetes causes a reduction in hepatic triglycerides, which is correlated with increases in insulin sensitivity. Moreover, increased release of adiponectin and reduced release of TNF-α, resistin, and FFAs may also be involved. The other theory proposes that TZDs act directly on insulin-sensitive target organs. The preponderance of current evidence suggests that it is the redistribution of tissue lipid, and alteration in release of adipocytokines is the major mechanism.

Two TZDs are currently approved for treatment of Type 2 diabetes in the United States—rosiglitazone and pioglitazone. Treatment with these agents leads to improvement in glycemic control (as reflected by HbA$_{1c}$ levels), reductions in insulin resistance, which are generally correlated with reductions in hepatic triglycerides (189), and improvements in β-cell function.

The improvements in glycemic control are best explained by changes in endogenous glucose production rather than improvements in peripheral glucose metabolism—similar to what has been observed with metformin. However, in contrast to metformin, TZDs appear to have a significant effect on pancreatic β-cell function independent of alleviation of glucose toxicity (191). Thus, one advantage of this class is β-cell preservation.

Drugs in this category differ from other agents in their slow onset of action (191). It generally takes about six months to achieve maximal effects, which argues in favor of the lipid transfer hypothesis. In general, if one looks at six-month results, the reduction in HbA$_{1c}$ levels with these agents is nearly equivalent to those achieved with metformin and insulin secretagogues. It is difficult at present to characterize this class regarding their effects on lipid metabolism and other parameters, because studies of the two available agents have revealed significant differences between them. In a recent meta-analysis (108), it was concluded that pioglitazone and rosiglitazone have similar efficacy in lowering HbA$_{1c}$ and similar effects on increases in weight, and are both generally neutral on blood pressure, but they differ in plasma lipid changes. Both increase plasma

HDL-cholesterol levels. Pioglitazone also tends to reduce plasma triglycerides; rosiglitazone causes a relative increase in LDL-cholesterol (see also Chapter 7). TZDs have been reported to have many nonantiglycemic actions that may reduce CVD (Table 9).

However, compared to the other insulin-sensitizing drug (metformin), this class appears to be less appealing because of its relative slow onset of action, increase in body weight, and, as a consequence, increased risk of heart failure (195), increased expense, and less dramatic effect on reducing macrovascular disease (182,195).

Table 9   Nonhypoglycemic Effects of Thiazolidinediones

Lower blood pressure
Increase cardiac output, stroke volume, and peripheral vascular resistance
Decrease cytosolic calcium and induce coronary artery relaxation
Reduce carotid intimal inflammation
Decrease in intimamedia compact thickness
Regulation of monocyte and macrophage function in atherosclerotic lesion
Decrease in calcium influx and attenuation of vascular contraction
Decrease vascular smooth muscle cell migration
Increase in forearm blood flow
Decrease in brachial artery vasoactivity
Decrease in renal artery/mesangial cell proliferation
Vasorelaxation of small arteries
Decrease intercellular adhesion molecule-1
Decrease vascular cell adhesion molecule-1
Decrease cyclooxygenase-2
Decrease endothelin
Decrease inducible nitric oxide synthase, tumor necrosis factor-α
Interleukin-6, tissue factor
Increase nuclear factor (B
Decrease C-reactive protein, oxidative stress
Decrease in microalbuminuria
Increase in high-density lipoprotein (HDL) cholesterol and low-density lipoprotein
   (LDL)-cholesterol levels
Increase LDL-cholesterol particle size
Decrease LDL-cholesterol oxidation
Increase fatty acid transport protein-1
Increase acyl-coenzyme A synthetase
Increase adiponectin
Increase intravascular lipolysis by increase in lipoprotein lipase activity
Decrease in plasminogen activator inhibitor-1 and fibrinogen levels
Increase in tissue plasminogen activator
Decrease in platelet aggregation
Decrease in intra-abdominal fat mass

Source: From Refs. 189, 192–194.

Pioglitazone and rosiglitazone lower HbA_{1c} by 0.5% to 1.5%, depending on the initial HbA_{1c}.

α-Glucosidase Inhibitors

Acarbose and miglitol improve HbA_{1c} levels 0.5% to 1.0% by delaying gastrointestinal absorption of complex carbohydrates and thus compensating for impaired insulin responses in people with IGT and Type 2 diabetes (110). They have no direct effects of β-cell function or insulin sensitivity and are neutral with respect to weight, lipids, and other components of the metabolic syndrome. These agents are not approved by the FDA for treating glucose intolerance, but acarbose has been shown to reduce development of and to prevent macrovascular events in people with IGT (196). Their major effects are on postprandial hyperglycemia and are therefore a logical choice for treatment of individuals with isolated postprandial hyperglycemia. Their major side effects are not serious, but are socially uncomfortable—flatulence. Generally this is related to overconsumption of high carbohydrate diets and is not a problem in countries such as Germany and Japan. Because of the benignity of their side effects, their demonstrated efficacy in reducing postprandial hyperglycemia, conversion to Type 2 diabetes of people with IGT, and diminishing cardiovascular events, this group of drugs should be considered as early treatment, along with weight loss drugs, for treatment of the metabolic syndrome in individuals with IGT.

Insulin Secretagogues

Insulin secretagogues are composed of two classes of drugs—sulfonylureas and meglitinides (197). The sulfonylureas have been available in the United States since 1954 (198). Glyburide (glibenclamide), glipizide, and glimepiride account for essentially all of the sulfonylurea market in the United States; gliclazide is popular in other countries such as the United Kingdom. The meglitinides— repaglinide and nateglinide—were recently introduced within the past five years. Although the drugs differ in their structures, both classes have similar mechanisms of action: their binding to a sulfonylurea receptor or pancreatic β-cell membranes closes adenosine triphosphate–sensitive K^+ channels. This causes depolarization of the cell membrane and an influx of Ca^{2+} through voltage-sensitive channels that leads to discharge of insulin-containing granules. Differences in their binding characteristics and retention within islets and half lives result in different patterns of insulin release (199–204). Glyburide and glipizide primarily affect late- or second-phase insulin release (205), whereas glimepiride, gliclazide, and repaglinide affect both phases (205), and nateglinide affects primarily early- or first-phase insulin release (200). As a consequence, glyburide and glipizide primarily affect fasting plasma glucose, and subsequent plasma glucose levels throughout the day are reduced to the extent that fasting plasma glucose levels are reduced (206). In contrast, glimepiride (207) and repaglinide (109) reduce postprandial plasma glucose levels to a greater extent than fasting plasma glucose levels, and nateglinide reduces postprandial plasma glucose levels without, in most instances as monotherapy, significantly reducing fasting plasma glucose levels (109). Extended release formulations of some sulfonylureas, e.g., glipizide and gliclazide, have led to modifications of their pharmacodynamics.

In general, one can expect reductions in footing plasma glucose of 50 to 60 mg/dL and in HbA_{1c} of approximately 1.5% to 2% depending on the baseline values (107).

All these insulin secretagogues are generally neutral in terms of nonglycemic cardiovascular risk factors (e.g., blood pressure and lipids) (153,198). However, with the exception of nateglinide, all are associated with weight gain and have the potential to cause severe hypoglycemia (153,197,198,208). With respect to efficacy in lowering HbA_{1c} levels in patients with Type 2 diabetes, as monotherapy all the sulfonylureas and repaglinide are comparable (152,153,198), whereas nateglinide is somewhat less effective (Table 5) (109,200). This characteristic would be relevant, however, only to patients with Type 2 diabetes, having the metabolic syndrome.

Most patients with the metabolic syndrome have IGT. Therefore, an agent, which primarily targets postprandial hyperglycemia, which does not cause weight gain, and, which does not have a risk for severe hypoglycemia, would be appropriate. Of all insulin secretagogues, only nateglinide fulfils these requirements. However, recall that no agents are currently approved by the FDA to treat IGT or the metabolic syndrome.

GLUCAGON-LIKE PEPTIDE 1 RECEPTOR AGONISTS AND DIPEPTIDYL PEPTIDASE IV INHIBITORS

When glucose is taken orally, insulin secretion is stimulated to a greater extent when comparable hyperglycemia is achieved by intravenous infusion (209,210). This increase in insulin secretion is called the incretin effect and is due to the release of two intestinal insulin-stimulating hormones, GLP-1, and glucose-dependent insulinotropic polypeptide (GIP) (211). GIP and GLP-1 are members of the glucagon peptide super-family (209). GIP is produced and secreted from intestinal K cells localized in the duodenum and proximal jejunum and is secreted in response to carbohydrate- and fat-rich meals. Its release stimulates insulin secretion in a glucose-dependent manner. GIP has other actions: it affects fat metabolism in adipocytes, but does not inhibit glucagon secretion or gastric emptying, as does GLP-1 (see below). Animal studies suggest that GIP may promote (-cell proliferation and survival (209,211). Currently, it is thought to be a less important factor than GLP-1 insofar as β-cell function is concerned (210,212,213). GLP-1 is synthesized in and secreted from enteroendocrine L cells located predominantly in the ileum and colon (214). Normally, circulating levels of GLP-1 rise rapidly within minutes of food ingestion. GLP-1 secretion is controlled by both neural and endocrine signals initiated by nutrient arrival into the proximal gastrointestinal tract. The incretin effect is impaired in patients with Type 2 diabetes (211,215,216). GLP-1 responses are reduced in people with Type 2 diabetes, whereas GIP responses are normal (209,215,216). Responses to infused GLP-1 are preserved in people with Type 2 diabetes, whereas responses to GIP are reduced (210,215,216). These results suggest that abnormalities in the incretin system may be involved in the pathogenesis of Type 2 diabetes and that agents, which increase the action or availability of GLP-1, may be useful. GLP-1 has numerous physiological and pharmacologic actions (Table 10).

These include glucose-dependent stimulation of insulin release, suppression of glucose secretion, decreased appetite, delaying gastric emptying, and trophic effects on pancreatic islets (210,214,215,217). Use of GLP-1 itself is limited by the fact that it has a short half-life and that it is a peptide (i.e., cannot be given orally). GLP-1 is rapidly inactivated and cleared from the circulation following secretion from L cells with a half-life in minutes due to enzymatic cleavage by a ubiquitously expressed serine protease dipeptidyl peptidase IV (DPP-IV). Pharmacological administration of GLP-1 in humans lowers plasma glucose, increases insulin release, suppresses glucagon release, and slows gastric emptying (209–211). Animal studies indicate that GLP-1 agonists promote β-cell proliferation and stimulate differentiation of exocrine cells or islet precursors to a more differentiated β-cell phenotype (212,218,219).

Given these theoretical benefits of GLP therapy, the pharmaceutical industry have embarked on a program to develop GLP-1 agonists resistant to degradation by DPP-IV and agents that block the degradation of endogenous GLP-1 production—DPP-IV inhibitors. In 2005, the FDA approved an analog of GLP-1 (exendin-4) for the treatment of Type 2 diabetes as add-on therapy to oral agents. Byetta® or exendin-4 (also called exenatide) was isolated from the venom of the Gila monster Heloderma suspectum and is a potent GLP-1 receptor agonist resistant to DPP-IV cleavage. Exenatide is a 39-amino acid peptide incretin mimetic that exhibits glucoregulatory activities by binding to the pancreatic GLP-1 receptor. It is similar in structure (52% homology) and function to GLP-1 but is more stable than GLP-1 avoiding degradation by DDP-IV (214). Byetta is administered subcutaneously twice daily (5 or 10 µg). During studies in nondiabetic and Type 2 diabetic patients, exenatide increased both first-phase and second-phase glucose-induced insulin secretion and reduced postprandial glucagon

Table 10 Major Biological Effects of GLP-1

Potentiates glucose-stimulated insulin secretion (211)
Enhances insulin biosynthesis (211)
Suppresses glucagon secretion (209)
Stimulates somatostatin secretion (209)
Increases β-cell mass (211)
Maintains β-cell function (211)
Improves insulin sensitivity (209,211)
Enhances glucose disposal (211)
Reduces food intake (209,210)
Slows gastric emptying (210,211)

Source: From Refs. 209–211.

release (220). When compared with placebo in trials lasting up to 30 weeks in patients with Type 2 diabetes treated with metformin and/or a sulfonylurea, the decrease in HbA_{1c} was approximately 0.8% to 1.0%, depending on baseline values. There was a substantial decrease in postprandial glycemic excursions and a modest decrease in fasting hyperglycemia and in weight (111–113). Currently, there is a considerable effort underway to develop additional GLP-1R agonists with longer duration of action, which can be administered weekly. A significant side effect of exenatide is nausea, which a significant percentage of patients cannot tolerate.

An alternative to GLP-1 agonists involves the development of inhibitors of DPP-IV, the principal enzyme responsible for incretin inactivation (221). DPP-IV is a circulating and cell-surface aminopeptidase as well as CD26 membrane protein involved in immune mechanisms. DPP-IV inhibition enhances the activity of both GLP-1 and GIP. DPP-IV inhibitors are orally active and lack the nausea side effects of GLP-1 agonists, but do not cause weight loss or weight gain. Two DPP-IV inhibitors, vildagliptin and sitagliptin, are currently being assessed in late-stage clinical trials. Vildagliptin (LAF237), taken once daily by patients inadequately controlled on metformin, lowered HbA_{1c} by approximately 0.5% from baseline, whereas HbA_{1c} increased in the placebo group by 0.5%, giving a placebo subtracted decrease of HbA_{1c} by approximately 1% over one year (222). In summary, DPP-IV inhibitors are somewhat less efficacious than GLP-1 agonists in lowering HbA_{1c} and in causing weight loss, but they lack the nausea of GLP-1 agonists, are effective orally, and still have positive effects on β-cell function.

Chronic hyperglycemia, which often precedes diagnosis of Type 2 DM, causes extensive vascular damage and leads to the early development of clinical complications (223). Therefore, it is recommended to treat patients intensively so as to achieve target HbA_{1c} < 6.5% within six months of diagnosis. After three months, if patients are not at target, HbA_{1c} less than 6.5% or fasting/postprandial glucose less than 110 mg/dL (6.0 mmol/L), one should consider combination therapy. The data in clinical studies demonstrates that adding a new agent to an existing regimen is typically better than using a new agent as monotherapy. Combination therapy or insulin should be initiated immediately for all patients with HbA_{1c} ≥9% at diagnosis.

While stepwise titration of monotherapy to the maximum recommended dose can be effective, it may also lead to an increased incidence of adverse effect without additional improvement of glycemic control. Early use of combination therapy using submaximal doses of agents in parallel with diet and exercise can improve glycemic control without significantly increasing side effects. Additional benefits are more likely to be achieved when chosen agents have complementary modes of action (224–227).

CONCLUSIONS

The metabolic syndrome represents a cluster of factors that increase the risk for atherothrombotic CVD. In genetically susceptible individuals, an imbalance between caloric intake and caloric expenditure leads to an accumulation of visceral fat. This leads to insulin resistance with a reduction in the beneficial effects of insulin on (i) carbohydrate and lipid metabolism, (ii) vascular health, and (iii) inflammatory mechanisms that lead to an increase in CVD in people whose insulin secretion cannot compensate for the increase in insulin resistance.

Given the role of obesity, it would appear that prevention and correction of obesity would be the logical target to prevent and treat the metabolic syndrome. On an individual basis, lifestyle interventions (diet and exercise) have been disappointing. Pharmacologic interventions to date (weight loss drugs) have also been disappointing in treating after the fact. The metabolic syndrome is a public health problem. The most effective approach, therefore, should be a public health approach—prevent obesity in the first place. Failing this, what does one do with the obese individual with the metabolic syndrome: treat the lipid abnormalities with lipid-modifying drugs; treat hypertension with anti-hypertensive drugs? What about subtle abnormalities of glucose metabolism? There is overwhelming data that hyperglycemia is a continuous and independent risk factor for CVD. Postprandial hyperglycemia is the earliest abnormality. It should be screened for and treated. However, at present, there are no FDA drugs approved for this purpose. Hopefully, this will change when results of current clinical trials with cardiovascular end points become available.

So what do we do given present day realities? There are multiple options: for the obese individual with IGT (the majority of people with the metabolic syndrome): in addition to referral to a dietician and an exercise physiologist, one could prescribe a weight reduction medication with minimal side effects, such as orlistat, rimonabant, or exenatide, and/or a combination of the above. It is likely that patients would prefer a pill. However, most would accept a once a week injection of a GLP-1 agonist. Early treatment of IGT should also consider the use of an α-glucosidase inhibitor because of its reduction of postprandial hyperglycemia, safety, and positive effects on cardiovascular endpoints. Nateglinide might also be considered because of its selective effects on postprandial hyperglycemia and lack of side effects. Other insulin secretagogueswould probably not be appropriate given their risk for hypoglycemia and weightgain. We currently have no data on the role of GLP-1 agonists or DPP-IV inhibitors in this context. People with Type 2 diabetes and other features of the metabolic syndrome should be treated according to current guidelines of the ADA, American Academy of Clinical Endocrinology, and World Health Organization as if they did not have the metabolic syndrome.

ACKNOWLEDGMENTS

We thank Mary Little for her excellent editorial assistance. The present work was supported in part by Division of Research Resources—GCRC Grant 5MO1 RR-00044 and the National Institute of Diabetes and Digestive and Kidney Diseases Grant DK-20411.

REFERENCES

1. Reaven G. Role of insulin resistance in human disease. Diabetes 1988; 37:1595–1607.
2. World Health Organization: Definition, Diagnosis and Classification of Diabetes Mellitus: Report of a WHO Consultation. Part I: Diagnosis and Classification of Diabetes Mellitus. Geneva, Switzerland: World Health Organization, 1999.
3. Balkau B, Charles MA. Comment on the provisional report from the WHO consultation. European Group for the Study of Insulin Resistance (EGIR). Diabet Med 1999; 16:442–443.
4. Executive Summary of The Third Report of The National Cholesterol Education Program (NCEP) Expert Panel on Detection, Evaluation, And Treatment of High Blood Cholesterol In Adults (Adult Treatment Panel III). JAMA 2001; 285:2486–2497.
5. Einhorn D, Reaven GM, Cobin RH, et al. American College of Endocrinology position statement on the insulin resistance syndrome. Endocr Pract 2003; 9:237–252.
6. Stern MP, Williams K, Gonzalez-Villalpando C, et al. Does the metabolic syndrome improve identification of individuals at risk of Type 2 diabetes and/or cardiovascular disease? Diabetes Care 2004; 27:2676–2681.
7. Bruno G, Merletti F, Biggeri A, et al. Metabolic syndrome as a predictor of all-cause and cardiovascular mortality in Type 2 diabetes: the Casale Monferrato Study. Diabetes Care 2004; 27:2689–2694.
8. Gale EA. The myth of the metabolic syndrome. Diabetologia 2005; 48:1679–1683.
9. Kahn R, Buse J, Ferrannini E, et al. The metabolic syndrome: time for a critical appraisal Joint statement from the American Diabetes Association and the European Association for the Study of Diabetes. Diabetologia 2005; 48:1684–1699.
10. Reaven GM. The metabolic syndrome: requiescat in pace. Clin Chem 2005; 51:931–938.
11. Meigs J, D'Agostino R, Wilson P, et al. Risk variable clustering in the insulin resistance syndrome. Diabetes 1997; 46:1594–1600.
12. Carr DB, Utzschneider KM, Hull RL, et al. Intra-abdominal fat is a major determinant of the National Cholesterol Education Program Adult Treatment Panel III criteria for the metabolic syndrome. Diabetes 2004; 53:2087–2094.
13. Garg A. Regional adiposity and insulin resistance. J Clin Endocrinol Metab 2004; 89:4206–4210.
14. St Onge MP, Janssen I, Heymsfield SB. Metabolic syndrome in normal-weight Americans: new definition of the metabolically obese, normal-weight individual. Diabetes Care 2004; 27:2222–2228.
15. Ferreira I, Twisk JW, van Mechelen W, et al. Development of fatness, fitness, and lifestyle from adolescence to the age of 36 years: determinants of the metabolic syndrome in young adults: the Amsterdam growth and health longitudinal study. Arch Intern Med 2005; 165:42–48:
16. Ford ES, Giles WH, Dietz WH. Prevalence of the metabolic syndrome among US adults: findings from the third National Health and Nutrition Examination Survey. JAMA 2002; 287:356–359.
17. Bouchard C. The genetics of obesity in humans. Curr Opin Endo Diabetes 1996; 3:29–35.

18. Bonora E, Bonadonna R, DelPrato S, et al. In vivo glucose metabolism in obese and type II diabetic subjects with or without hypertension. Diabetes 1993; 42:764–772.

19. Bonora E, Kiechi S, Willeit J, et al. Prevalence of insulin resistance in metabolic disorders—the Bruneck Study. Diabetes 1998; 47:1643–1649.

20. Ilanne-Parikka P, Eriksson JG, Lindstrom J, et al. Prevalence of the metabolic syndrome and its components: findings from a Finnish general population sample and the Diabetes Prevention Study cohort. Diabetes Care 2004; 27:2135–2140.

21. Nesto RW. Obesity: a major component of the metabolic syndrome. Tex Heart Inst J 2005; 32:387–389.

22. Yki-Jarvinen H. The PROactive study: some answers, many questions. Lancet 2005; 366:1241–1242.

23. Dormandy JA, Charbonnel B, Eckland DJ, et al. Secondary prevention of macrovascular events in patients with Type 2 diabetes in the PROactive Study (PROspective pioglitAzone Clinical Trial In macroVascular Events): a randomised controlled trial. Lancet 2005; 366:1279–1289.

24. Scheen AJ, Lefebvre PJ. Proactive study: secondary cardiovascular prevention with pioglitazione in Type 2 diabetic patients. Rev Med Liege 2005; 60:896–901.

25. Rizza R, Henry R, Kahn R. Commentary on the results and clinical implications of the PROactive study. Diabetes Care 2005; 28:2965–2967.

26. The DREAM (Diabetes REduction Assessment with ramipril and rosiglitazone Medication) investigators. Effect of rosiglitazone on the frequency of diabetes in patients with impaired glucose tolerance or impaired fasting glucose: a randomised controlled trial. Lancet 2006; 368:1096–1105.

27. Despres JP, Golay A, Sjostrom L. Effects of rimonabant on metabolic risk factors in overweight patients with dyslipidemia. N Engl J Med 2005; 353:2121–2134.

28. Van Gaal LF, Rissanen AM, Scheen AJ, et al. Effects of the cannabinoid-1 receptor blocker rimonabant on weight reduction and cardiovascular risk factors in overweight patients: 1-year experience from the RIO-Europe study. Lancet 2005; 365:1389–1397.

29. Stevens RJ, Coleman RL, Adler AI, et al. Risk factors for myocardial infarction case fatality and stroke case fatality in Type 2 diabetes: UKPDS 66. Diabetes Care 2004; 27:201–207.

30. Coutinho M, Gerstein H, Wang Y, et al. The relationship between glucose and incident cardiovascular events. A metaregression analysis of published data from 20 studies of 95:783 individuals followed for 12.4 years. Diabetes Care 1999; 22:233–240.

31. Gerich JE. Clinical significance, pathogenesis, and management of postprandial hyperglycemia. Arch Intern Med 2003; 163:1306–1316.

32. Selvin E, Marinopoulos S, Berkenblit G, et al. Meta-analysis: glycosylated hemoglobin and cardiovascular disease in diabetes mellitus. Ann Intern Med 2004; 141:421–431.

33. Tominaga M, Eguchi H, Manaka H, et al. Impaired glucose tolerance is a risk factor for cardiovascular disease, but not impaired fasting glucose. The Funagata Diabetes Study. Diabetes Care 1999; 22:920–924.

34. Khaw K-T, Wareham N, Luben R et al. Glycated haemoglobin, diabetes, and mortality in men in Norfolk cohort of European Prospective Investigation of Cancer and Nutrition (EPIC-Norfolk). BMJ 2001; 322:15–18.

35. Woerle HJ, Pimenta W, Meyer C, et al. Diagnostic and therapeutic implications of relationships between fasting, 2 hour postchallenge plasma glucose and HbA1c values. Arch Intern Med 2004; 164:1627–1632.

36. Torgerson JS, Hauptman J, Boldrin MN, et al. XENical in the prevention of diabetes in obese subjects (XENDOS) study: a randomized study of orlistat as an adjunct to lifestyle changes for the prevention of Type 2 diabetes in obese patients. Diabetes Care 2004; 27:155–161.

37. Knowler W, Barrett-Connor E, Fowler S, et al. Reduction in the incidence of Type 2 diabetes with lifestyle intervention or metformin. N Engl J Med 2002; 346:393–403.

38. Chiasson JL, Josse RG, Gomis R, et al. Acarbose for prevention of Type 2 diabetes mellitus: the STOP-NIDDM randomised trial. Lancet 2002; 359:2072–2077.

39. Buchanan TA, Xiang AH, Peters RK, et al. Preservation of pancreatic beta-cell function and prevention of Type 2 diabetes by pharmacological treatment of insulin resistance in high-risk hispanic women. Diabetes 2002; 51:2796–2803.

40. Standards of Medical Care in Diabetes. Diabetes Care 2005; 28:S4–S36.

41. American College of Endocrinology consensus statement on guidelines for glycemic control. Endocr Pract 2002; 8(suppl 1):5–11.

42. Standl E. International Diabetes Federation European Policy Group standards for diabetes. Endocr Pract 2002; 8(suppl 1):37–40.

43. Koro CE, Bowlin SJ, Bourgeois N, et al. Glycemic control from 1988 to 2000 among U.S. adults diagnosed with Type 2 diabetes: a preliminary report. Diabetes Care 2004; 27:17:20.

44. Blonde L. Best practices in diabetes management: getting more patients to goal. Am J Manag Care 2005; 11:S186–S188.

45. Lebovitz H. Effect of the postprandial state on nontraditional risk factors. Am J Cardiol 2001; 88:20H–25H.

46. Yamagishi S, Edelstein D, Du X, et al. Hyperglycemia potentiates collagen-induced platelet activation through mitochondrial superoxide overproduction. Diabetes 2001; 50:1491–1494.

47. Lipinski B. Pathophysiology of oxidative stress in diabetes mellitus. J Diabetes Complications 2001; 15:203–210.

48. Marfella R, Quagliaro L, Nappo F, et al. Acute hyperglycemia induces an oxidative stress in healthy subjects. J Clin Invest 2001; 108:635–636.

49. Vane J, Anggard E, Botting R. Regulatory functions of the vascular endothelium. N Engl J Med 1990; 323:27–36.

50. Williams S, Goldfine A, Timimi F, et al. Acute hyperglycemia attenuates endothelium-dependent vasodilation in humans in vivo. Circulation 1998; 97:1695–1701.

51. Title L, Cummings P, Giddens K, et al. Oral glucose loading acutely attenuates endothelium-dependent vasodilation in healthy adults without diabetes: an effect prevented by vitamins C and E. J Am Coll Cardiol 2000; 36:2185–2191.

52. Beckman J, Goldfine A, Gordon M, et al. Ascorbate restores endothelium-dependent vasodilation impaired by acute hyperglycemia in humans. Circulation 2001; 103:1618–1623.

53. Ting H, Timimi F, Boles K, et al. Vitamin C improves endothelium-dependent vasodilation in patients with non-insulin-dependent diabetes mellitus. J Clin Invest 1996; 97:22–28.

54. Meier M, King G. Protein kinase C activation and its pharmacological inhibition in vascular disease. Vasc Med 2000; 5:173–185.

55. King G, Wakasaki H. Theoretical mechanisms by which hyperglycemia and insulin resistance could cause cardiovascular diseases in diabetes. Diabetes Care 1999; 22 (suppl 3):C31–C37.

56. Tomkin G. Diabetic vascular disease and the rising star of Protein Kinase C. Diabetologia 2001; 44:657–658.
57. Stratton I, Adler A, Neil HA, et al. Association of glycaemia with macrovascular and microvascular complications of Type 2 diabetes (UKPDS 35: prospective observational study. BMJ 2000; 321:405–412.
58. Nathan DM, Cleary PA, Backlund JY, et al. Intensive diabetes treatment and cardiovascular disease in patients with type 1 diabetes. N Engl J Med 2005; 353:2643–2653.
59. Dinneen S, Gerich J, Rizza R. Carbohydrate metabolism in noninsulin-dependent diabetes mellitus. N Engl J Med 1992; 327:707–713.
60. Woerle HJ, Szoke E, Meyer C, et al. Mechanisms for abnormal postprandial glucose metabolism in Type 2 diabetes. Am J Physiol Endocrinol Metab 2006; 290:E67–E77.
61. Meyer C, Dostou J, Welle S, et al. Role of human liver, kidney and skeletal muscle in postprandial glucose homeostasis. Am J Physiol Endocrinol Metab 2002; 282:E419–E427.
62. Mitrakou A, Kelley D, Mokan M, et al. Role of reduced suppression of glucose production and diminished early insulin release in impaired glucose tolerance. N Engl J Med 1992; 326:22–29.
63. Meyer C, Woerle HJ, Dostou J, et al. Abnormal renal, hepatic and muscle glucose metabolism following glucose ingestion in Type 2 diabetes. Am J Physiol Endocrinol Metab 2004; 287:E1049–E1056.
64. Woerle HJ, Meyer C, Dostou JM, et al. Pathways for glucose disposal after meal ingestion in humans. Am J Physiol Endocrinol Metab 2003; 284:E716–E725.
65. Pratley R, Weyer C. The role of impaired early insulin secretion in the pathogenesis of type II diabetes mellitus. Diabetologia 2001; 44:929–945.
66. Kahn S, Prigeon R, McCulloch D, et al. Quantification of the relationship between insulin sensitivity and beta-cell function in human subjects. Evidence for a hyperbolic function. Diabetes 1993; 42:1663–1672.
67. Weyer C, Tataranni PA, Bogardus C, et al. Insulin resistance and insulin secretory dysfunction are independent predictors of worsening of glucose tolerance during each stage of Type 2 diabetes development. Diabetes Care 2000; 24:89–94.
68. Buchanan T, Catalano P. The pathogenesis of GDM: implications for diabetes after pregnancy. Diab Rev 1995; 3:584–601.
69. Efendic S, Hanson V, Persson B, et al. Glucose tolerance, insulin release and insulin sensitivity in normal-weight women with previous gestational diabetes. Diabetes 1987; 36:413–419.
70. Ward W, Johnston C, Beard J, et al. Insulin resistance and impaired insulin secretion in subjects with histories of gestational diabetes mellitus. Diabetes 1985; 34:861–869.
71. Chan S, Gelding S, McManus R, et al. Abnormalities of intermediary metabolism following a gestational diabetic pregnancy. Clin Endocrinol 1992; 36:417–420.
72. Ryan E, Imes S, Liu D, et al. Defects in insulin secretion and action in women with a history of gestational diabetes. Diabetes 1995; 44:506–512.
73. Dornhorst A, Edwards S, Nicholls J, et al. A defect in insulin release in women at risk of future non- insulin-dependent diabetes. Clin Sci 1991; 81:195–199.
74. Gerich J. The genetic basis of Type 2 diabetes mellitus: impaired insulin secretion versus impaired insulin sensitivity. Endocr Rev 1998; 19:491–503.

75. DeFronzo R. The triumvirate: B-cell, muscle, and liver: a collusion responsible for NIDDM. Diabetes 1988; 37:667–687.

76. Olefsky J. Diabetes mellitus (Type II): etiology and pathogenesis. In: DeGroot L, Besser M, Burger H, Jameson J, Loriaux D, Marshall J, O'Dell W, Potts J, Rubenstein A, eds. Endocrinology. Philadelphia: W. B. Saunders, 1995:1436–1463.

77. Kahn C. Insulin action, diabetogenes, and the cause of type II diabetes. Diabetes 1994; 43:1066–1084.

78. Perley J, Kipnis D. Plasma insulin responses to oral and intravenous glucose: studies in normal and diabetic subjects. J Clin Invest 1967; 46:1954–1962.

79. Grodsky G, Fanska R. The in vitro perfused pancreas. In: Hardman J, O'Malley B, eds. Methods in Enzymology. New York: Academic Press, 1975:364–372.

80. Van Haeften T, Pimenta W, Mitrakou A, et al. Relative contributions of b-cell function and tissue insulin sensitivity to fasting and postglucose-load glycemia. Metabolism 2000; 49:1318–1325.

81. Pimenta W, Kortytkowski M, Mitrakou A, et al. Pancreatic beta-cell dysfunction as the primary genetic lesion in NIDDM. JAMA 1995; 273:1855–1861.

82. Vaag A, Henriksen J, Madsbad S, et al. Insulin secretion, insulin action, and hepatic glucose production in identical twins discordant for non-insulin-dependent diabetes mellitus. J Clin Invest 1995; 95:690–698.

83. Weiss R, Caprio S, Trombetta M, et al. Beta-cell function across the spectrum of glucose tolerance in obese youth. Diabetes 2005; 54:1735–1743.

84. Bennet P. Epidemiology of diabetes mellitus. In: Rifkin H, Porte D, eds. Diabetes Mellitus. New York: Elsevier, 1990:357–377.

85. Jackson MB, Osei SY, Ahima RS. The endocrine role of adipose tissue: focus on adiponectin and resistin. Curr Opin Endocrinol Diabet 2005; 12:163–170.

86. Deng S, Vatamaniuk M, Huang X, et al. Structural and functional abnormalities in the islets isolated from Type 2 diabetic subjects. Diabetes 2004; 53:624–632.

87. U.K. Prospective Diabetes Study Group. U.K. prospective diabetes study 16: overview of 6 years' therapy of type II diabetes: a progressive disease. Diabetes 1995; 44:1249–1258.

88. Iozzo P, Beck-Nielsen H, Laakso M, et al. Independent influence of age on basal insulin secretion in nondiabetic humans. European Group for the Study of Insulin Resistance. J Clin Endocrinol Metab 1999; 84:863–868.

89. DeFronzo R, Ferrannini E. Insulin resistance: a multifaceted syndrome response for NIDDM, obesity, hypertension, dyslipidemia, and atherosclerotic cardiovascular disease. Diabetes Care 1991; 14:173–194.

90. American Diabetes Association. Consensus Development Conference on Insulin Resistance. Diabetes Care 1998; 21:310–314.

91. Tack CJ, Ong MK, Lutterman JA, et al. Insulin-induced vasodilatation and endothelial function in obesity/insulin resistance. Effects of troglitazone. Diabetologia 1998; 41:569–576.

92. Cummings M, Watts G, Umpleby A, et al. Acute hyperinsulinemia decreases the hepatic secretion of very-low-density lipoprotein apolipoprotein B-100 in NIDDM. Diabetes 1995; 44:1059–1065.

93. Malmberg K, Ryden L, Wedel H, et al. Intense metabolic control by means of insulin in patients with diabetes mellitus and acute myocardial infarction (DIGAMI 2): effects on mortality and morbidity. Eur Heart J 2005; 26:650–661.

94. Church TS, Cheng YJ, Earnest CP, et al. Exercise capacity and body composition as predictors of mortality among men with diabetes. Diabetes Care 2004; 27:83–88.

95. Rexrode KM, Carey VJ, Hennekens CH, et al. Abdominal adiposity and coronary heart disease in women. JAMA 1998; 280:1843–1848.
96. Svendsen OL, Hassager C, Christiansen C. Effect of an energy-restrictive diet, with or without exercise, on lean tissue mass, resting metabolic rate, cardiovascular risk factors, and bone in overweight postmenopausal women. Am J Med 1993; 95:131–140.
97. Jain A. Treating obesity in individuals and populations. BMJ 2005; 331:1387–1390.
98. Wadden TA, Berkowitz RI, Womble LG, et al. Randomized trial of lifestyle modification and pharmacotherapy for obesity. N Engl J Med 2005; 353:2111–2120.
99. Ratner R, Goldberg R, Haffner S, et al. Impact of intensive lifestyle and metformin therapy on cardiovascular disease risk factors in the diabetes prevention program. Diabetes Care 2005; 28:888–894.
100. Yusuf S, Hawken S, Ounpuu S, et al. Effect of potentially modifiable risk factors associated with myocardial infarction in 52: countries (the INTERHEART study): case-control study. Lancet 2004; 364:937–952.
101. Rosengren A, Hawken S, Ounpuu S, et al. Association of psychosocial risk factors with risk of acute myocardial infarction in 111119 cases and 13648 controls from 52 countries (the INTERHEART study): case-control study. Lancet 2004; 364:953–962.
102. Yusuf S, Hawken S, Ounpuu S, et al. Obesity and the risk of myocardial infarction in 27,000 participants from 52 countries: a case-control study. Lancet 2005; 366:1640–1649.
103. Grundy SM, Cleeman JI, Daniels SR, et al. Diagnosis and management of the metabolic syndrome: an American Heart Association/National Heart, Lung, and Blood Institute Scientific Statement. Circulation 2005; 112:2735–2752.
104. Brown JB, Nichols GA, Perry A. The burden of treatment failure in Type 2 diabetes. Diabetes Care 2004; 27:1535–1540.
105. Saydah SH, Fradkin J, Cowie CC. Poor control of risk factors for vascular disease among adults with previously diagnosed diabetes. JAMA 2004; 291:335–342.
106. Seufert J, Lubben G, Dietrich K, et al. A comparison of the effects of thiazolidinediones and metformin on metabolic control in patients with Type 2 diabetes mellitus. Clin Ther 2004; 26:805–818.
107. Inzucchi S, Maggs D, Spollett G, et al. Efficacy and metabolic effects of metformin and troglitazone in type II diabetes mellitus. N Engl J Med 1998; 338:867–872.
108. Chiquette E, Ramirez G, DeFronzo R. A meta-analysis comparing the effect of thiazolidinediones on cardiovascular risk factors. Arch Intern Med 2004; 164:2097–2104.
109. Rosenstock J, Hassman DR, Madder RD, et al. Repaglinide versus nateglinide monotherapy: a randomized, multicenter study. Diabetes Care 2004; 27:1265–1270.
110. Chiasson J, Josse R, Hunt J, et al. The efficacy of acarbose in the treatment of patients with non-insulin-dependent diabetes mellitus. A multicenter controlled clinical trial. Ann Intern Med 1994; 121:928–935.
111. DeFronzo RA, Ratner RE, Han J, et al. Effects of exenatide (exendin-4) on glycemic control and weight over 30 weeks in metformin-treated patients with Type 2 diabetes. Diabetes Care 2005; 28:1092–1100.
112. Fineman MS, Bicsak TA, Shen LZ, et al. Effect on glycemic control of exenatide (synthetic exendin-4) additive to existing metformin and/or sulfonylurea treatment in patients with Type 2 diabetes. Diabetes Care 2003; 26:2370–2377.
113. Kendall DM, Riddle MC, Rosenstock J, et al. Effects of exenatide (exendin-4) on glycemic control over 30 weeks in patients with Type 2 diabetes treated with metformin and a sulfonylurea. Diabetes Care 2005; 28:1083–1091.

114. Ahren B, Landin-Olsson M, Jansson PA, et al. Inhibition of dipeptidyl peptidase-4 reduces glycemia, sustains insulin levels, and reduces glucagon levels in Type 2 diabetes. J Clin Endocrinol Metab 2004; 89:2078–2084.

115. Stone NJ, Saxon D. Approach to treatment of the patient with metabolic syndrome: lifestyle therapy. Am J Cardiol 2005; 96:15E–21E.

116. Vazquez LA, Pazos F, Berrazueta JR, et al. Effects of changes in body weight and insulin resistance on inflammation and endothelial function in morbid obesity after bariatric surgery. J Clin Endocrinol Metab 2005; 90:316–322.

117. Guldstrand M, Ahren B, Adamson U. Improved beta-cell function after standardized weight reduction in severely obese subjects. Am J Physiol Endocrinol Metab 2003; 284:E557–E565.

118. Wadden TA. Treatment of obesity by moderate and severe caloric restriction. Results of clinical research trials. Ann Intern Med 1993; 119:688–693.

119. Watts NB, Spanheimer RG, DiGirolamo M, et al. Prediction of glucose response to weight loss in patients with non-insulin-dependent diabetes mellitus. Arch Intern Med 1990; 150:803–806.

120. Kelley DE, Kuller LH, McKolanis TM, et al. Effects of moderate weight loss and orlistat on insulin resistance, regional adiposity, and fatty acids in Type 2 diabetes. Diabetes Care 2004; 27:33–40.

121. Molitch ME, Fujimoto W, Hamman RF, et al. The diabetes prevention program and its global implications. J Am Soc Nephrol 2003; 14:S103–S107.

122. Beck-Nielsen H, Pedersen O, Lindskov H. Normalization of the insulin sensitivity and the cellular insulin binding during treatment of obese diabetics for one year. Acta Endocrinol.(Copenh) 1979; 90:103–112.

123. Eilat-Adar S, Eldar M, Goldbourt U. Association of intentional changes in body weight with coronary heart disease event rates in overweight subjects who have an additional coronary risk factor. Am J Epidemiol 2005; 161:352–358.

124. Haffner S, Temprosa M, Crandall J, et al. Intensive lifestyle intervention or metformin on inflammation and coagulation in participants with impaired glucose tolerance. Diabetes 2005; 54:1566–1572.

125. Yamaoka K, Tango T. Efficacy of lifestyle education to prevent Type 2 diabetes: a meta-analysis of randomized controlled trials. Diabetes Care 2005; 28: 2780–2786.

126. Dansinger ML, Gleason JA, Griffith JL, et al. Comparison of the Atkins, Ornish, Weight Watchers, and Zone diets for weight loss and heart disease risk reduction: a randomized trial. JAMA 2005; 293:43–53.

127. Franz MJ, Bantle JP, Beebe CA, et al. Nutrition principles and recommendations in diabetes. Diabetes Care 2004; 27 (Suppl 1):S36–S46.

128. www.glycemicindex.com.

129. Laaksonen DE, Toppinen LK, Juntunen KS, et al. Dietary carbohydrate modification enhances insulin secretion in persons with the metabolic syndrome. Am J Clin Nutr 2005; 82:1218–1227.

130. Alfenas RC, Mattes RD. Influence of glycemic index/load on glycemic response, appetite, and food intake in healthy humans. Diabetes Care 2005; 28:2123–2129.

131. Sacks FM, Svetkey LP, Vollmer WM, et al. Effects on blood pressure of reduced dietary sodium and the dietary approaches to stop hypertension (DASH) diet. DASH-Sodium Collaborative Research Group. N Engl J Med 2001; 344:3–10.

132. Svetkey LP, Sacks FM, Obarzanek E, et al. The DASH Diet, Sodium Intake and Blood Pressure Trial (DASH-sodium): rationale and design. DASH-Sodium Collaborative Research Group. J Am Diet Assoc 1999; 99:S96–104.

133. Obarzanek E, Sacks FM, Vollmer WM, et al. Effects on blood lipids of a blood pressure-lowering diet: the dietary approaches to stop hypertension (DASH) Trial. Am J Clin Nutr 2001; 74:80–89.

134. www.nih.gov.

135. Knoops KT, de Groot LC, Kromhout D, et al. Mediterranean diet, lifestyle factors, and 10-year mortality in elderly European men and women: the HALE project. JAMA 2004; 292:1433–1439.

136. Burani J, Longo PJ. Low-glycemic index carbohydrates: an effective behavioral change for glycemic control and weight management in patients with type 1 and 2 diabetes. Diabetes Educ 2006; 32:78–88.

137. Boden G, Sargrad K, Homko C, et al. Effect of a low-carbohydrate diet on appetite, blood glucose levels, and insulin resistance in obese patients with Type 2 diabetes. Ann Intern Med 2005; 142:403–411.

138. Kirk A, Mutrie N, MacIntyre P, et al. Effects of a 12-month physical activity counselling intervention on glycaemic control and on the status of cardiovascular risk factors in people with Type 2 diabetes. Diabetologia 2004; 47:821–832.

139. Petrella RJ, Lattanzio CN, Demeray A, et al. Can adoption of regular exercise later in life prevent metabolic risk for cardiovascular disease? Diabetes Care 2005; 28:694–701.

140. Tuomilehto J, Lindström J, Eriksson J, et al. Prevention of Type 2 diabetes mellitus by changes in lifestyle among subjects with impaired glucose tolerance. N Engl J Med 2001; 344:1343–1350.

141. Franco OH, de Laet C, Peeters A, et al. Effects of physical activity on life expectancy with cardiovascular disease. Arch Intern Med 2005; 165:2355–2360.

142. Duncan GE, Anton SD, Sydeman SJ, et al. Prescribing exercise at varied levels of intensity and frequency: a randomized trial. Arch Intern Med 2005; 165: 2362–2369.

143. Ahluwalia IB, Mack KA, Murphy W, et al. State-specific prevalence of selected chronic disease-related characteristics—Behavioral Risk Factor Surveillance System 2001; MMWR Surveill Summ 2003; 52:1–80:

144. Houston MC. The role of vascular biology, nutrition, and nutraceuticals in the prevention and treatment of hypertension. J Am Nutraceut Assoc 2002; 1:5–70:

145. Gregg EW, Gerzoff RB, Caspersen CJ, et al. Relationship of walking to mortality among US adults with diabetes. Arch Intern Med 2003; 163:1440–1447.

146. Brooks GA, Butte NF, Rand WM, et al. Chronicle of the Institute of Medicine physical activity recommendation: how a physical activity recommendation came to be among dietary recommendations. Am J Clin Nutr 2004; 79:921S–930S.

147. Hafidh S, Senkottaiyan N, Villarreal D, et al. Management of the metabolic syndrome. Am J Med Sci 2005; 330:343–351.

148. Pan X-R, Li G-W, Hu Y-H, et al. Effects of diet and exercise in preventing NIDDM in people with impaired glucose tolerance: the Da Qing IGT and Diabetes Study. Diabetes Care 1997; 20:537–544.

149. Anderssen SA, Hjermann I, Urdal P, et al. Improved carbohydrate metabolism after physical training and dietary intervention in individuals with the "atherothrombogenic syndrome." Oslo Diet and Exercise Study (ODES). A randomized trial. J Intern Med 1996; 240:203–209.

150. Liao D, Asberry PJ, Shofer JB, et al. Improvement of BMI, body composition, and body fat distribution with lifestyle modification in Japanese Americans with impaired glucose tolerance. Diabetes Care 2002; 25:1504–1510.
151. Krentz AJ, Bailey CJ. Oral antidiabetic agents: current role in Type 2 diabetes mellitus. Drugs 2005; 65:385–411.
152. Inzucchi S. Oral antihyperglycemic therapy for Type 2 diabetes: scientific review. JAMA 2002; 287:360–372.
153. DeFronzo R. Pharmacologic therapy for Type 2 diabetes mellitus. Ann Intern Med 1999; 131:281–303.
154. Bestermann W, Houston MC, Basile J, et al. Addressing the global cardiovascular risk of hypertension, dyslipidemia, diabetes mellitus, and the metabolic syndrome in the southeastern United States, part II: treatment recommendations formanagement of the global cardiovascular risk of hypertension, dyslipidemia, diabetes mellitus, and the metabolic syndrome. Am J Med Sci 2005; 329: 292–305.
155. Padwal R, Li SK, Lau DC. Long-term pharmacotherapy for overweight and obesity: a systematic review and meta-analysis of randomized controlled trials. Int J Obes 2003; 27:1437–1446.
156. DeRosa G, Cicero AF, Murdolo G, et al. Comparison of metabolic effects of orlistat and sibutramine treatment in Type 2 diabetic obese patients. Diabetes Nutr Metab 2004; 17:222–229.
157. Leung WY, Neil TG, Chan JC, et al. Weight management and current options in pharmacotherapy: orlistat and sibutramine. Clin Ther 2003; 25:58–80.
158. Damci T, Yalin S, Balci H, et al. Orlistat augments postprandial increases in glucagon-like peptide 1 in obese Type 2 diabetic patients. Diabetes Care 2004; 27:1077–1080.
159. Howlett AC. The cannabinoid receptors. Prostaglandins Other Lipid Mediat 2002; 68,69:619–631.
160. Gomez R, Navarro M, Ferrer B, et al. A peripheral mechanism for CB1 cannabinoid receptor-dependent modulation of feeding. J Neurosci 2002; 22:9612–9617.
161. Hanefeld M, Sachse G. The effects of orlistat on body weight and glycaemic control in overweight patients with Type 2 diabetes: a randomized, placebo-controlled trial. Diabetes Obes Metab 2002; 4:415–423.
162. Kelley DE, Bray GA, Pi-Sunyer FX, et al. Clinical efficacy of orlistat therapy in overweight and obese patients with insulin-treated Type 2 diabetes: a 1-year randomized controlled trial. Diabetes Care 2002; 25:1033–1041.
163. Vettor R, Serra R, Fabris R, et al. Effect of sibutramine on weight management and metabolic control in Type 2 diabetes: a meta-analysis of clinical studies. Diabetes Care 2005; 28:942–949.
164. Hundal RS, Inzucchi SE. Metformin: new understandings, new uses. Drugs 2003; 63:1879–1894.
165. Stumvoll M, Nurjhan N, Perriello G, et al. Metabolic effects of metformin in non-insulin-dependent diabetes mellitus. N Engl J Med 1995; 333:550–554.
166. Hundal RS, Krssak M, Dufour S, et al. Mechanism by which metformin reduces glucose production in Type 2 diabetes. Diabetes 2000; 49:2063–2069.
167. Cusi K, Consoli A, DeFronzo R. Metabolic effects of metformin on glucose and lactate metabolism in non-insulin-dependent diabetes mellitus. J Clin Endo & Metab 1996; 81:4059–4067.

168. Hundal H, Ramlal T, Reyes R, et al. Cellular mechanism of metformin action involves glucose transporter translocation from an intracellular pool to the plasma membrane in L6 muscle cells. Endocrinology 1992; 131:1165–1172.

169. Wulffele MG, Kooy A, de Zeeuw D, et al. The effect of metformin on blood pressure, plasma cholesterol and triglycerides in Type 2 diabetes mellitus: a systematic review. J.Intern.Med 2004; 256, 1–14:

170. Kirpichnikov D, McFarlane SI, Sowers JR. Metformin: an update. Ann Intern Med 2002; 137:25–33.

171. Grant PJ. Beneficial effects of metformin on haemostasis and vascular function in man. Diabetes Metab 2003; 29:6S44–6S52.

172. Beisswenger P, Ruggiero-Lopez D. Metformin inhibition of glycation processes. Diabetes Metab 2003; 29:6S95–6S103.

173. Mamputu JC, Wiernsperger NF, Renier G. Antiatherogenic properties of metformin: the experimental evidence. Diabetes Metab 2003; 29:6S71–6S76.

174. Pavlovic D, Kocic R, Kocic G, et al. Effect of four-week metformin treatment on plasma and erythrocyte antioxidative defense enzymes in newly diagnosed obese patients with Type 2 diabetes. Diabetes Obes Metab 2000; 2:251–256.

175. Faure P, Rossini E, Wiernsperger N, et al. An insulin sensitizer improves the free radical defense system potential and insulin sensitivity in high fructose-fed rats. Diabetes 1999; 48:353–357.

176. Wiernsperger NF. Membrane physiology as a basis for the cellular effects of metformin in insulin resistance and diabetes. Diabetes Metab 1999; 25: 110–127.

177. Bailey C, Turner R. Metformin. N Engl J Med 1996; 334:574–579.

178. Standeven KF, Ariens RA, Whitaker P, et al. The effect of dimethylbiguanide on thrombin activity, FXIII activation, fibrin polymerization, and fibrin clot formation. Diabetes 2002; 51:189–197.

179. Sirtori CR, Franceschini G, Gianfranceschi G, et al. Metformin improves peripheral vascular flow in nonhyperlipidemic patients with arterial disease. J Cardiovasc Pharmacol 1984; 6:914–923.

180. Wiernsperger NF, Bouskela E. Microcirculation in insulin resistance and diabetes: more than just a complication. Diabetes Metab 2003; 29:6S77–6S87.

181. Mather KJ, Verma S, Anderson TJ. Improved endothelial function with metformin in Type 2 diabetes mellitus. J Am Coll Cardiol 2001; 37:1344–1350.

182. UK Prospective Diabetes Study (UKPDS) Group. Effect of intensive blood-glucose control with metformin on complications in overweight patients with Type 2 diabetes (UKPDS 34). Lancet 1998; 352:854–865.

183. Padwal R, Majumdar SR, Johnson JA, et al. A systematic review of drug therapy to delay or prevent Type 2 diabetes. Diabetes Care 2005; 28:736–744.

184. Cryer DR, Nicholas SP, Henry DH, et al. Comparative outcomes study of metformin intervention versus conventional approach the COSMIC Approach Study. Diabetes Care 2005; 28:539–543.

185. Salpeter SR, Greyber E, Pasternak GA, et al. Risk of fatal and nonfatal lactic acidosis with metformin use in Type 2 diabetes mellitus: systematic review and meta-analysis. Arch Intern Med 2003; 163:2594–2602.

186. Misbin RI, Green L, Stadel BV, et al. Lactic acidosis in patients with diabetes treated with metformin. N Engl J Med 1998; 338, 265–266.

187. Orchard TJ, Temprosa M, Goldberg R, et al. The effect of metformin and intensive lifestyle intervention on the metabolic syndrome: the Diabetes Prevention Program randomized trial. Ann Intern Med 2005; 142:611–619.

188. Liberopoulos EN, Mikhailidis DP, Elisaf MS. Diagnosis and management of the metabolic syndrome in obesity. Obes Rev 2005; 6:283–296.

189. Yki-Jarvinen H. Thiazolidinediones. N Engl J Med 2004; 351:1106–1118.

190. Tiikkainen M, Hakkinen AM, Korsheninnikova E, et al. Effects of rosiglitazone and metformin on liver fat content, hepatic insulin resistance, insulin clearance, and gene expression in adipose tissue in patients with Type 2 diabetes. Diabetes 2004; 53:2169–2176.

191. Lebovitz HE, Banerji MA. Treatment of insulin resistance in diabetes mellitus. Eur J Pharmacol 2004; 490:135–146.

192. Parulkar A, Pendergrass M, Granda-Ayala R, et al. Nonhypoglycemic effects of thiazolidinediones. Ann Intern Med 2001; 134:61–71.

193. Granberry MC, Fonseca VA. Cardiovascular risk factors associated with insulin resistance: effects of oral antidiabetic agents. Am J Cardiovasc Drugs 2005; 5:201–209.

194. Fonseca VA. Management of diabetes mellitus and insulin resistance in patients with cardiovascular disease. Am J Cardiol 2003; 92:50J–60J.

195. Nesto RW, Bell D, Bonow RO, et al. Thiazolidinedione use, fluid retention, and congestive heart failure: a consensus statement from the American Heart Association and American Diabetes Association. Circulation 2003; 108:2941–2948.

196. Chiasson JL, Josse RG, Gomis R, et al. Acarbose treatment and the risk of cardiovascular disease and hypertension in patients with impaired glucose tolerance: the STOP-NIDDM trial. JAMA 2003; 290:486–494.

197. Smith T, Gerich JE. Insulin Secretogogues. In: Fonseca V, ed. Clinical Diabetes. Philadelphia: Elsevier Science, 2006;

198. Gerich J. Oral hypoglycemic agents. N Engl J Med 1989; 321:1231–1245.

199. Culy CR, Jarvis B. Repaglinide: a review of its therapeutic use in Type 2 diabetes mellitus. Drugs 2001; 61:1625–1660.

200. Dunn C, Faulds D. Nateglinide. Drugs 2000; 60:607–615.

201. Langtry H, Balfour J. Glimepiride. A review of its use in the management of Type 2 diabetes mellitus. Drugs 1998; 55:563–584.

202. Hu S, Boettcher BR, Dunning BE. The mechanisms underlying the unique pharmacodynamics of nateglinide. Diabetologia 2003; 46 (suppl 1), M37–M43.

203. Hu S, Wang S, Fanelli B, et al. Pancreatic beta-cell K_{ATP} channel activity and membrane-binding studies with nateglinide: a comparison with sulfonylureas and repaglinide. J Pharmacol Exp Ther 2000; 293:444–452.

204. Gribble FM, Reimann F. Differential selectivity of insulin secretagogues: mechanisms, clinical implications, and drug interactions. J Diabetes Complications 2003; 17:11–15.

205. Korytkowski M, Thomas A, Reid L, et al. Glimepiride improves both first and second phases of insulin secretion in Type 2 diabetes. Diabetes Care 2002; 25:1607–1611.

206. Simonson D, Ferrannini E, Bevilacqua S, et al. Mechanism of improvement in glucose metabolism after chronic glyburide therapy. Diabetes 1984; 33:838–845.

207. Schade D, Jovanovic L, Schneider J. A placebo-controlled, randomized study of glimepiride in patients with Type 2 diabetes mellitus for whom diet therapy is unsuccessful. J Clin Pharmacol 1998; 38:636–641.

208. Jawa AA, Fonseca VA. Role of insulin secretagogues and insulin sensitizing agents in the prevention of cardiovascular disease in patients who have diabetes. Cardiol Clin 2005; 23:119–138.

209. Drucker DJ. Enhancing incretin action for the treatment of Type 2 diabetes. Diabetes Care 2003; 26:2929–2940.

210. D'Alessio DA, Vahl TP. Glucagon-like peptide 1: evolution of an incretin into a treatment for diabetes. Am J Physiol Endocrinol Metab 2004; 286:E882–E890.

211. Sinclair EM, Drucker DJ. Proglucagon-derived peptides: mechanisms of action and therapeutic potential. Physiology (Bethesda.) 2005; 20:357–365.

212. List JF, Habener JF. Glucagon-like peptide 1 agonists and the development and growth of pancreatic beta-cells. Am J Physiol Endocrinol Metab 2004; 286:E875–E881.

213. Wang Q, Li L, Xu E, et al. Glucagon-like peptide-1 regulates proliferation and apoptosis via activation of protein kinase B in pancreatic INS-1 beta cells. Diabetologia 2004; 47:478–487.

214. Deacon CF. Therapeutic strategies based on glucagon-like peptide 1. Diabetes 2004; 53:2181–2189.

215. Vilsboll T, Holst JJ. Incretins, insulin secretion and Type 2 diabetes mellitus. Diabetologia 2004; 47:357–366.

216. Holst JJ, Gromada J. Role of incretin hormones in the regulation of insulin secretion in diabetic and nondiabetic humans. Am J Physiol Endocrinol Metab 2004; 287:E199–E206.

217. Sinclair EM, Drucker DJ. Glucagon-like peptide 1 receptor agonists and dipeptidyl peptidase IV inhibitors: new therapeutic agents for the treatment of Type 2 diabetes. Curr Opin Endocrinol Diabet 2005; 12:146–151.

218. Drucker DJ. Glucagon-like peptide-1 and the islet beta-cell: augmentation of cell proliferation and inhibition of apoptosis. Endocrinology 2003; 144:5145–5148.

219. Farilla L, Bulotta A, Hirshberg B, et al. Glucagon-like peptide 1 inhibits cell apoptosis and improves glucose responsiveness of freshly isolated human islets. Endocrinology 2003; 144:5149–5158.

220. Kolterman OG, Buse JB, Fineman MS, et al. Synthetic exendin-4 (exenatide) significantly reduces postprandial and fasting plasma glucose in subjects with Type 2 diabetes. J Clin Endocrinol Metab 2003; 88:3082–3089.

221. Drucker DJ. Therapeutic potential of dipeptidyl peptidase IV inhibitors for the treatment of Type 2 diabetes. Expert Opin Investig Drugs 2003; 12:87–100.

222. Ahren B, Gomis R, Standl E, et al. Twelve- and 52-week efficacy of the dipeptidyl peptidase IV inhibitor LAF237 in metformin-treated patients with Type 2 diabetes. Diabetes Care 2004; 27:2874–2880.

223. Bailey CJ, Del Prato S, Eddy D, et al. Earlier intervention in Type 2 diabetes: the case for achieving early and sustained glycaemic control. Int J Clin Pract 2005; 59:1309–1316.

224. Del Prato S, Felton AM, Munro N, et al. Improving glucose management: ten steps to get more patients with Type 2 diabetes to glycaemic goal. Int J Clin Pract 2005; 59:1345–1355.

225. Garber AJ. Using dose-response characteristics of therapeutics agents for treatment decisions in Type 2 diabetes. Diabetes Obes Metab 2000; 2:139–147.

226. Scheen AJ, Lefebvre PJ. Oral antidiabetic agents. A guide to selection. Drugs 1998; 55:225–236.

227. Kerenyi Z, Samer H, James R, et al. Combination therapy with rosiglitazone and glibenclamide compared with upward titration of glibenclamide alone in patients with Type 2 diabetes mellitus. Diabetes Res Clin Pract 2004; 63:213–223.

7

Dyslipidemia in the Metabolic Syndrome

Natalia B. Volkova

Department of Internal Medicine, University of California San Francisco, Fresno, California, U.S.A.

Prakash C. Deedwania

Cardiology Division, University of California San Francisco School of Medicine and Fresno Central San Joaquin Valley Medical Education Program, Fresno and Stanford University, Palo Alto, California, U.S.A.

SUMMARY

- The atherogenic lipid abnormalities associated with metabolic syndrome are comparable to dyslipidemia found in patients with type 2 diabetes.
- The increase in triglyceride-rich remnant particles in the postprandial state in patients with metabolic syndrome could play a major role in development of atherosclerosis and subsequent cardiovascular disease.
- The dyslipidemia is a central player in the development of atherosclerosis in the setting of insulin resistance and other components of the metabolic syndrome
- The treatment options currently available for patients with metabolic syndrome are similar to treatment strategies in patients with type 2 diabetes.
- Atherogenic dyslipidemia in metabolic syndrome is an important modifiable risk factor for coronary artery disease and the current pharmacologic approach to modify dyslipidemia includes statins, fibrates, niacin, and peroxisome proliferator–activated receptor agonists and, possibly in the future, endocannabinoid receptor blockers.

INTRODUCTION

An atherogenic dyslipidemia is an integral component of metabolic syndrome, and a major contributor to the cardiovascular risks in patients with the metabolic syndrome. A combination of various risk factors, noted in this condition can lead to significant increase in the risks of cardiovascular disease (CVD). For example, it was demonstrated that addition of dyslipidemia to the presence of diabetes or hypertension results in increased risk of myocardial infarction by 19-fold (1). An abnormal lipid profile has been demonstrated to be a more significant risk factor for CVD than either hypertension or diabetes alone (1).

Although, the typical lipid abnormalities defined in patients with the metabolic syndrome consist of a triad: increased triglycerides, decreased high-density lipoprotein (HDL) cholesterol, and increased small, dense low-density lipoprotein (LDL) cholesterol, there are several additional abnormalities that might play an important role in atherosclerosis.

The role of LDL-cholesterol (LDL-C) in the development of CVD is indisputable; however, despite this fact, it is necessary to emphasize that patients with the metabolic syndrome have far more complex lipid abnormalities. The atherogenic lipid abnormalities associated with the metabolic syndrome are comparable to dyslipidemia found in patients with type 2 diabetes.

PATHOPHYSIOLOGIC MECHANISMS OF DYSLIPIDEMIA IN THE METABOLIC SYNDROME

The initiating step responsible for producing dyslipidemia in patients with the metabolic syndrome starts from the insulin resistance at the level of adipose tissue leading to increased release and decreased clearance of free (nonesterified) fatty acids (FFAs). Visceral adipocytes release their FFA into the portal venous system and are taken up by the liver in proportion to their circulating concentration (2).

Increased hepatic secretion of very low-density lipoprotein (VLDL) is considered to be one of the important mechanisms of atherogenic dyslipidemia in patients with the metabolic syndrome and leads to hypertriglyceridemia, which is often one of the earliest manifestations of insulin resistance (2–4).This can also lead to increased level of apolipoprotein B (Apo B), regulated at the posttranslational stage by the availability of lipids for synthesis of VLDL particle core. Increased VLDL concentrations could be also due to decreased degradation or inhibition of microsomal triglyceride transfer protein activity, a protein, which is a main component of the VLDL-assembly process (2,5). Cholesterol ester transfer protein (CETP) exchanges excessive VLDL triglycerides for cholesterol esters with HDL and LDL. HDL particles become triglyceride-rich and hydrolyzed by hepatic lipase, leading to the reduction in the particle size (Fig. 1) (6).

HDL particles are varied in size, and are classified as small, dense HDL_3 or large HDL_2 particles (7). Typical changes in HDL particle size in patients with the metabolic syndrome are similar to those observed in diabetics including

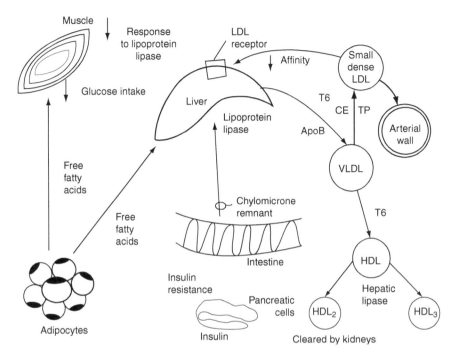

Figure 1 Pathophysiologic mechanisms of dyslipidemia in metabolic syndrome. *Abbreviations*: LDL, low density lipoprotein; VLDL, very low density lipoprotein; HDL, high density lipoprotein; CETP, cholesterol ester transfer protein.

reduction in the HDL_2 subspecies with an increase in HDL_3 subfraction. This trend toward a smaller HDL particle size is considered a risk factor for atherogenesis; in contrast, the larger particles of HDL_2 subfraction are thought to be cardioprotective and antiatherogenic (8). The increased concentrations of VLDL in patients with the metabolic syndrome result in the increased production of small, dense LDL particles. Currently, seven different subtypes of LDL have been identified (9). There is direct correlation between increased levels of VLDL with increased density and decreased size of LDL particles. The increased concentrations of small, dense LDL particles have been shown to be closely associated with high triglycerides levels (10–12). The reduced affinity of small, dense LDL in plasma to LDL receptor leads to prolongation of circulation time for this particle (9).

Insulin resistance has another mechanism that leads to abnormal lipid profiles in the metabolic syndrome patients. It includes impaired clearance of lipid and lipoprotein particles. Insulin resistance is associated with increase in hepatic lipase activity, leading to fast removal of HDL particles, especially HDL_2 subfraction. Activity of lipoprotein lipase synthesized in muscle and adipose tissue is also impaired in the state of insulin resistance. This results in decreased hydrolysis of triglyceride-rich VLDL in capillary endothelial cell beds and conversion of triglycerides into FFAs, which are cleared by the liver (13–15). Increases in FFA concentrations due to increased adipose tissue efflux and impaired insulin-mediated skeletal muscle uptake are frequently found in patients with the metabolic syndrome and diabetes mellitus (16,17). Elevated FFA concentrations can also influence glucose metabolism and impair glucose uptake by the skeletal muscle (18). In patients with insulin resistance and type 2 diabetes, intravenous infusion of lipid emulsions and heparin that leads to increased FFA levels has been shown to increase gluconeogenesis and balanced by reduction in glycogenolysis leading to unchanged net glucose production (3,19). Elevated levels of FFAs in plasma also impair hepatic insulin extraction and may contribute to peripheral hyperinsulinemia in patients with the metabolic syndrome (20).

Chronic exposure of pancreatic β-cell to FFAs impairs insulin secretion, though acute exposure increases glucose-stimulated insulin secretion (21). In patients with the metabolic syndrome, esterified fatty acids in the form of triglycerides are deposited in muscle, liver, heart, and pancreas leading to impaired function of these organs (22). The fatty deposits in the liver can lead to the serious complication of nonalcoholic steatoto-hepatitis (NASH). There is preliminary evidence that NASH might be amenable to treatment with thiazolidinediones, which lower elevated levels of FFAs by improving insulin sensitivity in muscle, liver, and adipose tissue (23,24).

Another abnormality of lipid metabolism attracting interest, and may contribute to increased risk of CVD in patients with the metabolic syndrome, is postprandial hyperlipidemia. In the postprandial state, i.e., after food digestion, the plasma concentration of chylomicrons increases. These triglyceride-rich remnant particles compete with endogenous triglyceride-rich proteins (VLDL-triglyceride) to be cleared by the liver resulting in exaggerated and prolonged postprandial circulating lipid levels. It is known that such postprandial hyperlipidemia is associated with endothelial dysfunction. Thus, the increase in triglyceride-rich remnant particles in the postprandial state in patients with the metabolic syndrome could play a major role in the development of atherosclerosis and subsequent CVD (25).

In summary, high levels of VLDL and high triglycerides, coupled with low levels of HDL-cholesterol (HDL-C), with a predominance of small, dense LDL-C particles are typical features of dyslipidemia seen in the metabolic syndrome. In patients with the metabolic syndrome, the suppression of FFA release from adipose tissue is impaired, secondary to insulin resistance (26). This translates into increased influx of FFAs into the liver, the consequences of which are: an increase in hepatic production and release of VLDL and triglycerides, associated with decreased clearance of these substances, resulting in increase in circulating levels of these lipids. Transportation of cholesterol and triglyceride ester among HDL, LDL, and VLDL leads to formation of triglyceride-rich LDL and HDL particles, which become the preferred substrate for hepatic lipase. Due to impaired activity of hepatic lipase, there is poor clearance of small, dense particles of HDL-C, which are more atherogenic and have higher susceptibility to oxidation. Elevated levels of triglyceride-rich lipoproteins lower HDL-C by inducing cholesterol exchange from

HDL to VLDL via CETP. A high proportion of small, dense LDL particles have been classified as a LDL subclass B, or atherogenic lipoprotein phenotype (27).

The atherogenic dyslipidemia of the metabolic syndrome is similar to the common form of combined hyperlipidemia, and there appears to be an overlap of these two phenotypes (28). The cardiovascular outcomes associated with the atherogenic dyslipidemia typical in the metabolic syndrome patients are much worse, compared to clinical outcomes in patients with isolated elevation of LDL-C (29). The patients with this lipid triad are more likely to have other features of the metabolic syndrome, e.g., hypertension and glucose intolerance, which puts them at greater risk for cardiovascular event (30).

Despite complex pathophysiology of the lipid abnormalities in the metabolic syndrome, it is crucial for clinicians to recognize associated cardiovascular risks and manage them effectively. In the following section, we will discuss the association between dyslipidemia and CVD risk and the effective management of atherogenic dyslipidemia in the metabolic syndrome.

DYSLIPIDEMIA AND CARDIOVASCULAR DISEASE RISK IN PATIENTS WITH THE METABOLIC SYNDROME

Elevated triglycerides levels and decreased HDL-C levels are included in the criteria for the diagnosis of the metabolic syndrome according to the National Cholesterol Education Program (NCEP) and World Health Organization (WHO) definitions (31). As already discussed, these lipid abnormalities are recognized as risk factors for atherosclerotic CVD (32,33). More than half of the patients diagnosed with the metabolic syndrome have elevated LDL (34). A meta-analysis of seventeen population-based prospective studies demonstrated that after adjustment for HDL-C levels and other risk factors increases in plasma triglycerides levels were linked to increases in coronary artery disease (CAD) in men of 14% and in women of 37% (35). Triglyceride-rich VLDL particles play an important role in atherogenic effects of elevated triglycerides level leading to increase in CAD risk (3,36,37). It is well known that diminished levels of HDL-C are associated with increases in the risk of heart disease (38,39). Effects on cholesterol efflux on cellular level, anti-inflammatory properties, and direct antioxidative properties are well-described functions of HDL-C. Mediated by CETP, reduced HDL-C levels are often associated with elevated triglycerides in patients with the metabolic syndrome (40,41).

A number of prospective clinical trials have demonstrated that the combination of high triglyceride levels with decreased HDL-C is strongly associated with an enhanced risk of CAD (42–44). The Veterans Affairs HDL Intervention Trial conducted in men with HDL-C levels below 40 mg/dL (1.03 mmol/L) demonstrated decreased coronary events associated with increased HDL_3 particles after treatment with gemfibrozil (45). As a consequence, of the increased transfer of HDL-C for triglyceride-rich VLDL mediated by CETP, patients with the metabolic syndrome have small HDL particles typical of individuals with visceral obesity and insulin resistance (7). There is also important evidence that, in vitro, small, dense LDL-C particles typically encountered in patients with the metabolic syndrome contributes to arterial damage. This subclass of particles has reduced LDL receptor affinity, greater propensity for transport into subendothelial space, and demonstrate increased binding to arterial wall proteoglycans; small-dense LDL particles have an increased susceptibility to oxidative modifications (46–50). Analysis of the biomarker data indicated that individuals with small dense LDL had a 3.6-fold increase in risk for heart attack as compared to individuals with large, buoyant LDL with five years follow up as demonstrated by Quebec Cardiovascular Study (51). The NCEP Adult Treatment Panel III (ATP) III emphasized the importance of recognition and focused attention to the metabolic syndrome. The major risk factors leading to the epidemic of this syndrome in the United States are visceral obesity, physical inactivity, and an atherogenic diet.

Recent studies suggest that some of the changes leading to the metabolic syndrome may originate in utero and continue to progress during childhood and adolescence, reaching in prevalence in severely obese youngsters almost 50% (52–56). It is estimated that about 47 million U.S. residents have the metabolic syndrome (including those with diabetes), corresponding to 22% of men and 24% of women aged 20 years and above, and it rises to more than 40% in patients older than 60 years of age (57). Based on the NCEP definition, the unadjusted prevalence of the metabolic syndrome was recently found to be as high as 35%, and if the new International Diabetes Federation definition was used, the unadjusted prevalence of the metabolic syndrome was 39.0% (58). The environmental factors and changes in the lifestyle are considered the major contributors to the global epidemic of obesity and the metabolic syndrome. It is possible that changes in people's behavior, which lead to consumption of high calorie, refined food in association with decreased levels of physical activity mainly responsible for obesity and the metabolic syndrome (59).

The growth in prevalence of the metabolic syndrome parallels the dramatic rise in prevalence of obesity, which highlights the need of attention focus among health professionals to warranty aggressive treatment of the multiple components of this condition (60,61).

Individuals with the metabolic syndrome are at a threefold greater risk of CAD and stroke, and more than a fourfold greater risk of cardiovascular mortality (60,62). This group of patients requires specific attention to minimize their risks by treating aggressively each component of the metabolic syndrome.

MANAGEMENT OF DYSLIPIDEMIA IN PATIENTS WITH THE METABOLIC SYNDROME

The Importance of Therapeutic Lifestyle Changes

Visceral or abdominal obesity, which presents clinically as an increase in waist circumference due to the increased amount of visceral adipose tissue, is strongly associated with the metabolic syndrome and the related cardiovascular risk factors (Table 1). However, the absolute waist circumference criteria as described by ATP III guidelines may not be suitable for certain populations, such as South and East Asians and other immigrant groups. In these individuals, WHO criteria, which utilize the waist-to-hip ratio, might be more appropriate in identifying patients with the metabolic syndrome (Table 2). Waist circumference was shown independently to predict obesity-related CVD even in patients with normal weight (63). In the International Diabetes Federation recommendations from 2005, the diagnosis of visceral obesity can be made based on the waist circumference in Europeans: male more than 94 cm and female more than 80 cm, in contrast to ATP III recommendations for male more than 102 cm and for female more than 88 cm. ATP III described the "obesity epidemic" to be primarily responsible for the rising prevalence of the metabolic syndrome (64). Increased visceral adipose tissue is considered a major factor responsible for many of the abnormalities associated with the metabolic syndrome including insulin resistance. Adipocyte is now recognized as an important secretory organ (Fig. 2) (65). Adipocyte-secreted molecules are called adipocytokines, one of which is adiponectin, and it is considered an important mediator for insulin sensitivity (66). Current evidence suggests that low levels of adiponectin are not only a marker of cardiovascular risk but also a significant contributor to the pathophysiological process involving atherosclerosis. Modest weight reduction of 10% led to significant increase in serum adiponectin levels in overweight diabetic and nondiabetic patients (67). Similar result were observed in another study evaluating obese patients undergoing gastric bypass surgery (68,69). However, the removal of subcutaneous fat by liposuction did not significantly improve obesity-related metabolic abnormalities and could not achieve the metabolic benefits of weight loss (70). This emphasizes the pivotal

Table 1 Modified ATP III (AHA/NHLBI)/Definition of Metabolic Syndrome[a]

Risk factor	Characteristic
Waist circumference	Men > 102 cm (>40 in.)
	Women > 88 cm (>35 in.)
Triglycerides	≥150 mg/dL (≥1.69 mmol/L) or on medication to lower triglycerides
High-density lipoprotein (HDL)- cholesterol (C)	Men < 40 mg/dL (<1.03 mmol/L) Women <50 mg/dL (<1.29 mmol/L), or on medication to raise HDL-C
Blood pressure	≥ 130 or ≥85 mmHg, or on antihypertensive medication
Fasting glucose	≥100 mg/dL (≥5.55 mmol/L), or on antidiabetic agents

[a]The diagnosis of metabolic syndrome is made when three or more of these risk factors are present.
Abbreviation: AHA/NHLBI, American Heart Association/National Heart Lung and Blood Institute.
Source: From Refs. 31 and 94.

Table 2   World Health Organization Criteria for the Metabolic Syndrome

Essential component:
  Impaired glucose regulation or diabetes and/or insulin resistance (under hyperinsulinemic
    conditions, glucose uptake below lowest quartile for background population)

Plus two of the following:
  Raised arterial pressure (≥ 140/90 mmHg)
  Raised plasma triglycerides (≥ 1.7 mmol/L; 150 mg/dL) and/or low HDL-cholesterol
    (<0.9 mmol/L; 35 mg/dL in men: <1.0 mmol/L, 39 mg/dL in women)
  Central obesity (males: waist-to-hip ratio >0.90; females: waist-to-hip ratio > 0.85)
    and/or BMI > 30 kg/m²
  Microalbuminuria (urinary albumin excretion rate ≥ 20 g/min or albumin:creatinine
    ratio ≥ 30 mg/g)

Abbreviations: HDL, high-density lipoprotein; BMI, body mass index.

role of visceral adipose tissue in the pathophysiological mechanisms of insulin resistance and related cytokines abnormalities.

Therefore, the initial goal for the treatment should be mainly directed toward the reduction in visceral fat by physiological means such as weight modifying diet and physical activity. To achieve successful weight loss, an individual has to spend more energy than consumed on a daily basis. No specific diet is currently recommended for patients with the metabolic syndrome in the absence of diabetes. Diets incorporating reduction of caloric intake and increased caloric expenditure have

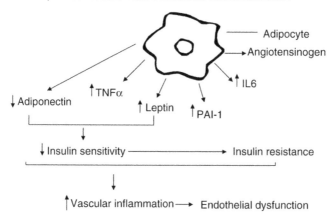

Figure 2   Role of adipocyte in visceral obesity and metabolic syndrome. *Abbreviations*: IL, interleukin; PAI, Plasiminogen activator inhibitor; TNFα tissue necrosis factor alpha.

demonstrated success in losing weight. To achieve long-term diet induced changes in weight management, it is important to increase servings of fruits, vegetables, low-fat dairy products and high-fiber whole grains, which are considered low-energy nutrient-dense food in combination with a decrease in low-nutrient, high-caloric food, e.g., "fast food," along with regular physical activity (70). In the recent large prospective study of 42,504 U.S. professional men, who were followed for up to 12 years, two major dietary patterns were identified—a prudent pattern, characterized by a high consumption of vegetables, fruits, fish, poultry, and whole grains; and a Western pattern, characterized by a high consumption of red meat, processed meat, high-fat dairy products, French fries, refined grains, and sweets and desserts. The prudent diet was associated with a modestly lower risk for type 2 diabetes (relative risk 0.84, CI 0.70–1.00). The Western pattern, however, was associated with a substantially higher risk for type 2 diabetes (relative risk 1.59, CI 1.32–1.90). This association was stronger than that for individual foods and was independent of body mass index (BMI), physical activity, family history of diabetes, and age. The combination of a Western dietary pattern with a low level of physical activity or obesity was associated with a particularly high risk for type 2 diabetes (relative risk for low level of physical activity 1.96, CI 1.35–2.84; and relative risk for obesity 11.2, CI 8.07–15.6) (71). It is important to note that physician needs to focus on each patient's specific metabolic requirements and dietary habits in order to provide appropriate and sustainable dietary modifications. Furthermore, sustained dietary changes will require continued physician-counseling and nutritionist support to maintain the weight loss without compromising electrolyte balance and adequate vitamin intake.

Therapeutic lifestyle changes are a crucial part of the management strategy in the metabolic syndrome. Current evidence suggests that the longer the behavior therapy program, the better the long-term weight loss outcome compared with standard treatment. As recently suggested, models of therapeutic lifestyle changes, which could be utilized in the metabolic syndrome, describes visits intervals and goals for follow up (Fig. 3) (72). Structured meal plans, which provide adequate nutrition with portion size restriction for at least two meals a day may improve the risk factors for the metabolic syndrome and assist with healthy meal choices. Strategies for optimizing lifestyle interventions are discussed in more detail in Chapter 10.

Based on current evidence, patients with the metabolic syndrome should benefit from regular physical activity. The exercise program is an important component of successfully maintaining weight loss in the longer term; the effect of exercise alone on weight loss is not as powerful as when combined with caloric restriction. Although the previously recommended 30 minutes of physical activity a day five times a week was considered adequate, after the recent review of the data and the results of epidemiologic studies, the recent multidisciplinary expert panel recommends 60 minutes of daily physical activity for adults and children (73). It is recommended that every patient should have an individual readiness evaluation by his or her primary care physician. Obstacles to daily exercise should

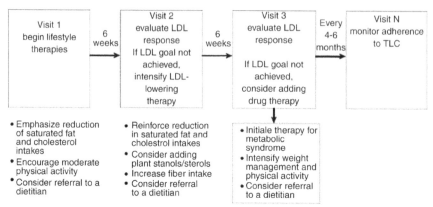

Figure 3   Model of steps in TLC. *Abbreviations*: LDL, low-density lipoprotein; TLC, therapeutic lifestyle changes. *Source*: From Ref. 31.

be discussed and modified to implement the exercise program. Patients need to be given advice regarding the importance of warm-up and cool-down periods and the incorporation of the exercise into daily life activities. The exercise recommendations should include setting certain goals as improving cardiovascular fitness, increasing strength with resistance training, and enhancing flexibility through a wide range of motion.

Pharmacologic Approaches to Weight Management

There are currently few medications available for the treatment of obesity. For patients who have a BMI (≥ 27 kg/m^2 with complications of obesity, e.g., diabetes, or patients with an increased BMI ≥ 30 kg/m^2 without such complications), the U.S. Food and Drug Administration (FDA) has approved two drugs for long-term weight management: sibutramine (Meredia$^\circledR$) and orlistat (Xenical$^\circledR$). Sibutramine therapy induced greater body weight loss than placebo in hypertensive obese patients in Brazilian study, though no clinically significant change in lipid profile was observed in both groups (74). Orlistat is inhibitor of pancreatic lipase, which leads to decreased fat absorption in the intestine. Steatorrhea is a common side effect, as well as reduction in fat-soluble vitamins (vitamin D and E), and supplementation of these vitamins while on orlistat is sometimes recommended. Results in routine clinical practice are variable; safety issues with sibutramine and tolerability issues with orlistat must be borne in mind. Weight loss in response to a reduced calorie diet and orlistat administration in obese hypercholesterolemic patients was associated with a significant decrease in plasma LDL cholesterol levels and the improvement was greatest in patients with combined dyslipidemia (type IIB) (75). A recently published study from Greece with six months follow-up showed that treatment with orlistat and hypocaloric diet in patients with the metabolic syndrome and type 2 diabetes had favorable effects on cardiovascular risk factors with statistically significant reduction in total cholesterol and LDL-C, though no difference was found in triglycerides and HDL-C (76).

There is growing interest regarding the role of drugs that modify the endocannabinoid system; such drugs may have applications in the treatment of obesity and the metabolic syndrome. It has been shown that endocannabinoid receptors are present not only in the limbic area of the brain, but are also located in gastrointestinal tract and adipose tissue. Endocannabinoid receptor activity has been shown to be a key to the appetite stimulation and aspects of motivation in eating, possible mediating the craving for and enjoyment of the most desired, and most fattening, foods (77). Fat and glucose metabolism have been found to be modulated by endocannabinoids (77). Selective pharmacological endocannabinoid receptor blockade have been demonstrated to suppress the motivation to eat, and results in reduced consumption of energy-dense foods. Endocannabinoid antagonists may influence adiposity through direct metabolic mechanisms as well as via alterations in food intake (77). Selective endocannabinoid receptor blockers not only help in achieving weight reduction, but they are also associated with favorable changes in dyslipidemia. One of the first cannabinoid-1 receptor blockers—rimonabant, 20 mg daily—produced statistically significant decreases in insulin resistance and circulating triglycerides levels; these effects were accompanied by an increase in HDL-C levels of 23.4% with 20mg and a 15.6% increase with 5mg of rimonabant (p=0.017) compared to placebo; thus, several components of the metabolic syndrome were favorably altered, notably aspects of the characteristic dyslipidemia. No statistically significant changes in triglycerides were noted with a 5 mg dose of rimonabant but a 20 mg dose led to a 15.8% reduction with p-value <0.001. Changes in levels of HDL cholesterol translated into a dose-dependent reduction in the total cholesterol:HDL cholesterol ratio of −15.2% with 20 mg and (78,79). Despite the fact, that no change in levels of LDL cholesterol was observed, the distribution of LDL particles shifted toward larger size in the group receiving 20 mg of rimonabant, as compared with placebo (80). Another important finding was increase in plasma adiponectin level with rimonabant treatment (at a dose of 20 mg) by 57.7%—an increase significantly greater than that observed in the placebo group (79). The drug was generally well tolerated with only mild and transient side effects observed over a one-year treatment period. If this recently developed cannabinoid-1 receptor blocker is approved for clinical use it might prove a useful addition to the presently limited treatment options in patients with the metabolic syndrome (78,79).

Surgical therapy of obesity may achieve the most profound and long-lasting weight loss, leading to improvement in the comorbidities related to obesity, including diabetes, hypertension, hyperlipidemia, and insulin resistance. Gastric bypass surgery is considered the most effective bariatric procedure and may help achieve permanent weight loss of excess body weight in many patients. Two hundred thirty-two morbidly obese patients had a 12 month follow up after gastric bypass surgery in Chile. During follow up, BMI decreased from 44 to 29.3 kg/m^2. Total and HDL cholesterol, blood glucose, and insulin resistance significantly decreased from the third month after surgery. Diabetes disappeared in

97% of diabetic subjects, blood pressure normalized in 53% of subjects, with hypertension and serum lipid levels returned to normal in 88% of subjects with dyslipidemia (80). It is also important to note that patients after surgery need to be managed with the help of nutritionist as well as physical and occupational therapists to achieve sustained weight loss.

Insulin Resistance

There is a widely held view that the central abnormality responsible for many of the features of the metabolic syndrome that increase cardiovascular risk is insulin resistance. Insulin resistance can be defined as an inability to respond normally to various actions of insulin. However, insulin resistance and the metabolic syndrome are not synonymous. In the insulin resistant state, cells are deprived from glucose, which is critical for metabolic activity. The fasting plasma glucose concentration is the variable with the greatest positive predictive value for insulin resistance and hyperinsulinemia, especially when between 110 and 126 mg/dL (6.05 and 6.93 mmol/L). Despite the above, the currently recommended fasting plasma glucose concentration is not as sensitive an indicator due to the fact that majority of insulin resistant individuals have glucose concentrations less than 110 mg/dL (6.05 mmol/L) (81). Due to these limitations, recent American Diabetic Association statement defines plasma glucose concentration higher than 100 mg/dL (5.5 mmol/L) the new cutpoint for defining impaired fasting glucose (Table 1).

Postprandial hyperglycemia has been considered by some investigators as an early marker of insulin resistance that may have prognostic implications. The Collaborative Analysis of Diagnostic Criteria in Europe (DECODE) study, which summarized the results of 22 large, European population-based studies, revealed that increasing fasting plasma glucose and two-hour postchallenge glucose were associated with increasing risk of cardiovascular death. In this study, insulin resistance, which was indicated indirectly by increased two-hour postchallenge blood glucose concentrations, was better predictor of cardiovascular mortality in subjects without diabetes than elevated fasting glucose levels (82). Associated metabolic abnormalities, e.g., postprandial dyslipidemia and oxidative stress, may be relevant mechanistically (83). The potential clinical importance of targeting postprandial hyperglycemia was supported by the results of a recent placebo-controlled mutlicenter study, which suggested a reduction in the risk of incident CVD in insulin resistant patients, who were taking an α-glucosidase inhibitor (acarbose), decreasing postprandial hyperglycemia (84). The mean serum lipid profiles did not differ among the four groups and were not affected by acarbose treatment during the 12-month study period (84). These results require confirmation.

The study of 3234 individuals with impaired glucose tolerance randomly assigned to receive intensive lifestyle intervention, metformin, or placebo. Triglyceride levels fell in all treatment groups, but fell significantly more with intensive lifestyle intervention. Total cholesterol and LDL cholesterol levels were similar among treatment groups. Intensive lifestyle intervention significantly increased the HDL cholesterol level and reduced the cumulative incidence of the proatherogenic LDL phenotype B (85).

In the open-label extension study of 828 patients with type 2 diabetes with 52 weeks follow up, treatment with glyburide/metformin had a durable, favorable effect on lipid levels, particularly in those with poor glycemic control and dyslipidemia at baseline (86).

Exercise and weight loss ameliorate insulin resistance and may in some cases help prevent or delay onset of the metabolic syndrome or diabetes mellitus. However, drug treatment that improves insulin resistance in those who cannot change their lifestyle for one reason or another is also needed. Current pharmacologic approaches are only partially successful at improving the consequences of insulin resistance. These include hyperglycemia, dyslipidemia, abnormal coagulation and fibrinolysis, and hypertension; each risk factor may require the use of at least one specific medication. Thus, the recent introduction of drugs that may help reverse the hypothesized fundamental cause of the metabolic syndrome, i.e., insulin resistance, is regarded as an important step. The insulin-sensitizing agents known as thiazolidinediones, which are selective ligands of the nuclear transcription factor peroxisome proliferator–activated receptor-γ (PPAR-γ), are the first drugs to address the basic defect (87). The two currently available PPAR-γ agonists, rosiglitazone and pioglitazone consistently lower fasting and postprandial glucose concentrations, insulin concentrations as well as FFA concentrations. These drugs are currently licensed for treatment of type 2 diabetes. Thiazolidinediones also improve aspects of the complex dyslipidemia of diabetes. Pioglitazone has been shown to consistently reduce circulating triglyceride concentrations and to increase HDL-C levels (87). Both pioglitazone and rosiglitazone have effects on the buoyancy of LDL particles that are thought to offset increases in the levels of LDL-C, these medication reduce visceral fat and increase subcutaneous fat as well as increase adiponectin levels (87). A recent clinical trial—the PROactive study—studied the impact of pioglitazone add-on therapy versus placebo in patients with type 2 diabetes and established CVD (88). This trial, aspects of which have been criticized, provides some support for a beneficial cardiovascular effect of pioglitazone, albeit at the expense of a higher incidence of reported heart failure, a side effect that was not adjudicated (89). The mechanisms of benefit in this trial may reflect the combined effects of the drug on glycemia, dyslipidemia, and blood pressure; it remains unclear whether targeting insulin resistance per se is advantageous.

Although NASH is not currently a recognized part of the metabolic syndrome diagnostic criteria, it is not infrequently encountered in obese individuals who have other features of the syndrome. More common still are lesser degrees of fatty infiltration without a significant inflammatory component, i.e., nonalcoholic fatty-liver disease (NAFLD) (90).

Since a proportion of patients with NASH progress to hepatic fibrosis and even cirrhosis, this is a potentially important public health issue. Preliminary data suggest that thiazolidinediones can improve not only laboratory markers of NASH but also improve the histological status of these patients (91). Further studies are required, not least since the progenitor drug in this class—troglitazone—was withdrawn because of reports of serious, sometimes fatal, idiosyncratic hepatotoxicity (87). None of the thiazolidinediones has been licensed for the treatment of NASH. The importance of rigorously controlling any associated dyslipidemia in patients with NAFLD or NASH has not been adequately studied.

Agonists of the PPAR-α, such as fenofibrate and gemfibrozil have cardioprotective effect due to the lipid-lowering action. This, coupled with the aforementioned glucose-lowering effects of PPAR-γ agonists, have led to a search for dual PPAR agonists—compounds that might combine the therapeutic effects of PPAR-α and -γ activation (87). According to the Food, Drug, and Cosmetic Act report of new drug applications, as many as eight dual PPAR agonists are currently under clinical development, including two in phase 3 trials (87). The FDA advisory board has recently recommended approval for the first dual PPAR agonist—muraglitazar. However, concerns have been raised regarding the benefit versus safety of this agent; accordingly, it has been recommended that there is a need for a large randomized prospective clinical trial to evaluate the effects of muraglitzar on the morbidity and mortality.

SPECIFIC MANAGEMENT OF DYSLIPIDEMIA IN THE METABOLIC SYNDROME

The Role of Dietary Modification

Despite the complex pathophysiology of the lipid abnormalities in metabolic syndrome, it is crucial for clinicians to recognize and manage them effectively in the hope to reduce increased risks of cardiovascular events. As previously discussed, weight reduction and lifestyle modification are crucial in the general management of metabolic syndrome including dyslipidemia. However, it is important to note, that the previously recommended American Heart Association diet consisting of low-calorie, low-fat, high-carbohydrates diets can lead to elevated triglycerides levels and reduce HDL-C. The clinical relevance of these changes is not clear and in general long-term effect of low-fat diet is relatively minor and will lead to reduction of HDL-C by 5% to 7% only. It is prudent to avoid diets which might reduce levels of HDL-C due to its cardioprotective role (91). Individuals with metabolic syndrome should reduce the intake of saturated fat and carbohydrates, and increase the proportion of protein in their diet (92). Although the precise amount of protein which is recommended in the diet for patients with metabolic syndrome has not been established, substituting soy for animal protein may help reduce LDL-C and triglyceride levels (92).

It has also been shown that both plant-derived and marine-derived omega-3 fatty acids can reduce the incidence of cardiovascular events. Also omega-3 fatty acids from fish oil, if consumed in the dose of 4 g a day, can reduce triglycerides by 25% to 30% with accompanying minor elevations of LDL-C of 5% to 10% and HDL-C of 1% to 3%. The triglyceride-lowering effect of the omega-3 fatty acids is dose related though low doses as 2g a day could be effective in some individuals. In the Gruppo Italiano per 10 Studio della Sopravvivenza nell' Infartomiocardico (GISSI) Prevenzione Trial, the use of the omega-3 fatty acids was shown to reduce the risk of cardiovascular events and sudden cardiac death particularly in patients with impaired systolic function (93). However, additional research is needed to define the role and the optimal dose of omega-3 fatty acids and its specific role, if any in the management of dyslipidemia in metabolic syndrome.

The Role of Statins

The current ATP guidelines recommend the use of 3-hydroxy-3-methylglutaryl coenzyme A reductase inhibitors (statins) as first-line drug therapy in the treatment of high-risk patients with metabolic syndrome. It has been suggested that statins may have multiple indirect effects on the vasculature, beside their direct-cholesterol lowering effect. These positive actions, commonly referred to as pleiotropic effects, include anti-inflammatory actions, improved endothelial function, reduced oxidative stress, decreased risk of thrombosis and platelet aggregation, reduced levels of cell-adhesion molecules and stabilization of vulnerable plaques (94).

Because of the increased risk of cardiovascular events in patients with diabetes and/or the metabolic syndrome, it is important to set aggressive LDL-C goals. The recent results from the Collaborative Atorvastatin Diabetes Study (CARDS) and Anglo-Scandinavian Cardiac Outcomes Trial—Lipid Lowering Arm (ASCOT-LLA) clinical trials have clearly demonstrated the favorable impact of statin therapy on cardiovascular events in patients with diabetes and metabolic syndrome (95,96). Recent clinical trial data suggest that the incidence of coronary events is reduced when LDL-C levels are lowered to approximately 70 mg/dL (1.79 mmol/L) in patients who are at the highest risk (97,98). This level has been recommended as an optional target in patients with overt CVD, who have diabetes or are under threat from multiple cardiovascular risk factors.

In patients with metabolic syndrome, the selection of the statin should be not only based on its efficacy in reducing the LDL-C, but also the overall effect on non-HDL-C. The latter is calculated as total cholesterol minus HDL-C and is regarded as being representative of all the circulating atherogenic lipoproteins. Non-HDL-C level could be utilized in patients with metabolic syndrome-I although data are presently sparse. In a recently published study, non-HDL-C was found to be as good as or better than Apo fractions in the prediction of future cardiovascular events in women (99). Non-HDL-C was found to be useful in patients with type 2 diabetes in predicting cardiovascular events (100). Target levels for non-HDL-C could be easily calculated by adding 30 mg/dL (0.77 mmol/L) to the HDL-C target levels. As recommended by the recent update from the ATP III group, the goal for non-HDL-C in patients with metabolic syndrome should be set at 100 to 130 mg/dL (2.56–3.33 mmol/L). However, this target is not based on clinical trials with cardiovascular outcomes. It is important to note that the currently available statins have different effects not only on LDL-C, but also on triglycerides and HDL-C (97). Comparison of the effects of rosuvastatin to atorvastatin, simvastatin, and pravastatin on atherogenic dyslipidemia in patients with metabolic syndrome demonstrated that while all of the statins had favorable effects on the atherogenic dyslipidemia, rosuvastatin had more favorable effects on atherogenic lipid profile in patients with metabolic syndrome (Table 3) (101). However, whether these differential effects of various statins translate into different clinical outcomes remain to be established.

It is also important to consider that, although in general statins are well tolerated by most patients, there is the potential risk of adverse reactions. Gastrointestinal upset, muscle aches and elevated hepatic transaminase levels are among the most common adverse effects of statins. Serious hepatotoxicity is very rare and usually seen mostly in patients taking high doses; rhabdomyolysis is also very uncommon (97). Despite the low incidence of rhabdomyolysis, or lesser degrees of myositis, the incidence of myalgia attributed to statin therapy can range anywhere between 5% to 10%. However, it is often difficult to establish a cause and effect relationship (97). Patients with metabolic syndrome can be at risk for potential complications due to the fact that they frequently take multiple medications and could have NASH, but benefits of statins in these patients outweigh the potential risks.

The Role of Combination Therapy

Combination therapy using a statin plus a drug from another class of lipid-modifying agents may often be necessary to combat the mixed lipid abnormalities in metabolic syndrome (102). Bile acid–binding resins are now only rarely used as adjuncts to statin therapy in patients for whom additional reduction in LDL-C by 10% to 20% is desired and level of triglycerides is not elevated. Currently available bile acid–resins include cholestyramine, colesevelam, and colestipol. These medications are usually given in doses 4 to 10 g twice a day with meals, as a suspension in juice or water. The increase in triglyceride concentrations induced by bile acid–resins can be a problem especially in patients already prone to hypertriglyceridemia such as that associated with the metabolic syndrome. Due to their mechanism of action based on binding to bile acids in the small intestine and leading to interruption of the entero-hepatic circulation of bile acids and an increase in the conversion of cholesterol to bile in the liver, these agents can inhibit the intestinal absorption of fat-soluble vitamins, warfarin, digoxin, levothyroxin, thiazide diuretics, folic acid, and even statins. Also up to 30% of patients develop abdominal fullness, gas, and constipation while taking bile acid–resins, which could be corrected with dose adjustment and the use of fiber or prune juice in daily diet. Because of the high incidence of undesirable side-effects associated with bile acid–binding resins, they are falling out of favor and their use is largely being replaced by ezetimibe. The latter is the first of a new class of lipid-lowering drugs known as intestinal cholesterol absorption

Table 3 Comparison of the Effects of Statins on Lipids

	Rosuvastatin	Atorvastatin	Simvastatin	Pravastatin
10 mg (*n>*)	49	56	57	69
20 mg (*n>*)	55	48	49	59
40 mg (*n>*)	61	51	59	58
80 mg (*n>*)	NA	65	62	NA
Low-density lipoprotein-cholesterol				
10 mg				
Baseline, mg/dL	191 ± 22	189 ± 16	188 ± 19	188 ± 18 (*See note*)
Percentage change	−43.9 ± 1.7	−36.6 ± 1.6	−27.6 ± 1.6[a]	−20.0 ± 1.5[a]
20 mg				
Baseline, mg/dL	189 ± 18	191 ± 20	191 ± 21	185 ± 14
Percentage change	−53.4 ± 1.7	−41.1 ± 1.8[b]	−37.0 ± 1.7[b]	−23.0 ± 1.6[ab]
40 mg				
Baseline, mg/dL	193 ± 17	191 ± 21	186 ± 16	190 ± 20
Percentage change	−55.3 ± 1.6	−49.6 ± 1.7	−39.4 ± 1.6[bc]	−28.6 ± 1.6[abc]
80 mg				
Baseline, mg/dL	NA	192 ± 20	190 ± 20	NA
Percentage change	NA	−48.8 ± 1.5	−46.6 ± 1.6[c]	NA
Triglycerides				
10 mg				
Baseline, mg/dL	198 ± 56	211 ± 56	201 ± 59	220 ± 59
Percentage change	−22.3 ± 2.9	−22.9 ± 2.7	−15.2 ± 2.7	−12.5 ± 2.5
20 mg				
Baseline, mg/dL	224 ± 68	222 ± 54	217 ± 59	217 ± 58
Percentage change	−24.1 ± 2.8	−24.7 ± 3.0	−22.5 ± 2.9	−12.9 ± 2.7
40 mg				
Baseline, mg/dL	217 ± 51	222 ± 54	209 ± 56	211 ± 60
Percentage change	−33.8 ± 2.6	−30.8 ± 2.9	−21.5 ± 2.7[c]	−15.3 ± 2.7[c]
80 mg				
Baseline, mg/dL	NA	214 ± 54	221 ± 64	NA
Percentage change	NA	−33.3 ± 2.5	−23.0 ± 2.6	NA
High-density lipoprotein cholesterol				
10 mg				
Baseline, mg/dL	47 ± 10	43 ± 9	45 ± 9	45 ± 9
Percentage change	+7.6 ± 1.6	+7.2 ± 1.5	+8.3 ± 1.5	+3.3 ± 1.3
20 mg				
Baseline, mg/dL	45 ± 8	43 ± 8	45 ± 8	44 ± 9
Percentage change	+11.1 ± 1.5	+9.4 ± 1.6	+9.5 ± 1.6	+6.9 ± 1.4
40 mg				
Baseline, mg/dL	44 ± 8	46 ± 8	45 ± 10	45 ± 8
Percentage change	+10.4 ± 1.4	+5.0 ± 1.6	+8.0 ± 1.5	+6.4 ± 1.5

(*Continued*)

Table 3   Comparison of Statins Effects *(Continued)*

	Rosuvastatin	Atorvastatin	Simvastatin	Pravastatin
80 mg				
Baseline, mg/dL	NA	45 ± 11	43 ± 9	NA
Percentage change	NA	+4.7 ± 1.4[b]	+10.0 ± 1.4	NA

[a]$p<0.002$ compared with [a]rosuvastatin 10 mg, [b]rosuvastatin 20 mg, and [c]rosuvastatin 40 mg.
Note: Mean ± SD baseline and least-squares mean ± SE percent changes from baseline in lipids and total cholesterol/HDL-cholesterol ratio in patients with metabolic syndrome receiving rosuvastatin 10–40 mg, atorvastatin 10–80 mg, simvastatin 10–80 mg, or pravastatin 10–40 mg for 6 wk.
Source: From Ref. 101.

inhibitors. Ezetimibe is administered in a once-daily dose of 10 mg and to date its use has generally been free of any major side effects. The coadministration of ezetimibe with stains offers a well-tolerated and efficacious treatment of hypercholesterolemia that produces a degree of LDL-C lowering that is comparable to, or exceeds, the effects of titrating a statin to its maximum recommended dose (103). Combination of atorvastatin with ezetimibe in 628 patients with primary hypercholesterolemia provided significant incremental reductions in LDL-C and triglycerides and increases in HDL-C (104). In some cases, the combination of statin and ezetimibe may result in a small increase in the incidence of elevated liver enzyme levels, although cases of severe hepatotoxicity have not been demonstrated (103).

Based on the current evidence, the European Consensus Panel recommends that the minimum target for HDL-C should be 40 mg/dL (1.03 mmol/L) in patients with metabolic syndrome (105).

Nicotinic acid inhibits the mobilization of FFAs from peripheral tissue, thereby reducing hepatic synthesis of triglycerides and secretion of VLDL-cholesterol and its conversion to LDL-C. Nicotinic acid has a unique ability to decrease triglycerides level by up to 30%. The effects of nicotinic acid on triglycerides is accompanied by an increase in cardioprotective HDL-C (97). Higher doses of nicotinic acid may not be well tolerated—facial flushing being the main clinical problem. The administration of aspirin 325 mg 30 to 60 minutes before each dose of nicotinic acid for a few days, taking nicotinic acid at the end of a meal and avoiding taking the drug with hot liquids can minimize the flushing, which around 10% of patients taking nicotinic acid find intolerable (105). The starting dose is 250 to 500 mg and should be increased monthly to by 500 to 1000 mg to a maximum of 3000 mg a day. Combination of niacin and statin may correct most forms of complex dyslipidemias (106,107). Liver function abnormalities are more frequent in patients who are taking nicotinic acid in combination with stains, especially in the doses 2000 to 3000 mg. Niacin extended-release (Niaspan® or Advicor®) is efficacious and safe and can be the niacin product used to improve dyslipidemias in metabolic syndrome patients, but patients should be closely monitored by physicians during the treatment (108). Other side effects include conjunctivitis, nasal stuffiness, loose bowel movements or diarrhea, acanthosis nigricans, and ichthyosis (97). The use of nicotinic acid in patients with metabolic syndrome is controversial, because it is well known that at higher doses nicotinic acid increases fasting plasma glucose concentrations and has the potential to convert a patient with insulin resistance and glucose intolerance to clinical diabetes. Although it is important to consider this aspect, the clinician should weigh the risk versus benefit in the given individual patient. As discussed above, the fibric-acid derivates (gemfibrozil, clofibrate, fenofibrate) are agonists for hepatic PPAR-α. The fibrates are considered the most effective triglyceride-lowering drugs producing as much as 50% reduction. The two most commonly used fibrate preparations in the United States are gemfibrozil and fenofibrate. Currently fenofibrate is the preferred agent, because it is more effective and causes fewer gastro-intestinal symptoms, myalgias and rhabdomyolysis than gemfibrozil. All fibrates are excreted via the kidney and can therefore accumulate in patients with renal failure and there is a possible increased risk of rhabdomyolysis. Due to their complementary effects, statin and fibrate combinations can improve the complex dyslipidemia of metabolic syndrome, more than either drug alone (109,110). However, the combination of these two agents leads to an increase in the risk of myotoxicity. Gemfibrozil has been found to inhibit statin glucoronidation leading to inhibition of statin elimination. This drug also inhibits the cytochrome P450 enzyme CYP2C8, which can increase the plasma concentration of statins (110–114). In clinical trials using a statin-fibrate combination, myalgia or other muscle symptoms were reported in 1.9% of patients, and elevated creatine kinase levels were reported in 2.1% (110–114). It is also very important to note, that the majority of reports of statin-fibrate—associated myopathy have involved gemfibrozil, and that fenofibrate appears to be associated with much lower risk of this complications when combined with statin, as this combination does not appear to increase statin concentrations (110,111,114). Cerivastatin was withdrawn from U.S. markets because of reports of fatal rhabdomyolysis side effects which happen mainly in combination with gemfibrozil.

SUMMARY

The metabolic syndrome represents a clustering of several coronary risk factors linked with an increased risk of cardiovascular events and development of diabetes. Insulin resistance has been linked to each of the ATP III criteria needed for diagnosis of metabolic syndrome (Table 1). Since insulin resistance is an independent risk factor for CVD, its presence has been thought to be associated with development of atherosclerosis, long before the development of diabetes or manifestation of other features of metabolic syndrome (the "ticking clock hypothesis") (115). Currently, visceral or central adiposity is considered by many investigators to be a key defect linked with whole-body insulin resistance. Increases in visceral adipose tissue mass leads to an elevated FFA influx in portal and systemic circulations. In turn, this initiates a cascade of events that are thought to be responsible for insulin resistance and an atherogenic dyslipidemia (52). Dyslipidemia is a central player in the development of atherosclerosis in the setting of insulin resistance and other components of the metabolic syndrome. The treatment options currently available for patients with metabolic syndrome are similar to treatment strategies in patient with type 2 diabetes. These are centered on therapeutic lifestyle changes and the treatment of the individual components of the syndrome. The overall strategy should include physiological approaches that include regular physical exercise, weight loss, and a prudent diet. The latter should focus on substitution of saturated and trans-fats to non-hydrogenated unsaturated fats, higher consumption of omega-3 fatty acids from fish, fish oil supplements or plant sources, and higher consumption of a diet rich in fruits, vegetables, nuts, and whole grains, and low in refined grain products.

The atherogenic dyslipidemia in metabolic syndrome is an important modifiable risk factor for CHD and the current pharmacologic approach to modify dyslipidemia includes statins, fibrates, niacin, and PPAR agonists and, possibly in the future, endocannabinoid receptor blockers (94). The evidence epidemiological and observational studies outlined in this chapter highlight the importance of increasing awareness among clinicians regarding the strong relationship between dyslipidemia and CVD in metabolic syndrome patients. This evidence also underscores the urgency of intervention and modification of the fatal cascade of events in these patients that lead to a significant increase in mortality and morbidity. The scene is set for the metabolic syndrome to have a major public health impact worldwide in the coming years. There is an urgent need for clinical trials to evaluate and compare the benefits of various therapeutic approaches in the management of the atherogenic dyslipidemia and other modifiable components of the syndrome.

REFERENCES

1. Assmann G, Schulte H. The Prospective Cardiovascular Munster Study: prevalence and hyperlipidemia in persons with hypertension and/or diabetes mellitus and relationship to coronary heart disease. Am Heart J 1988; 116:1713–1724.
2. Lebovitz HE. Insulin Resistance. London: Science press Ltd., 2002:16–18.
3. Krauss RM, Siri PW. Dyslipidemia in type 2 diabetes. Med Clin N Am 2004; 88:897–909.
4. Reynisdottir S, Angelin B, Landgin D, et al. Adipose tissue lipoprotein lipase and hormone-sensitive lipase. Contrasting findings in familial combined hyperlipidemia and insulin resistance syndrome. Arterioscler Thromb Vasc Biol 1997; 17:2287–2292.
5. Fisher EA, Ginsberg HM. Complexity in the secretory pathway: the assembly and secretion of apolipoprotein B-containing lipoproteins. J Biol Chem 2002; 277(20):17377–17380.
6. Hopkins GJ, Barter PJ. Role of triglyceride-rich lipoproteins and hepatic lipase in determining the particle size and composition of high-density lipoproteins. J Lipid Res 1986; 27(12):1265–1277.

7. Pascot A, Lemieux I, Prud'homme D, et al. Reduced HDL particle size as an additional feature for the atherogenic dyslipidemia of abdominal obesity. J Lipid Res 2001; 42(12):2007–2014.

8. Lamarche B, Moorjani S, Cantin B, et al. Associations of HDL_2 and HDL_3 subfractions with ischemic heart disease in men. Prospective results from the Québec Cardiovascular study. Arterioscler Thromb Vasc Biol 1997; 17:1098–1105.

9. Berneis KK, Krauss RM. Metabolic origins and clinical significance of LDL heterogeneity. J Lipid Res 2002; 43(9):1363–1379.

10. McNamara JR, Campos H, Ordovas JM, et al. Effect of gender, age, and lipid status on low density lipoprotein subfraction distribution. Results of Framingham Offspring Study. Arteriosclerosis 1987; 7(5):483–490.

11. Mc Namara JR, Jenner JL, Li Z, et al. Change in LDL particle size is associated with change in plasma triglyceride concentration. Arterioscler Thromb 1992; 12(11):1284–1290.

12. Krauss RM, Williams PT, Lindgren FT, et al. Coordinate changes in levels of human serum low and high density lipoprotein subclasses in healthy men. Arteriosclerosis 1988; 8(2):155–162.

13. Tan CE, Foster L, Caslake MJ, et al. Relations between plasma lipids and postheparin plasma lipases and VLDL and LDL subfraction patterns in normolipemic men an women. Arterioscler Thromb Vas Biol 1995; 15(11):1839–1848.

14. Watson TD, Caslake MJ, Freeman DJ, et al. Determinants of LDL subfraction distribution and concentrations in young normolipidemic subjects. Arterioscler Thromb 1994; 14(6):902–910.

15. Zambon A, Austin MA, Brown BG. Effect of hepatic lipase on LDL in normal men and those with coronary artery disease. Arterioscler Thromb Vas Biol 1993; 13(2):147–153.

16. Boden G. Role of fatty acids in the pathogenesis of insulin resistance and NIDDM. Diabetes 1997; 46(1):3–10.

17. Kelley DE, Simoneau JA. Impaired free fatty acid utilization by skeletal muscle in non–insulin-dependent diabetes mellitus. J Clin Invest 1994; 94(6):2349–2356.

18. Dresner A, Laurent D, Marcucci M, et al. Effects of free fatty acids on glucose transport and IRS-1 associated phosphatidylinositol 3-kinase activity. J Clin Invest 1999; 103(2):253–259.

19. Lewis GF, Carpentier A, Adeli K, et al. Disordered fat storage and mobilization in the pathogenesis of insulin resistance and type 2 diabetes. Endocr Rev 2002; 23(2):201–229.

20. Wiesenthal SR, Sandhu H, McCall RH, et al. Free fatty acid impair hepatic insulin extraction in vivo. Diabetes 1999; 48(4):766–774.

21. Carpentier A, Mittelman SD, Lamrche B, et al. Acute enhancement of insulin secretion by FFA in humans is lost with pronged FFA elevation. Am J Physiol 1999; 276(Pt 1):E1055–E1066.

22. Unger RH, Orci L. Diseases of liporegulation: new perspective on obesity and related disorders. FASEB J 2001; 15(2):312–321.

23. Mayerson AB, Hundal RS, Dufour S, et al. The effects of rosiglitazone on insulin sensitivity, lipolysis, and hepatic and skeletal muscle triglyceride content in patient with type 2 diabetes. Diabetes 2002; 87(6):2784–2791.

24. Miyazaki Y, Mahankali A, Matsuda M, et al. Effect of piogitazone on abdominal fat distribution and insulin sensitivity in type 2 diabetic patients. J Clin Endocrinol Metab 2002; 87(6):2784–2791.

25. Mamo JC, Yu KC, Elsegood CL, et al. Is atherosclerosis exclusively a postprandial phenomenon? Clin Exp Pharmacol Physiol 1997; 24:288–293.
26. Reynisdottir S, Angelin B, Landgin D, et al. Adipose tissue lipoprotein lipase and hormone-sensitive lipase. Contrasting findings in familial combined hyperlipidemia and insulin resistance syndrome. Arterioscler Thromb Vasc Biol 1997; 17:2287–2292.
27. Davy BM, Melby LC. The effect of fiber-rich carbohydrates on features of Syndrome X. J Am Diet assoc 2003; 103(1):86–96.
28. Eckel RH. Familial combined hyperlipidemia and insulin resistance: distant relatives linked by intraabdominal fat? Arterioscler Thromb Vasc Biol 2001; 21:469–470.
29. Castelli WP. Epidemiology of triglycerides: a view from Framingham. Am J Cardiol 1992; 70:3H–9H.
30. Ballantyne CM, Olsson AG, Cook TJ, et al. Influence of low high-density lipoprotein cholesterol and elevated triglyceride on coronary heart disease events and response to simvastatin therapy in 4S. Circulation 2001; 18:3046–3051.
31. Executive summary of the Third Report of the National Cholesterol Education Program (NCEP) Expert Panel on Detection, Evaluation, and Treatment of High Blood Cholesterol in Adults (Adult Treatment Panel III). JAMA 2001; 285:2486–2497.
32. Austin MA, Rodriguez BL, Mc Knight B, et al. Low-density lipoprotein particle size, triglycerides, and high-density lipoprotein cholesterol as a risk factors for coronary heart disease in older Japanese-American men. Am J Cardiol 2000; 86:412–416.
33. Buring JE, O'Connor CT, Goldhaber SZ, et al. Decreased HDL2 and HDL3 cholesterol, Apo A-I and Apo A-II, and increased risk of myocardial infarction. Circulation 1992; 85:22–29.
34. Wong ND, Pio J, Franklin SS, L'Italien GJ, Kamath T, Williams R. Preventing heart disease by nominal and optimal control of blood pressure and lipids in persons with the metabolic syndrome. Am J Cardiol 2003; 91:1421–1426.
35. Hokanson JE, Austin MA. Plasma triglyceride level is a risk factor for cardiovascular disease independent of high-density lipoprotein cholesterol level: a meta-analysis of population based prospective studies. J Cardiovasc Risk 1996; 3(2):213–219.
36. Krauss R. Triglycerides and atherogenic lipoproteins: rationale for lipid management. J Med 1998; 105(suppl 1A):S58–62.
37. Krauss RM. Atherogenicity of triglyceride-rich lipoproteins. Am J Cardiol 1998; 81(suppl 4A):B13–17.
38. Rader DJ. High-density lipoproteins as an emerging therapeutic target for atherosclerosis. JAMA 2003; 290:2322–2324.
39. Gordon DJ, Probstfield JL, Garrison RJ, et al. High-density lipoprotein cholesterol and cardiovascular disease. Four Prospective American Studies. Circulation 1989; 79(1):8–15.
40. Lamarche B, Despres JP, Moorjani S, et al. Triglycerides HDL-cholesterol as risk factor for ischemic heart disease. Results from Quebec cardiovascular study. Atherosclerosis 1996; 119(2):235–245.
41. Tall A. Plasma lipid transfer proteins. Annu Rev Biochem 1995; 64:235–257.
42. Assman G, Schulte H. Relation of high-density lipoprotein cholesterol and triglycerides to incidence of atherosclerotic coronary artery disease (the PROCAM experience). Prospective Cardiovascular Munster study. Am J Cardiol 1992; 70(7):733–737.

43. Jeppesen J, Hein HO, Suadicani P, et al. Relation of high TG-low HDL-cholesterol and LDL cholesterol to the incidence of ischemic heart disease. An 8-year follow-up in the Copenhagen Male Study. Arterioscler Thromb Vas Biol 1997; 17(6):1114–1120.
44. Manninen V, Tenkanen L, Koskinen P, et al. Joint effects of serum triglyceride and LDL cholesterol and HDL cholesterol concentrations on coronary heart disease risk in the Helsinki heart study. Implications for treatment. Circulation 1992; 85(1):37–45.
45. Rubins HG, Robins SJ, Collins D. Gemfibrozil for the secondary prevention of coronary heart disease in men with low levels of high-density lipoprotein cholesterol. Veterans Affairs High–Density Lipoprotein Cholesterol Intervention Trial Study Group. N Engl J Med 1999; 341(6):410–418.
46. Campos H, Arnold KS, Balestra ME, et al. Differences in receptor binding of LDL subfractions. Arterioscler Thromb Vasc Biol 1996; 16(6):794–801.
47. Galeano NF, Milne R, Marcel YL, et al. Apoprotein B structure and receptor recognition of triglyceride-rich low density lipoprotein (LDL) is modified in small LDLD but not in triglyceride-rich LDL of normal size. J Biol Chem 1994; 269(1):511–519.
48. Bjornheden T, Babyi A, Bondjers G, et al. Accumulation of lipoprotein fractions and subfractions in the arterial wall, determined in an in vitro perfusion system. Atherosclerosis 1996; 123(1–2):43–56.
49. Chait A, Brazg RL, Tribble DL, et al. Susceptibility of small, dense, low-density lipoprotein to oxidative modification in subjects with the atherogenic lipoprotein phenotype B. Am J Med 1993; 94(4):350–356.
50. de Graaf J, Hak-Lemmers HL, Hectors MP, et al. Enhanced susceptibility to in vitro oxidation of the sense low density lipoprotein subfraction in healthy subjects. Arterioscler Thromb 1991; 11(2):298–306.
51. Lamarche B, Tchernof A, Moorjani S, et al. Lipid Research Center, CHUL Research Center, Ste-Foy, Quebec, Canada. Small, dense, low-density lipoprotein particles as a predictor of the risk of ischemic heart disease in men. Prospective results from the Quebec Cardiovascular Study. Circulation 1997; 95(1):69–75.
52. Volkova N, Deedwania PC. Current treatment options for patients with metabolic syndrome. Curr Treat Options Cardiovasc Med 2005; 7:61–74.
53. Caprio S. Insulin resistance in childhood obesity. J Pediatr Endocrinol Metab 2002; 15(suppl 1):487–492.
54. Weiss R, Dziura J, Burgert T, et al. Obesity and metabolic syndrome in children adolescents. N Engl J Med 2004; 350:2362–2374.
55. Sinha R, Fisch G, Teague B, et al. Prevalence of impaired glucose tolerance among children and adolescents with marked obesity. N Engl J Med 2002; 346(11):802–810.
56. Strauss RS, Pollack HA. Epidemic increase in childhood overweight, 1986–1998. JAMA 2001; 286(22):2845–2848.
57. Ford ES, Giles WH, Dietz WH. Prevalence of metabolic syndrome among U.S. adults: findings from the third National Health and Nutrition Examination Survey. JAMA 2002; 287:356–359.
58. Ford ES. Prevalence of the metabolic syndrome defined by the International Diabetes Federation among adults in the U.S. Diabetes Care 2005; 28:2745–2749.
59. Deedwania PC. Metabolic syndrome and vascular disease. Is nature or nurture leading the new epidemic of cardiovascular disease. Circulation 2004; 109:2–4.

60. Isomaa B, Almgren P, Tuomi T, et al. Cardiovascular morbidity and mortality associated with the metabolic syndrome. Diabetes Care 2001; 24:683–689.

61. Cook S, Witzman M, Auinger P, et al. Prevalence of a metabolic syndrome phenotype in adolescents. Arch Pediatr Adolesc Med 2003; 157:821–827.

62. Lakka HM, Laaksonen DE, Lakka TA, et al. The metabolic syndrome and total and cardiovascular disease mortality in middle-aged men. JAMA 2002; 25:2709–2716.

63. Janssen I, Katzmarzyk, Ross R. Body mass index, waist circumference and health risk. Arch Intern Med 2002; 162:2074–2079.

64. Grundy SM, Brewer HB, Cleeman JI, et al. Definition of metabolic syndrome. Circulation 2004; 109:433–438.

65. Frayn KN. Adipose tissue and the insulin resistance syndrome. Proc Nutr Soc 2001; 60:375–380.

66. Yamauchi T, Kamon J, Waki H, et al. The fat-derived hormone adiponectin reverses insulin resistance associated with both lipoatrophy and obesity. Nat Med 2001; 7:941–946.

67. Hotta K, Funahashi T, Arita Y, et al. Plasma concentrations of novel, adipose-specific protein, adiponectin, in type 2 diabetic patients. Arterioscler Thromb Vas Biol 2000; 20:1595–1599.

68. Yang WS, Lee WJ, Funahashi T, et al. Weight reduction increases plasma levels of adipose-derived anti-inflammatory protein, adiponectin. J Clin Endocrinol Metab 2001; 86:2815–2819.

69. Klein S, Fontana L, Young L, et al. Absence of an effect of liposuction on insulin action and risk factors for coronary heart disease. N Engl J Med 2004; 350:2549–2557.

70. Bonow RO, Eckel RH. Diet, obesity, and cardiovascular risk. N Engl J Med 2003; 348:2057–2058.

71. Van Dam RM, Rimm EB, Willett WC, et al. Dietary patterns and risk for type 2 diabetes mellitus in U.S. Men. Ann Intern Med 2002; 136:201–209.

72. Executive Summary of the Third Report of the National Cholesterol Education Program (NCEP) Expert Panel on Detection, Evaluation, and Treatment of High Blood Cholesterol in Adults (Adult Treatment Panel III) Expert Panel on Detection, Evaluation, and Treatment of High Blood Cholesterol in Adults. JAMA 2001; 285:2486–2497.

73. Brooks GA, Butte NF, Rand WM, et al. Chronicle of the Institute of Medicine physical activity recommendation: how a physical activity recommendation came to be among dietary recommendations. Am J Clin Nut 2004; 79(5):921S–930S.

74. Faria AN, Ribeiro Filho FF, Kohlmann NE, et al. Effects of sibutramine on abdominal fat mass, insulin resistance and blood pressure in obese hypertensive patients. Diabetes Obes Metab 2005; 7(3):246–253.

75. Lucas CP, Boldrin MN, Reaven GM. Effect of orlistat added to diet (30% of calories from fat) on plasma lipids, glucose, and insulin in obese patients with hypercholesterolemia. Am J Cardiol 2003; 91(8):961–964.

76. Didangelos T, Thanopoulou A, Bousboulas, et al. The orlistat and cardiovascular risk profile inpatients with metabolic syndrome and type 2 diabetes (ORLICARDIA) study. Curr Med Res Opin 2004; 20(9):1393–1401.

77. Kirkham TC, Williams CM. Endocannabinoid receptor antagonists. Potential for obesity treatment. Treat Endocrinol 2004; 3(6):345–360.

78. Van Gaal LF, Rissanen AM, Scheen AJ, et al; RIO-Europe Study Group. Effects of the cannabinoid-1 receptor blocker rimonabant on weight reduction and cardiovas-

cular risk factors in overweight patients: 1-year experience from the RIO-Europe study. Lancet 2005; 365(9468):1389–1397.

79. Despres JP, Golay A, Sjostrom L. Rimonabant in Obesity-Lipid Study Group. Effects of rimonabant on metabolic risk factors in overweight patients with dyslipidemia. N Engl J Med 2005; 353:2121–2134.

80. Papapietro K, Diaz E, Csendes A, et al. Effects of gastric bypass on weight, blood glucose, serum lipid levels and arterial blood pressure in obese patients. Rev Med Chil 2005; 133(5):511–516.

81. Reaven G. Metabolic syndrome: pathophysiology and implications for management of cardiovascular disease. Circulation 2002; 106:286–288.

82. The DECODE Study Group on behalf of the European Diabetes Epidemiology Group. Is current definition for diabetes relevant to mortality risk from all causes and cardiovascular and non-cardiovascular diseases? Diabetes Care 2003; 26:688–696.

83. Takeda E, Arai H, Yamamoto H, et al. Control of oxidative stress and metabolic homeostasis by the suppression of postprandial hyperglycemia. J Med Invest 2005; 52(suppl):259–265.

84. Chiasson JL, Josse RG, Gomis R, et al. Acarbose treatment and the risk of cardio-vascular disease and hypertension in patients with impaired glucose tolerance. The Stop-NIDDM trial. JAMA 2003; 290(4):486–494.

85. The Diabetes Prevention Program Research Group. Impact of intensive lifestyle and metformin therapy on cardiovascular disease risk factors in the diabetes prevention program. Diabetes Care 2005; 28:888–894.

86. Dailey GE 3rd, Mohideen P, Fiedorek FT. Lipid effects of glyburide/metformin tablets in patients with type 2 diabetes mellitus with poor glycemic control and dyslipidemia in an open-label extension study. Clin Ther 2002; 24(9):1426–1438.

87. Yki-Järvinen H. Thiazolidinediones. N Engl J Med 2004; 351(11):1106–1118.

88. Dormandy JA, Charbonnel B, Eckland DJ, et al. Secondary prevention of macrovas-cular events in patients with type 2 diabetes in the PROactive Study (PROspective pioglitazone Clinical Trial In macrovascular Events): a randomised controlled trial. Lancet 2005; 366(9493):1279–1289.

89. Yki-Jarvinen H. The PROactive study: some answers, many questions. Lancet. 2005; 366(9493):1241–1242.

90. Grant LM, Lisker-Melman M. Nonalcoholic fatty liver disease. Ann Hepatol 2004; 3(3):93–99.

91. Bravata DM, Sanders L, Huang J, et al. Efficacy and safety of low-carbohydrate diets: a systemic review. JAMA 2003; 289:1837–1850.

92. Aude YW, Mego P, Mehta J. Metabolic syndrome: dietary interventions. Curr Opin Cardiol 2004; 19:453–459.

93. Macchia A, Levantesi G, Franzosi MG, et al. GISSI-Prevenzione Investigators. Left ventricular systolic dysfunction, total mortality, and sudden death in patients with myocardial infarction treated with n-3 polyunsaturated fatty acids. Eur J Heart Fail 2005; 7(5):904–909.

94. Grundy SM, Cleeman JI, Daniels SR, et al. Diagnosis and management of the meta-bolic syndrome. An American Heart Association/National Heart, Lung, and Blood Institute Scientific Statement. Circulation 2005; 112:2735–2752.

95. Sever PS, Dahlof B, Poulter NR, et al; ASCOT investigators. Prevention of coro-nary and stroke events with atorvastatin in hypertensive patients who have average

or lower-than-average cholesterol concentrations, in the Anglo-Scandinavian Cardiac Outcomes Trial—Lipid Lowering Arm (ASCOT-LLA): a multicentre randomised controlled trial. Lancet 2003; 361(9364):1149–1158.

96. Colhoun HM, Betteridge DJ, Durrington PN, et al. CARDS investigators. Primary prevention of cardiovascular disease with atorvastatin in type 2 diabetes in the Collaborative Atorvastatin Diabetes Study (CARDS): multicentre randomised placebo-controlled trial. Lancet 2004; 364(9435):685.

97. Knopp RH. Drug treatment of lipid disorders. N Engl J Med 1999; 341(7):498–511.

98. Deedwania PC, Shephard J, Barter P, et al. Intensive lipid lowering treatment with atorvastatin in patients with metabolic syndrome. Circulation 2005; 112(17):II-662

99. Ridker PM, Rifai N, Cook NR, et al. Non–HDL cholesterol, apolipoproteins A-I and B100 , standard lipid measures, lipid ratios, and CRP as risk factors for cardiovascular disease in women. JAMA 2005; 294:326–333.

100. Lu W, Resnick HE, Jablonski KA, et al. Non-HDL cholesterol as a predictor of cardiovascular disease in type 2 diabetes: the strong heart study. Diabetes Care 2003; 26(1):16–23.

101. Deedwania PS, Hunninghake DB, Bays HE. et al; STELLAR Study Group. Effects of rosuvastatin, atorvastatin, simvastatin, and pravastatin on atherogenic dyslipidemia in patients with characteristics of the metabolic syndrome. Am J Cardiol 2005; 95:360–366.

102. Deedwania PS, Hunninghake DB, Bays H. Effects of lipid-altering treatment in diabetes mellitus and the metabolic syndrome. Am J Cardiol 2004; 93(suppl):18c–26c.

103. Dimons L, Tonkon M, Masana L, et al. Effects of ezetimibe added to on-going stain therapy on lipid profile of hypercholesterolemic patients with diabetes mellitus or metabolic syndrome. Curr Med Res Opin 2004; 20(9):1437–1445.

104. Ballantyne CM, Houri J, Notarbartolo A, et al. Effect of ezetimibe coadministered with atorvastatin in 628 patients with primary hypercholesterolemia: a prospective, randomized, double-blind trial. Circulation 2003; 107(19):2409–2415.

105. Chapman MJ, Assmann G, Fruchart JC, et al. Raising high-density lipoprotein cholesterol with reduction of cardiovascular risk: the role of nicotinic acid–a position paper developed by the European Consensus Panel on HDL-C. Curr Med Res Opin 2004; 20(8):1253–1268.

106. Van JT, Pan J, Wasty T, et al. Comparison of extended-release niacin and atorvastatin monotherapies and combination treatment of the atherogenic lipid profile in diabetes mellitus. Am J Cardiol 2002; 89:1306–1308.

107. Morse JS, Brown BG, Zhao X-Q, et al. Niacin plus simvastatin protect against atherosclerosis progression and clinical events in CAD patients with low HDLc and diabetes mellitus or impaired fasting glucose [abstract]. J Am Coll Cardiol 2001; 37(suppl A):262A.

108. McKenney JM, Proctor JD, Harris S, Chinchili VM. A comparison of the efficacy and toxic effects of sustained-vs. immediate-release niacin in hypercholesterolemic patients. JAMA 1994; 271:672–677.

109. Gavish D, Leibovitz E, Shapira I, et al. Bezafibrate and simvastatin combination therapy for diabetic dyslipidaemia: efficacy and safety. J Intern Med 2000; 247:563–569.

110. Athyros VG, Papageorgiou AA, Athyrou W, et al. Atorvastatin and micronized fenofibrate alone and in combination in type 2 diabetes with combined hyperlipidemia. Diabetes Care 2002; 25:1198–1202.

111. Grundy SM, Vega GL, Yuan Z, et al. Effectiveness and tolerability of simvastatin plus fenofibrate for combined hyperlipidemia. (The SAFARI trial) Am J Cardiol 2005; 95:462–468.
112. Pasternak RC, Smith SC, Bairey-Merz CN, et al. ACC/AHA/NGLBI clinical advisory on the use and safety of statins. J Am Coll Cardiol 2002; 40:567–572.
113. Shek A, Ferril MJ. Statin-fibrate combination therapy. Ann of Pharmacother 2001; 35:908–917.
114. Jones PH, Davidson MH. Reporting rate of rhabdomyolysis with fenofibrate+statin versus gemfibrozil+any statin. Am J Cardiol 2005; 95:120–122.

8

Hypertension in the Metabolic Syndrome

Stanley S. Franklin

Heart Disease Prevention Program, Department of Medicine, University of California, Irvine, California, U.S.A.

SUMMARY

- Elevated blood pressure, although weakly linked to lipid and glucose metabolism, is considered an important component of the metabolic syndrome.
- Hypertension is the leading metabolic syndrome risk factor that predisposes to increased cardiovascular morbidity and mortality.
- Persons with the metabolic syndrome and treatment-resistant hypertension have a significant risk of having hyperaldosteronism and/or obstructive sleep apnea.
- Postmenopausal women who gain appreciable weight have a high prevalence of the metabolic syndrome and systolic hypertension, and an increased propensity for developing diabetes and cardiovascular disease.
- Hypertension is an important risk factor for development of chronic kidney disease in the presence of obesity, the metabolic syndrome, and microalbuminuria.

INTRODUCTION

There is general agreement that the metabolic syndrome describes a cluster of clinical characteristics whose components vary considerably among different individuals and different racial and ethnic groups (1). Elevated blood pressure

(BP), a cardinal risk factor for cardiovascular disease (CVD), has been included as a component of the metabolic syndrome in all guidelines that define this entity. The World Health Organization (WHO) (2) report defined elevated BP as ≥140/90 mmHg, for defining the metabolic syndrome whereas the National Cholesterol Education Program Adult Treatment Panel III (ATP III) guidelines (3) used a cut point of ≥130/85 mmHg (high-normal BP).

Some investigators have been reluctant to link elevated BP with the metabolic syndrome because factor analysis has shown a weak relation between hypertension and other metabolic abnormalities that define the syndrome (4,5). On the other hand, the linkage of elevated BP with the metabolic syndrome is strong through the causative pathway of obesity, although only about half of the persons with hypertension or obesity have the metabolic syndrome (6). Indeed, hypertension is multifactorial in origin, with increased peripheral vascular resistance intrinsically linked to hypertension in young adults and arterial stiffness playing an important hemodynamic role in the development of isolated systolic hypertension (ISH) in the middle-aged and elderly (7). However, the presence of abdominal obesity at any age, defined as a waist circumference of > 40 inches. (>102 cm) in men or >35 inches. (>88 cm) in women or to a lesser extent by a body mass index (BMI) of 30 kg/m^2 or greater in either sex, greatly increases the likelihood of having one or more of the metabolic abnormalities [high-normal BP or hypertension, decreased levels of high-density lipoprotein (HDL)–cholesterol, elevated serum triglycerides, and impaired fasting glucose] that define the metabolic syndrome (1,8,9). Indeed, optimal BP, <120/80 mmHg, is infrequently associated with the metabolic syndrome as currently defined by ATP III criteria of three or more risk factor abnormalities (3).

NEUROBIOLOGY OF HYPERTENSION AND OBESITY

Role of Fat Cells

Adipocytes, both visceral and perhaps to a lesser extent in peripheral subcutaneous depots, function as an endocrine organ that produces a variety of cytokines and hormones, many of which regulate BP homeostasis (6). These include leptin, adiponectin, and angiotensinogen. Adipocytes may release other substances that affect the sympathetic nervous system (SNS) indirectly, such as free (nonesterified) fatty acids (FFAs) and an aldosterone-releasing factor. The magnitude of the production and release of these substances may be directly proportional to the overall mass of adipose tissue, although many studies point to a preferential endocrine role of the visceral adipocytes (6).

Sympathetic Nervous System

Chief among the links between obesity and elevated BP is hyperactivity of the SNS (Fig. 1) (6). The potential causative pathways between obesity and a hyperactive SNS are many and have not been completely delineated. Leptin, an

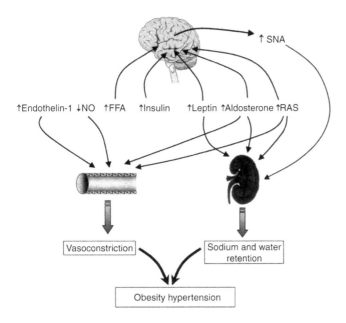

Figure 1 Summary of mechanisms and hormonal systems involved in obesity-associated hypertension. *Abbreviations*: FFA, free fatty acids; SNA, sympathetic nerve activity. *Source*: From Ref. 6.

adipocyte-derived hormone, not only regulates appetite but also plays an important role in energy expenditure by way of activating the SNS. Serum leptin levels are grossly elevated in obesity and thus play an important role in causing SNS hyperactivity. In contrast, receptors in the appetite center of the brain in obese persons are resistant to downregulation by increased blood levels of leptin. The site of leptin action in upregulating the SNS appears to be in the ventromedial and dorsomedial hypothalamus (6). Norepinephrine spillover as a measure of regional SNS activity in obese individuals has implicated the kidney as the major effector organ of sympathetic overactivity (10). Increased renal efferent sympathetic outflow results in salt and water retention and ultimately a rise in BP. Huggett et al. (11) have shown SNS hyperactivity by the microneurography technique in normotensive nondiabetic individuals with the metabolic syndrome. In individuals with the metabolic syndrome who were hypertensive, there was even greater SNS hyperactivity; this finding suggests that hypertension adds significantly to the cardiovascular risk associated with the metabolic syndrome (11). Compression of the kidney from perirenal fat deposition and the resulting changes in the renal structure may also contribute to further rises in BP, perhaps in part by stimulation of renal afferent sympathetic nerves and in part by initiation of renovascular hypertension—analogous to the experimental model of wrapped kidneys (12).

The causative relation between obesity and hypertension may be bidirectional. In individuals predisposed to developing hypertension, increased SNS activity is associated with downregulation of β-adrenergic receptors, thereby resulting in impaired thermoregulation and the tendency to gain weight (13). In age- and sex-matched individuals from the community-based Framingham Heart Study, those with the higher BP gained more weight than those with the lower BP (14). Allemann et al. (15) found that young, lean male offspring of essential hypertension parents were more prone to develop increased central body fat followed by the onset of hypertension during a five-year follow-up, as compared with matched individuals without a positive family history of hypertension. Thus, both genetic and environmental factors may link obesity with hypertension through SNS hyperactivity.

Insulin resistance and hyperinsulinemia may be associated with a hyperactive SNS and a rise in BP in certain rat models; however, in humans this association remains controversial (16,17). In some studies, the relation between hyperinsulinemia and hypertension disappears after adjusting for BMI, suggesting that obesity is a confounding factor (17). Indeed, the Framingham Heart Study showed that insulin sensitivity was confounded not only by BMI but also by age and baseline BP, thereby making insulin resistance a poor predictor of a future rise in BP (18).

The high-circulating FFAs released into the portal vein of individuals with visceral adiposity may induce SNS overactivity and hypertension in association with other elements of the metabolic syndrome (6). Similarly, the peptides adiponectin, released from fat cells, and ghrelin, released from the stomach, in alliance with hypothalamic neurons, act to downregulate the SNS activity and hence to lower BP. The role of adiponectin and ghrelin in obesity, hypertension, and the metabolic syndrome is not clear from the limited data at hand (6).

Renin–Angiotensin System

The adipose renin–angiotensin system (RAS) is characterized by fat cell secretion of angiotensinogen into the blood stream in amounts directly proportional to the size of the fat mass (6,19). This activation of the RAS, both by circulating and tissue paracrine stimulation and by cross-talk with the SNS, results in the development of increased BP. Increased renin and angiotensin II levels are typically found in obese individuals with hypertension, despite the presence of salt retention and volume expansion. Hyperactivity of the RAS is usually associated with increased reactive oxygen species, diminished nitric oxide levels, insulin resistance, coagulation abnormalities, increased inflammatory markers, and endothelial dysfunction—all of which are frequently found in patients with obesity, hypertension, and the metabolic abnormalities that help define the metabolic syndrome (19). Engeli et al. (20) studied the effect of weight reduction in obese postmenopausal women with the metabolic syndrome; they found that a 5% reduction in body weight resulted in a significant decrease in plasma and tissue renin, angiotensin II, and angiotensinogen gene expression, along with a significant reduction in systolic BP (SBP). These findings suggest that the RAS may play an important role in the pathophysiology of the common obesity–hypertension complex and that blockade of the RAS may have therapeutic value in treating patients with the metabolic syndrome.

Hyperaldostronism

Plasma aldosterone levels are frequently elevated in obese hypertensives, especially in patients with abdominal (visceral) adiposity and hypertension (21). The mechanisms responsible for this association are unclear; the presence of a suppressed plasma renin activity suggests volume expansion and would rule out secondary causes of hyperaldosteronism. Possible primary causes of hyperaldosteronism are secretion of mineralocorticoid-releasing factor from adipocytes or oxidized derivatives of linoleic acid acting directly on the adrenal glands to secrete excessive aldosterone (22); functioning adrenal adenomas are found rarely in association with the metabolic syndrome. Although the mechanism underlying aldosterone secretion is speculative, there is strong evidence that hyperaldosteronism is associated with resistant hypertension, occurring as often as 20% in one series, often without hypokalemia, and is frequently associated with obesity and other elements of the metabolic syndrome (23).

Obstructive Sleep Apnea

The presence of obesity, most often central visceral adiposity, together with obstructive sleep apnea (OSA) and resistant hypertension is a recently described one that is associated with insulin resistance, endothelial dysfunction, and many elements of the metabolic syndrome (Fig. 2). When OSA and obesity coexist, they have an additive effect in contributing to treatment-resistant hypertension, and this may be mediated by further stimulation of the SNS (25). Calhoun et al. (26) found that primary hyperaldosteronism was almost twice as prevalent in individuals at high risk compared to those at low risk for OSA, on the basis of the Berlin questionnaire, a validated algorithm for identification of subjects at risk for this entity. They hypothesized, therefore, that OSA may contribute to resistant hypertension in part by stimulating excess adrenal secretion of aldosterone.

DEMOGRAPHIC FACTORS: HYPERTENSION, OBESITY, AND THE METABOLIC SYNDROME

Aging and Hypertensive Subtypes

The prevalence of both hypertension and the metabolic syndrome are strongly age dependent (27–29). However, BP levels have increased significantly over the past decade among children and adolescents in association with the obesity epidemic.

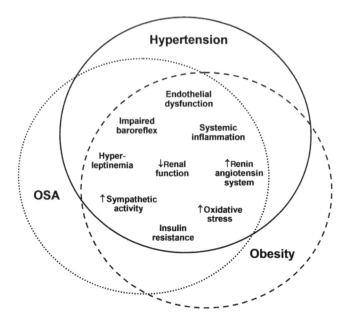

Figure 2 Putative pathophysiological mechanisms involved in the interactions between obesity, obstructive sleep apnea (OSA), and hypertension. *Source*: From Ref. 24.

Weiss et al. (30) have observed a parallel increase in prevalence rates of the metabolic syndrome and obesity, with values as high as 50% in severely obese children. In the third National Health and Nutrition Survey (NHANES III, 1988–1991) (29), hypertensive subtypes, as intermediate phenotypes, showed age dependency: isolated diastolic hypertension (IDH) was the most frequent form of diastolic hypertension in adults less than age 40 years and comparable in prevalence to systolic–diastolic hypertension (SDH) from age 40 to 49 years (Fig. 3) (29). By contrast, ISH was by far the most common subtype of hypertension from age 50 to 59 and beyond. The development of IDH and SDH subtypes in young adults is consistent with increased peripheral vascular resistance (7,31). In contrast, the development of ISH in older persons is consistent with increased large artery stiffness (31). It has been unclear, however, if different hemodynamic patterns are related to the likelihood of metabolic syndrome.

Interestingly, the Framingham Heart Study has shown that new-onset IDH developed primarily from normal and high-normal BP and largely evolved into SDH during a 10-year follow-up (7). In addition to BP, predictors of IDH were increased BMI at baseline, weight gain over time, and being a young adult male. In a recent NHANES 1999–2002 study, persons with IDH were almost 15 times as likely to have the metabolic syndrome as individuals with optimal BP (32). These findings, therefore, provide further compelling evidence to refute earlier

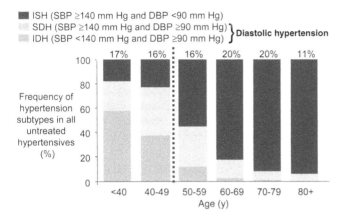

Figure 3 Frequency distribution of untreated individuals by age and hypertension sub-type of all subtypes of untreated hypertension in that age group. Analysis based on National health and Nutrition Examination Survey (NHANES) III, 1988–1991. *Abbreviations*: SBP, systolic blood pressure; DBP, diastolic blood pressure; ISH, isolated systolic hypertension; SDH, systolic-diastolic hypertension; IDH, isolated diastolic hypertension. *Source*: From Ref. 29.

studies that concluded that IDH was an artifact of diastolic measurement (33) or without increased cardiovascular risk (34–38). Interestingly, an early investigation by Julius et al. (39) in the Tecumseh Blood Pressure Study identified a group of young adults with so-called borderline hypertension (mean BP of 138.0/96.1 mmHg) and various metabolic abnormalities including being overweight or obese, which by contemporary definitions would classify them as persons with IDH and the metabolic syndrome. Thus, obesity at an early age "trumps" aging in predisposing to hypertension in combination with the metabolic syndrome. Because subjects with IDH and the metabolic syndrome were, on average, 11 years younger than those with SDH and 19 years younger than those with ISH, they will have a prolonged period of exposure to cardiovascular risk factors that could result in a significant increase in cardiovascular events and the development of diabetes as compared to normotensive persons of the same age. Undoubtedly, the current epidemic of obesity in adolescents and young adults has contributed to the substantial prevalence of the metabolic syndrome and IDH. While prospective studies are needed to confirm these results, these cross-sectional findings in U.S. adults support close monitoring of young adults with IDH and appropriate lifestyle and pharmacologic intervention as indicated by the type and severity of the metabolic risk burden (40,41). However, due to its high frequency in the hypertensive population, ISH is the most common hypertensive subtype in persons with the metabolic syndrome, and thus, attention to identifying and controlling systolic hypertension cannot be ignored.

Gender

Young adult women as compared to their male counterparts have some natural protection from developing hypertension during the childbearing age. Furthermore, young women with the metabolic syndrome rarely have a 10-year, 20% risk for cardiovascular events, whereas as many as 20% of young men with the metabolic syndrome are at this risk level (42). This situation changes drastically in middle age and beyond: there is a sex-related reversal whereby more women than men develop hypertension, primarily of the ISH phenotype (29). Postmenopausal women who gain appreciable weight, regardless of the level of physical activity, have a high prevalence of the metabolic syndrome with ISH, an increased propensity for developing diabetes, and a greatly increased risk for CVD (43). In a large Danish study of postmenopausal women followed up for a mean of 8.5 years, cardiovascular mortality was strongly related to abdominal obesity and to all elements of the metabolic syndrome, especially elevated serum triglycerides (44).

Race and Ethnicity

Populations vary in their susceptibility to the complications of obesity. South Asians, Chinese, and Japanese develop the metabolic syndrome in association with only moderate weight gain (45). The new International Diabetes Federation consensus definition of the metabolic syndrome in Asians uses as a measure of obesity a waist circumference of $\geq$90 cm for men and $\geq$80 cm for women (45). In South Asians, the increased coronary artery disease (CAD) risk is twofold greater than can be explained by standard risk factors; insulin resistance is thought to be the emerging risk factor that predisposes to premature CAD and Type 2 diabetes (46). In contrast, Blacks of African origin are prone to early and severe development of hypertension when they gain weight (47). Blacks are more resistant to developing low HDL-cholesterol and high serum triglycerides with the same degree of weight gain, suggesting that these atherogenic dyslipidemic factors are not reliable markers of insulin resistance (48). Lastly, obese Native Americans and Hispanics are more susceptible to the development of Type 2 diabetes and less so to hypertension (49). This heterogeneity in body habitus and susceptibility to different elements of the metabolic syndrome may well be the result of variation in genetic makeup as well as environmental influences.

CVD: HYPERTENSION, OBESITY, AND THE METABOLIC SYNDROME

The pathways from obesity to hypertension to CAD and ultimately heart failure represent a "vicious triangle" that most often includes the metabolic syndrome (50). As discussed earlier, not only is there cross-talk between obesity and hypertension, but renal disease increases the severity of hypertension and produces nocturnal nondipping of BP; this results in a more treatment-resistant form of hypertension (50). Thomas et al. (51) showed in a large, French population with a 14-year follow-up that hypertension was the most important risk factor that resulted in increased cardiovascular mortality among overweight and obese individuals with the metabolic syndrome (Fig. 4). This same group showed in an earlier study that moderate systolic hypertension combined with the metabolic syndrome could identify persons at increased risk for developing new-onset diabetes (52). Moreover, Schillaci et al. (53) have shown that hypertensive patients without clinically evident CVD had cardiovascular event rates directly related to the number of metabolic syndrome risk factors; moreover, those with versus those without the metabolic syndrome had nearly a twofold greater risk for developing cardiovascular events after adjustment for age, sex, and other risk factors. Further evidence that hypertension is of paramount importance as a cardiovascular risk factor was provided by another Italian study that showed that subjects with the metabolic syndrome and elevated BP have increased carotid atherosclerosis compared with subjects with metabolic syndrome but without elevated BP (54). On the other hand, the presence of the metabolic syndrome, as compared to its absence, contributes to increased left ventricular hypertrophy (LVH) and increased microalbuminuria after correcting for 24-hour levels and nighttime ambulatory BP values (55). Similarly, in the Losartan Intervention for Endpoint (LIFE) reduction in hypertension study, subjects with significant hypertension and LVH showed an increase in cardiovascular end points when stratified by BMI (56). Thus, it is the combination of hypertension and obesity on a background of atherosclerotic dyslipidemia and impaired fasting glucose that contributes greatly to future cardiovascular risk.

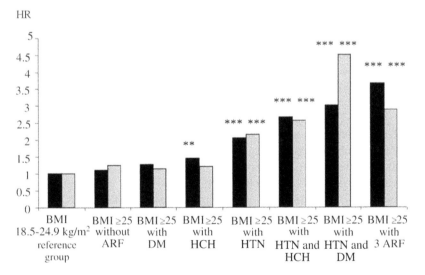

Figure 4 Hazard ratios for cardiovascular disease mortality according to body mass index and other ARF [men (*black bars*), women (*gray bars*); **$p < 0.001$, ***$p < 0.0001$]. *Abbreviations*: ARF, associated risk factors; DM, diabetes; HCH, hypercholesterolemia; HTN, hypertension. *Source*: From Ref. 51.

Ischemic Stroke

The Women's Health Study (57), a 10-year follow-up of postmenopausal women, showed that obesity was related to the incidence of ischemic stroke. This association was mediated by hypertension, diabetes, and the other risk factors that characterize the metabolic syndrome. In a Swiss study (58) of ischemic stroke patients, 69% had evidence of OSA, which was associated with higher 24-hour BP values. The stroke severity and stroke outcome, however, were more related to the nocturnal nondipping status than to the 24-hour BP value (58). Thus, being overweight or obese can predispose to stroke by multiple pathways that include metabolic syndrome–associated risk factors, OSA, and not only daytime but also nighttime BP levels.

Chronic Kidney Disease

There is strong evidence favoring an association in nondiabetic patients between the metabolic syndrome and an increased risk for chronic kidney disease (CKD). Indeed, stage 3 CKD, defined as a glomerular filtration rate (GFR) of <60 mL/min, is becoming increasingly common in the United States, with as many as 8 million people being identified in the NHANES III Survey (59). Some of these individuals will develop end-stage renal disease, but many more will die prematurely from cardiac disease and stroke. A significant number of individuals with stage 3 CKD are overweight or obese and have many elements of the metabolic syndrome (60). Several cross-sectional studies have shown a correlation between the metabolic syndrome and microalbuminuria. Chen et al. (61) also showed a significant relation between the number of positive metabolic syndrome risk factors and a GFR of <60 mL/min, with hypertension and hyperglycemia showing the highest individual correlations. The Atherosclerosis Risk in Communities Study (62), over a nine-year follow-up period, clearly showed an association between an increasing number of metabolic syndrome risk factors and incident CKD; this relation remained significant after adjusting for diabetes and BP. However, it should be kept in mind that clinical BP may not be as sensitive as 24-hour ambulatory BP in recording significant periods of elevated BP. Furthermore, hyperglycemia, obesity, and aging have been shown to interfere with renal autoregulation of renal blood flow and GFR, thus allowing the injurious transmission of what has been considered mild elevation of BP to the microcirculation of the kidney (63). The combination of prolonged obesity, inappropriate vasodilation and hyperfiltration, neurohumoral activation, impairment in renal-pressure natriuresis, and further worsening of hypertension may all contribute to a gradual loss of renal function (Fig. 5) (64). Other possible mechanisms that could make the kidneys more susceptible to damage are the aforementioned effects of compression of the kidney from adipose tissue, reduced birth weight leading to decreased nephron numbers, and adverse effects of hyperuricemia. Clearly, there is much still to be learned regarding the adverse effects of the metabolic syndrome and CKD.

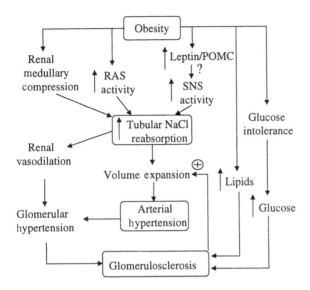

Figure 5 Summary of mechanisms by which obesity increases renal tubular sodium reabsorption, impairs pressure natriuresis, and causes hypertension as well as progressive glomerular injury. *Abbreviations*: RAS, renin angiotensin system; NaCl, Sodium chloride *Source*: From Ref. 64.

MANAGEMENT OF HYPERTENSION IN THE METABOLIC SYNDROME

The two main clinical goals in the management of the metabolic syndrome are prevention of Type 2 diabetes and atherosclerotic CVD.

Lifestyle Intervention

The first-line treatment strategy to achieve these goals, as outlined in the Seventh Report of the Joint National Committee on Prevention, Detection, Evaluation, and Treatment of High Blood Pressure (JNC-7) (40), is the reversal of the underlying causes of hypertension in the metabolic syndrome: being overweight or obese and physically inactive. A variety of lifestyle interventions have been shown to lower BP, the most effective being successful weight reduction in overweight and obese hypertensives (Table 1) (65). Even a reduction of 10 to 15 lb (~4.5–7 kg) can have a significant benefit in lowering BP. Unfortunately, most patients are refractory to successful weight reduction and even when partially successful, tend to have a high percentage of recidivism within a year of losing weight. The more recent use of the Dietary Approaches to Stop Hypertension (DASH) diet (67), rich in fruits, vegetables, and high-calcium but low animal–fat foods, has been successful in reducing BP even more than a sodium-restrictive diet. Avoidance of sedentary lifestyles and increased physical activity is important in any successful weight reduction program, especially when combined with successful dieting. In addition, daily physical

Table 1 Lifestyle Interventions for Prevention or
Treatment of Hypertension

Intervention	Blood pressure effect
Exercise	5–10 mm Hg (≥30 min ≥3x/wk)
Weight reduction	1–2 mm Hg/Kg ↓
Alcohol intake reduction	1 mm Hg/drink/d ↓
Sodium intake reduction	1–3 mm Hg/40 mmol/d ↓
DASH diet	3–10 mm Hg ↓

Source: Adapted from Refs. 65 and 66.

activity is critical in maintaining an ideal weight. Successful lifestyle intervention
may reduce the need for extensive antihypertensive therapy and minimize associated cardiovascular risk factors. It should be emphasized that lifestyle intervention
is more likely to be successful in preventing the development of hypertension when
initiated at the normal or high-normal BP level than in reversing existing hypertension (40). Ideally, therefore, early identification of at-risk individuals and institution
of preventive measures are likely to bring most benefit.

Antihypertensive Therapy

There are no definitive outcome studies on the benefit of drug treatment in persons with high-normal BP (as defined in JNC-7) (40) and metabolic syndrome or
on the selection of specific antihypertensive agents in the management of hypertension in the presence of the metabolic syndrome. However, there are specific
directives for the treatment of hypertension, such as the JNC-7 report (40) and
WHO guidelines (2) for the optimal reduction of BP to achieve maximum benefit from antihypertensive therapy. These guidelines, based on observational studies as well as on outcome trials, suggest that low-risk patients be treated to a
target goal of <140 mm Hg Systolic BP and <90 mm Hg Diastolic BP. For high-
risk subjects with diabetes, renal impairment, or heart failure, the therapeutic target goals are <130 mm Hg Systolic BP and <80 mm Hg Diastolic BP.

The Blood Pressure Treatment Trialists Collaboration (68), a meta-analysis of
29 trials involving 162,341 persons with a mean age of 65 years, concluded that all
classes of commonly used antihypertensive agents were equally successful in reducing the risk of CAD and stroke events. Moreover, the reduction in risk was directly
proportional to the reduction in SBP. An updated Trialists Collaboration study (69),
involving 27 randomized trials that included 33,395 individuals with diabetes, also
concluded that all BP-lowering regimens studied were comparable for patients with
and without diabetes. These conclusions were supported by the Antihypertensive
and Lipid-Lowering Treatment to Prevent Heart Attack Trial (ALLHAT) (70), an
outcome trial of 33,357 high-risk subjects with a mean age of 67 years. The ALL-
HAT study showed that a thiazide-type diuretic (chlorthalidone) was equally effective

in reducing the primary end points of nonfatal myocardial infarction and CAD deaths when compared to the calcium channel blocker (CCB) amlodipine or the angiotensin-converting enzyme inhibitor (ACEI) lisinopril (70). The meta-regression analysis of Verdecchia et al. (71) updated the Trialists Collaboration study by adding five new trials published since 2003. This new analysis not only confirmed the primary importance of lowering BP in reducing cardiovascular events, but also showed specific class effects beyond BP control: ACEIs were superior to CCBs in preventing CAD, whereas CCBs were superior to ACEIs in preventing stroke.

Perhaps β-blockers represent an exception to the dictum that the benefit of an antihypertensive agent is directly proportional to its brachial BP-lowering capability. This was shown in the LIFE (72), a trial of patients with hypertension and LVH and with a high frequency of the metabolic syndrome, in which losartan [an angiotensin II receptor blocker (ARB)] was superior to atenolol (a β-blocker) in preventing fatal and nonfatal strokes, independent of any significant difference in brachial BP lowering between the two therapeutic arms (72). However, peripheral brachial BP recordings can overestimate the hemodynamic benefit of β-blocker–based treatment and underestimate the hemodynamic benefit of drugs that affect the RAS in reducing central aortic pressures, as was recently shown in the Conduit Artery Functional Evaluation (CAFÉ) study (73) of the Anglo-Scandinavian Cardiac Outcomes Trial (ASCOT) (74).

It should be noted also that a diuretic was an add-on drug in more than 77% of both therapeutic arms in the LIFE study, suggesting that the combination of a diuretic and an ARB was an effective modality of treatment for stroke prevention in this high-risk group of older hypertensive patients. The LIFE study reinforces an earlier meta-analysis of 10 geriatric hypertension outcome studies that showed the inferiority of β-blockers to diuretics in reducing cardiovascular events (75). Interestingly, β-blockers with intrinsic α_1-blocking properties, such as carvedilol, could have beneficial BP-lowering effects in patients with the metabolic syndrome and diabetes, perhaps because of a favorable effect on metabolic risk factors secondary to arterial vasodilatation (76); however, outcome studies will be required to prove this thesis.

What is the potential risk of developing diabetes with various antihypertensive drug classes in nondiabetic individuals with the metabolic syndrome? Lindholm et al. (77) in the Antihypertensive treatment and Lipid Profile in a North of Sweden Efficacy Evaluation (ALPINE) study found that many patients receiving diuretic antihypertensive therapy for one year, often combined with a b-blocker when needed, were more prone to develop an abnormal metabolic pattern—either metabolic syndrome or frank diabetes—than those patients receiving ARBs. Mason et al. (78) in a meta-analysis of seven hypertensive clinical trials concluded that patients exposed to treatment regimens combining thiazides and b-blockers were at a greater risk of developing diabetes than those with regimens avoiding this combination of drugs. Furthermore, Abuissa et al. (79) in a meta-analysis of 12 randomized clinical trials (including the LIFE trial), showed a reduction in new-onset diabetes by 27% in patients receiving

ACEI–diuretic combinations and by 23% in those receiving an ARB–diuretic combination (Fig. 6) In contrast to ACEIs and ARBs that protect against new-onset diabetes, CCBs have a neutral effect (80); however, they fail to protect against new-onset heart failure and they should only be used in conjunction with ACEIs or ARBs in proteinuric kidney disease because when used alone, they are less protective against progressive CKD (80).

In summary, current evidence suggests that drugs that block the RAS, taken with or without a low-dose thiazide diuretic, would be considered first-line treatment in patients with the metabolic syndrome to prevent new-onset diabetes, although definitive outcome studies are lacking. Indeed, there are two prospective trials in progress, the Diabetes Reduction Approaches with Ramipril and Rosiglitazone Medications (DREAM) (81) trial utilizing ACEIs and the Nateglinide and Valsartan in Impaired Glucose Tolerance Outcomes Research (NAVIGATOR) (82) trial using ARBs, which will address the important issue of preventing patients with impaired glucose tolerance from progressing to new-onset diabetes and assessing the possible beneficial effect of these antihypertensive agents beyond BP control on cardiovascular morbidity and mortality.

How do ACEIs and ARBs compare with other antihypertensive classes and with each other in protecting against cardiovascular events in patients with the metabolic syndrome and diabetes, and is there an advantage in combining these

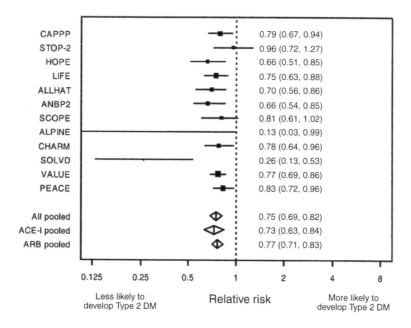

Figure 6 Pooled risk estimates of the different angiotensin-converting enzyme (ACE) inhibitor and angiotensin receptor blocker (ARB) trials. *Source*: From Ref. 79.

two classes of drugs that block the RAS? Burnier and Zanchi (83), in a recent review, concluded that blocking the RAS with either an ACEI or an ARB reduces cardiovascular events in patients with diabetes and delays the progression of diabetic nephropathy toward end-stage renal failure beyond reduction in BP. However, Casas et al. (84), in an extensive meta-analysis of diabetic and nondiabetic renal disease, concluded that there were no significant ACEI or ARB reno-protective effects beyond BP control. Thus, there is still uncertainty in regard to the role of ARBs and ACEIs when used alone or as a combination in high-risk populations with controlled hypertension. The Ongoing Telmisartan Alone and in Combination with Ramipril Global Endpoint Trial (ONTARGET) (85) will address these important questions in 23,000 high-risk patients with diabetes and/or CVD who are randomized to telmisartan, ramipril, or the combination of the two drugs.

The recognition that hypertension and dyslipidemia coexist more often than would be expected by chance and that their combination increases the risk for CVD has important therapeutic implications. Indeed, since persons with the metabolic syndrome frequently have atheromatous dyslipidemia and about 60% also have low-density lipoprotein–cholesterol values of ≥130 mg/dL (42) (>3.4 mmol/L), the use of combined antihypertensive and statin therapy can be justified on the basis of overall high cardiovascular risk. This therapeutic approach was supported by the ASCOT trial (74), which showed that in addition to good BP control, the use of lipid-lowering therapy resulted in impressive reductions in both CAD and stroke events.

Treatment Algorithm

Even though the American Diabetes Association and the European Association for the Study of Diabetes published a statement in 2004 (86) to the effect that the metabolic syndrome is imprecisely defined and is not worthy of being called a syndrome, the current ATP III definition of the metabolic syndrome may be useful in improving our decision making in the treatment of elevated BP. On the basis of what we know (or think we know), a provisional BP treatment algorithm can be constructed for patients with the metabolic syndrome, as follows:

1. Patients with high-normal BP (Systolic BP 130–139 mm Hg or Diastolic BP 85–89 mm Hg) qualify only for lifestyle modification therapy as per JNC-7 recommendations (40). However, the European Society of Hypertension guidelines (41) supplement lifestyle modification with antihypertensive drug therapy in the presence of a total of at least three cardiovascular risk factors, supposedly because this would often equate to a 10-year >20% risk for sustaining a cardiovascular event. Risk factors consist of the following: men >55 years, women >65 years, dyslipidemia, smoking, family history of premature CVD, LVH, and microalbuminuria. Many persons with the metabolic syndrome

would qualify for antihypertensive drug therapy on the basis of these guidelines. An ACEI or ARB would be the preferred antihypertensive drug class for initial therapy.

2. Patients with stage 1 hypertension (Systolic BP 140–159 mm Hg or Diastolic BP 90–99 mm Hg) need no additional risk factors to qualify for antihypertensive drug therapy to reach the goal of BP <140/90 mmHg. A low-dose diuretic (hydrochlorothiazide, 12.5–25 mg QD) or a CCB would be a suitable add-on second drug to an initial ACEI or ARB therapy. Presently, we have no head-to-head comparison of diuretics versus CCBs when added to ACEI or ARBs in terms of BP lowering, protection from cardiovascular events, or safety; the Avoiding Cardiovascular events through COMbination therapy in Patients Living with Systolic Hypertension trial (87), a randomized and blinded comparison of benazepril/HCTZ versus benazepril/amlodipine in progress, is designed to answer some of these questions.

3. Patients with stage 2+ hypertension (Systolic BP ≥160 mmHg or Diastolic BP ≥ 100 mmHg) will require polypharmacy with two or more drugs to reach a goal of <140/90 mmHg. Two-drug combinations can be started simultaneously for most patients to hasten BP control, and thus minimize cardiovascular events, as shown in the Valsartan Antihypertensive Long-term Use Evaluation (VALUE) trial (88). A low-dose diuretic and/or CCBs would be suitable second- and/or third-choice drugs.

4. Patients with diabetes and the metabolic syndrome, with or without concurrent CKD, qualify as having a coronary risk equivalent and require aggressive polypharmacy with two or three drugs to reach a target goal BP value <130/80 mmHg. A low-dose diuretic and CCB would be a suitable add-on second and third choice drugs.

5. Patients with resistant hypertension to triple therapy (ACEI/ARB, diuretic, and CCB) should be evaluated for possible primary hyperaldosteronism; even if not present, an aldosterone inhibitor (spironolactone and eplerenone) may be added as a fourth drug unless contraindicated by the presence of hyperkalemia (89,90). In addition, OSA should be considered in the presence of treatment-resistant hypertension. If the diagnosis of OSA is confirmed, effective treatment with continuous positive airway pressure can result in a decrease in both daytime and nighttime BP (24).

CONCLUSIONS

The association of elevated BP with the metabolic syndrome is strongly linked through the causative pathway of obesity. Adipocytes, in proportion to the size of the fat mass, function as an endocrine organ that produces a variety of cytokines and hormones, including leptin and angiotensinogen. The resulting hyperactivity of the SNS and renin–angiotensin–aldosterone system is associated with elevated BP, insulin resistance, and endothelial dysfunction—all of which are frequently found in patients with the metabolic syndrome. Furthermore, the elements of the metabolic syndrome, including the presence and severity of elevated BP, can vary by gender, age, and ethnicity. There is a twofold increased risk for cardiovascular events in the presence of the metabolic syndrome, although the event rate is directly related to the number of positive metabolic risk factors present. The two main clinical goals in the management of the metabolic syndrome are prevention of Type 2 diabetes and atherosclerotic cardiovascular events. The primary modality of treatment is lifestyle intervention with reduced caloric intake and increased physical activity. Pharmacologic intervention is indicated on the basis of the severity of BP elevation, associated cardiovascular risk factors, and the presence of target organ damage. Although hypertension is the most important metabolic syndrome risk factor contributing to increased cardiovascular morbidity and mortality, definitive outcome studies to determine optimal drug management of hypertension are lacking.

REFERENCES

1. Grundy SM, Cleeman JI, Daniels SR, et al. Diagnosis and management of the metabolic syndrome. An American Heart Association/National Heart, Lung, and Blood Institute Scientific Statement. Circulation 2005; 112:2735–2752.
2. Guidelines Sub-Committee. 1999 World Health Organization-International Society of Hypertension guidelines for the management of hypertension. J Hypertens 1999; 17:151–183.
3. Grundy SM, Cleeman JI, Daniels SR, et al. Diagnosis and management of the metabolic syndrome: an American Heart Association/National Heart, Lung, and Blood Institute Scientific Statement. Circulation 2005; 112:2735–2752.
4. Shen BJ, Todaro JF, Niaura R, et al. Are metabolic risk factors one unified syndrome? Modeling the structure of the metabolic syndrome X. Am J Epidemiol 2003; 157:701–711.
5. Ford ES. Factor analysis and defining the metabolic syndrome. Ethn Dis 2003; 13:429–437.
6. Rahmouni K, Correia MLG, Hayes WG, et al. Obesity-associated hypertension. New insights into mechanisms. Hypertension 2005; 45:9–14.
7. Franklin SS, Pio JR, Wong ND, et al. Predictors of new-onset diastolic and systolic hypertension. The Framingham Heart Study. Circulation 2005; 111:1121–1127.
8. Poirier P, Lemieux I, Mauriege P, et al. Impact of waist circumference on the relationship between blood pressure and insulin. The Quebec Health Survey. Hypertension 2005; 45:363–367.
9. Hayashi T, Boyko EJ, Leonetti DL, et al. Visceral adiposity and the prevalence of hypertension in Japanese Americans. Circulation 2003; 108:1718–1723.
10. Eikelis N, Schlaich M, Aggarwal A. Interactions between leptin and the human sympathetic nervous system. Hypertension 2003; 41:1071–1079.

11. Huggett RJ, Burns J, Mackintosh AF, et al. Sympathetic neural activation in nondiabetic metabolic syndrome and its further augmentation by hypertension. Hypertension 2004; 44:847–852.

12. Hall JE, Crook ED, Jones DW, et al. Mechanisms of obesity-associated cardiovascular and renal disease. Am J Med Sci 2002; 324:127–137.

13. Julius S, Valentine M, Palatini P. Overweight and hypertension. A 2-way street? Hypertension 2000; 35:807–813.

14. Kannel WB, Brand N, Skinner JJ Jr, et al. The relation between adiposity to blood pressure and development of hypertension. Ann Intern Med 1967; 67:48–59.

15. Allemann Y, Hutter D, Aeschbacher BC, et al. Increased central body fat deposition precedes a significant rise in blood pressure in male offspring of essential hypertensive parents: a 5 year follow-up study. J Hypertens 2001; 19:2143–2148.

16. Saad MF, Rewers M, Selby J, et al. Insulin resistance and hypertension. The Insulin Resistance Atherosclerosis Study. Hypertension 2004; 43:1324–1331.

17. Hu FB, Stampfer MJ. Insulin resistance and hypertension. The chicken-egg question revisited. Circulation 2005; 112:1678–1680.

18. Amlov J, Pencina MJ, Nam BH, et al. Relations of insulin sensitivity to longitudinal blood pressure tracking. Variations with baseline age, body mass index, and blood pressure. Circulation 2005; 112:1719–1727.

19. Prasad A, Quyyumi AA. Renin-angiotensin system and angiotensin receptor blockers in the metabolic syndrome. Circulation 2004; 110:1507–1512.

20. Engeli S, Bohnke J, Gorzelniak K, et al. Weight loss and the renin-angiotensin-aldosterone system. Hypertension 2005; 45:356–362.

21. Pratt-Ubunama MN, Nishizaka MK, Calhoun DA. Aldosterone antagonism: an emerging strategy for effective blood pressure lowering. Curr Hypertens Rep 2005; 7:186–192.

22. Goodfriend TL, Calhoun DA. Resistant hypertension, obesity, sleep apnea, and aldosterone. Theory and therapy. Hypertension 2004; 43:518–524.

23. Calhoun DA, Nishizaka MK, Zaman MA, et al. Hyperaldostronism among Black and White subjects with resistant hypertension. Hypertension 2002; 40:892–896.

24. Wolk R, Shamsuzzaman SM, Somers VK. Obesity, sleep apnea, and hypertension. Hypertension 2003; 42:1067–1074.

25. Grassi GF, Facchini A, Trevano FQ, et al. Obstructive sleep apnea—dependent and independent adrenergic activation in obesity. Hypertension 2005; 45:321–325.

26. Calhoun DA, Nishizaka MK, Zaman MA, et al. Aldosterone excretion among subjects with resistant hypertension and symptoms of sleep apnea. Chest 2004; 125:112–117.

27. Ford ES, Giles Wh, Dietz WH. Prevalence of the metabolic syndrome among U.S. adults: findings for the third National Health and Nutrition Examination Survey. JAMA 2002; 287:356–359.

28. Burt VL, Whelton P, Roccella EJ, et al. Prevalence of hypertension in the U.S. adult population. Results from the third National Health and Nutrition Examination Survey, (1988–1991). Hypertension 1995; 25:305–313.

29. Franklin SS, Milagros J, Wong ND, et al. Predominance of isolated systolic hypertension among middle-aged and elderly U.S. hypertensives. Analysis based on National health and Nutrition Examination Survey (NHANES) III. Hypertension 2001; 37:869–874.

30. Weiss M, Dziura J, Burgert, et al. Obesity and the metabolic syndrome in children and adolescents. N Engl J Med 2004; 350:2362–2374.

31. Franklin SS, Gustin W IV, Wong ND, et al. Hemodynamic pattern of age-related changes in blood pressure. The Framingham Heart Study. Circulation 1997; 96:308–315.

32. Franklin SS, Barboza M, Pio J, Wong ND. Blood pressure categories, hypertensive subtypes and the metabolic syndrome. J Hypertens 2006; 24:2009–2016.

33. Blank SG, Mann SJ, James GD, et al. Isolated elevation of diastolic blood pressure. Real or artifactual? Hypertension 1995; 26:383–389.

34. Pickering TG. Isolated diastolic hypertension. J Clin Hypertens 2003; 5:411–413.

35. Fang J, Madhavan S, Cohen H, et al. Isolated diastolic hypertension. A favorable finding among young and middle-aged hypertensive subjects. Hypertension 1995; 25:377–382.

36. Petrovitch H, Curb JD, Bloom-Marcus E. Isolated systolic hypertension and risk of stroke in Japanese American men. Stroke 1995; 26:25–29.

37. Nielsen WB, Lindenstrom E, Vestbo J, et al. Is diastolic hypertension an independent risk factor for stroke in the presence of normal systolic blood pressure in the middle-aged and elderly? Am J Hypertens 1997; 10:634–639.

38. Strandberg TE, Saloman VV, Vanhanen HT, et al. Isolated diastolic hypertension, pulse pressure, and mean arterial pressure as predictors of mortality during a follow-up of up to 32 years. J Hypertens 2002; 20:399–404.

39. Julius S, Jamerson K, Mejia A, Krause L, Schork N, Jones K. The association of borderline hypertension with target organ changes and higher coronary risk. Tecumseh Blood Pressure Study. JAMA 1990; 264:354–358.

40. Chobanian AV, Bakris GL, Black HR, et al. The Seventh Report of the Joint National Committee on Prevention, Detection, Evaluation, and Treatment of High Blood Pressure: the JNC 7 report. JAMA 2003; 289:2560–2572.

41. 2003 European Society of Hypertension-European Society of Cardiology guidelines for the management of arterial pressure. J Hypertens 2003; 21:1011–1053.

42. Wong ND, Pio JR, Franklin SS, et al. Preventing coronary events by optimal control of blood pressure and lipids in patients with the metabolic syndrome. Am J Cardiol 2003; 91:1421–1426.

43. Carr MC. The emergence of the metabolic syndrome with menopause. J Clin Endocrinol Metab 2003; 88:2404–2411.

44. Tanko LB, Bagger YZ, Qin G, et al. Enlarged waist combined with elevated triglycerides is a strong predictor of accelerated atherogenesis and related cardiovascular mortality in postmenopausal women. Circulation 2005; 111:1883–1890.

45. Zimmet P, Alberti KG, Rios S. A new International Diabetes Federation worldwide definition of the metabolic syndrome: the rationale and the results. Rev Esp Cardiol 2005; 58:1371–1376.

46. Miller GJ, Beckles GL, Maude GH, et al. Ethnicity and other characteristics predictive of coronary heart disease in a developing community: principal results of the St. James Survey. Trinidad Int J Epidemiol 1989; 18:808–817.

47. Lteif AA, Han K, Mather KJ. Obesity, insulin resistance, and the metabolic syndrome. Determinants of endothelial dysfunction in Whites and Blacks. Circulation 2005; 112:32–38.

48. Sumner AE, Finley KB, Genovese DJ, et al. Fasting triglyceride and the triglyceride-HDL cholesterol ratio are not markers of insulin resistance in African Americans. Arch Intern Med 2005; 165:1395–1400.

49. Gonzalez-Villalpando C, Stern MP, Haffner SM, et al. Prevalence of hypertension in a Mexican population according to the Sixth Report of the Joint National committee on Prevention, Detection, Evaluation and Treatment of High Blood Pressure. J Cardiovasc Risk 1999; 6:177–181.

50. Montani JP, Antic V, Yang Z, et al. Pathways from obesity to hypertension: from the perspective of a vicious triangle. Int J Obes 2002; 26(suppl 2):S28–S38.

51. Thomas F, Bean K, Pannier B, et al. Cardiovascular mortality in overweight subjects. The key role of associated risk factors. Hypertension 2005; 46:654–659.

52. Henry P, Thomas F, Benetos A, et al. Impaired fasting glucose, blood pressure and cardiovascular disease mortality. Hypertension 2002; 40:458–463.

53. Schillaci G, Pirro M, Vaudo G, et al. Prognostic value of the metabolic syndrome in essential hypertension. J Am Coll Cardiol 2004; 43:1817–1822.

54. Irace C, Cortese C, Fiaschi E, et al. Components of the metabolic syndrome and carotid atherosclerosis. Role of elevated blood pressure. Hypertension 2005; 45:597–601.

55. Cuspidi C, Meani S, Fusi V, et al. Metabolic syndrome and target organ damage in untreated essential hypertensives. J Hypertens 2004; 22:1991–1998.

56. de Simone G, Wachtell K, Palmieri V, et al. Body build and risk of cardiovascular hypertrophy. The LIFE (Losartan Intervention For Endpoint reduction in hypertension) Study. Circulation 2005; 111:1924–1931.

57. Kurth T, Gaziano JM, Rexrode KM, et al. Prospective study of body mass index and risk of stroke in apparently healthy women. Circulation 2005; 111:1992–1998.

58. Selic C, Siccole MM, Hermann DM, et al. Blood pressure evolution after acute ischemic stroke in patients with and without sleep apnea. Stroke 2005; 36:2614–2618.

59. Coresh J, Astor BC, Greene T, et al. Prevalence of chronic kidney disease and decreased kidney function in adult US populations: Third National Health and Nutrition Examination Survey. Am J Kidney Dis 2003; 41:1–12.

60. Schelling JR, Sedor JR. The metabolic syndrome as a risk factor for chronic kidney disease: more than a fat chance? J Am Soc Nephrol 2004; 15:2773–2774.

61. Chen J, Muntner P, Hamm LL, et al. The metabolic syndrome and chronic kidney disease in US adults. Ann Intern Med 2004; 140:167–174.

62. Kurella M, Lo JC, Chertow GM. Metabolic syndrome and the risk for chronic kidney disease among nondiabetic adults. J Am Soc Nephrol 2005; 16:2134–2140.

63. Henegar JR, Bigler SA, Henegar LK, et al. Functional and structural changes in the kidney in the early stages of obesity. J Am Soc Nephrol 2001; 12:1211–1217.

64. Hall JE. The kidney, hypertension and obesity. Hypertension 2003; 41(part 2):625–633.

65. Cushman W, Dubbert P. Nonpharmacologic approaches to therapy of hypertension. Endocr Pract 1997; 3:106–111.

66. Sacks FM, Svetkey LP, Vollmer WI, et al. Effects on blood presure of reduced dietary sodium and the dietary approaches to stop hypertension (DASH) diet. N Engl J Med 2001; 344:3–10.

67. Appel LJ, Moore TJ, Obarzanek E, et al. The effect of dietary patterns on blood pressure: results from the Dietary Approaches to Stop Hypertension (DASH) randomized clinical trial. N Engl J Med 1997; 336:1117–1124.

68. Blood Pressure Lowering Treatment Trialists' collaboration. Effects of different blood pressure-lowering regimens on major cardiovascular events: results of

prospectively-designed overviews of randomized trials. Lancet 2003; 362:1527–1535.

69. Blood Pressure Lowering Treatment Trialists' Collaboration. Effects of different blood pressure-lowering regimens on major cardiovascular events in individuals with and without diabetes mellitus. Arch Intern Med 2005; 165:1410–1419.

70. The ALLHAT Officers and Coordinators for the ALLHAT Collaborative Research Group. Major outcomes in high-risk hypertensive patients randomized to angiotensin-converting enzyme inhibitor or calcium channel blockers vs diuretic. The Antihypertensive and Lipid-Lowering Treatment to Prevent Heart Attack Trial (ALLHAT). JAMA 2002; 288:2981–2997.

71. Verdecchia P, Reboldi G, Angeli Fabio, et al. Angiotensin-converting enzyme inhibitors and calcium channel blockers for coronary heart disease and stroke prevention. Hypertension 2005; 46:386–392.

72. Dahlöf B, Devereux RB, Kjeldsen SE, et al. LIFE Study Group. Cardiovascular morbidity and mortality in the Losartan Intervention For Endpoint reduction in hypertension study (LIFE): a randomized trial against atenolol. Lancet 2002; 359:995–1003.

73. The CAFÉ investigators, for the ASCOT investigators. Differential impact of blood pressure lowering drugs on central aortic pressure and clinical outcomes—principal results of the conduit artery function evaluation study: The CAFE Study. Circulation 2006; 113. In press.

74. Dahlof B, Sever PS, Poulter NR, et al. Prevention of cardiovascular events with an antihypertensive regimen of amlodipine adding perindopril as required versus atenolol adding bendroflumethiazide as required, in the Anglo-Scandinavian Cardiac Outcomes Trial-Blood Pressure Lowering Arm (ASCOT-BPLA): a multicenter randomized controlled trial. Lancet 2005; 366:895–906.

75. Messerli FH, Grossman E, Goldbourt U. Are beta-blockers efficacious as first-line therapy for hypertension in the elderly? A systematic review. JAMA 1998; 279:1903–1907.

76. Bakris GL, Fonseca V, Katholi RE, et al. Metabolic effects of carvedilol vs metoprolol in patients with Type 2 diabetes mellitus and hypertension. A randomized controlled trial. JAMA 2004; 292:2227–2236.

77. Lindholm LH, Persson M, Alaupovic P, et al. Metabolic outcome during 1 year in newly detected hypertensives: results of the Antihypertensive treatment and Lipid Profile in a North of Sweden Efficacy Evaluation (ALPINE study). J Hypertens 2003; 21:1563–1574.

78. Mason JM, Dickinson HO, Nicolson DJ, et al. The diabetogenic potential of thiazide-type diuretic and beta-blocker combinations in patients with hypertension. J Hypertens 2005; 23:1777–1781.

79. Abuissa H, Jones PG, Marso SP, et al. Angiotensin-converting enzyme inhibitors or angiotensin receptor blockers for prevention of Type 2 diabetes. A meta-analysis of randomized clinical trials. J Am Coll Cardiol 2005; 46:821–826.

80. Nathan S, Peping CJ, Bakris GL. Calcium antagonists. Effects on cardio-renal risk in hypertensive patients. Hypertension 2005; 45:637–642.

81. Gerstein HC, Yusuf S, Holman R, et al. Rationale, design and recruitment characteristics of a large, simple international trial of diabetic prevention: the DREAM trial. Diabetologia 2004; 47:1519–1627.

82. Tsujii S. NAVIGATOR trial (nateglinide). Nippon Rinsho 2005; 63(suppl 2):483–487.

83. Burnier M, Zanchi A. Blockade of the renin-angiotensin-aldosterone system: a key therapeutic strategy to reduce renal and cardiovascular events in patients with diabetes. J Hypertens 2006; 24:11–25.

84. Casas JP, Loukogeorgakis CS, Vallance P, et al. Effects of inhibitors of the renin-angiotensin system and other antihypertensive drugs on renal outcomes: systematic review and meta-analysis. Lancet 2005; 366:2026–2033.

85. Sleight P. The ONTARGET/TRANSCEND trial PROGRAMME: baseline data. Acta Diabetol 2005; 42(suppl 1):S50–S56.

86. Kahn R, Buse J, Ferrannini E, et al. The metabolic syndrome: time for a clinical appraisal. Diabetes Care 2005; 28:2289–2389.

87. Jamerson KA, Bakris GL, Wun CC, et al. Rationale and design of the Avoiding Cardiovascular events through COMbination therapy in Patients Living with Systolic Hypertension (ACCOMPLISH) trial. Am J Hypertens 2004; 17:793–801.

88. Julius S, Kjeldsen SE, Weber M, et al. Outcomes in hypertensive patients at high cardiovascular risk treated with regimens based on valsartan or amlodipine; the VALUE randomised trial. Lancet 2004; 363:2022–2031.

89. Nishizaka MK, Zaman MA, Calhoun DA. Efficacy of low-dose spironolactone in subjects with resistant hypertension. Am J Hypertens 2003; 16:925–930.

90. de Paula RB, da Silva AA, Hall JE. Aldosterone antagonism attenuates obesity-induced hypertension and glomerular hyperfiltration. Hypertension 2004; 43:41–47.

9

Obesity, Physical Activity, and Nutrition in the Metabolic Syndrome

Gang Hu

Department of Epidemiology and Health Promotion, National Public Health Institute, and Department of Public Health, University of Helsinki, Helsinki, Finland

Timo A. Lakka

Department of Physiology, Institute of Biomedicine, University of Kuopio, and Kuopio Research Institute of Exercise Medicine, Kuopio, Finland

Hanna-Maaria Lakka

Department of Public Health and Clinical Nutrition, University of Kuopio, Kuopio, Finland

Jaakko Tuomilehto

Department of Epidemiology and Health Promotion, National Public Health Institute, and Department of Public Health, University of Helsinki, Helsinki, Finland and South Ostrobothnia Central Hospital, Seinäjoki, Finland

SUMMARY

■ Overweight, obesity, or weight gain has been shown to be an important risk factor for the development of Type 2 diabetes and an important component of the metabolic syndrome. Physical inactivity is another important risk factor for the development of Type 2 diabetes.

241

■ Data from prospective studies have shown that at least 30 minutes per day of moderate-to-vigorous physical activity can prevent Type 2 diabetes. Moderate or high levels of physical fitness are effective in preventing Type 2 diabetes.

■ Results from clinical trials have indicated that lifestyle changes, including dietary modification and an increase in physical activity, can prevent Type 2 diabetes.

■ Analyses from prospective studies have confirmed that healthy diets are effective and safe ways to prevent Type 2 diabetes and the metabolic syndrome.

■ Public health messages, healthcare professionals, and the healthcare system should aggressively promote physical activity and responsible nutritional habits during occupation, leisure time, and daily life to prevent overweight and obesity.

INTRODUCTION

Sedentary lifestyle and overweight are major public health and clinical problems. They are the most prevalent risk factors for common chronic diseases and premature mortality. More than half of the adults in the United States do not engage in physical activity at the level currently recommended for health promotion, e.g., 30 minutes or more of moderate-intensity physical activity on most days of the week (1,2). Two in three adults in the United States are currently classified as overweight [body mass index (BMI) 25.0–29.9 kg/m^2] or obese (BMI ≥30 kg/m^2), compared with fewer than one in four adults in the early 1960s (3,4). This trend is similar for all age, gender, and race groups (4). More than half of the adults in most developed countries are overweight or obese, and the prevalence of obesity is increasing rapidly in these countries (5). Overweight in childhood and adolescence has more than doubled over the past decades in the United States (6), some European countries, and Japan (5). Overweight is increasing in many developing countries as well (5).

The worldwide epidemic of excess weight is a consequence of positive energy balance due to both reduced energy expenditure and increased energy intake. Urbanization and automation in recent decades has resulted in a progressive reduction in the level of habitual physical activity associated with work and chores of daily living, as well as a growing amount of time spent in very sedentary activities such as watching TV, working on the computer, and playing video games (5,7). The almost unlimited availability of highly palatable, energy-dense foods and drinks and increased portion sizes are undoubtedly contributing to the current epidemic of overweight and obesity (5,8–10).

The epidemic of sedentary lifestyle and overweight has serious public health and economical consequences. Physical inactivity increases the incidence of coronary artery disease (CAD), stroke, hypertension, obesity, Type 2 diabetes, osteoporosis, cancers of the breast and colon, depression, and premature mortality (1,2). Overweight and obesity increase the risk of CAD, hypertension, Type 2 diabetes, dyslipidemia, gout, osteoarthritis, gallbladder disease, cancers of the breast, endometrium, and colon, psychosocial problems, sleep apnea, disability, and premature mortality (5,11,12). Physical inactivity, unhealthy diet, and obesity have been estimated to account for about 14% of all deaths in the United States (13,14). If current trends continue, these modifiable risk factors will overtake smoking as the primary preventable cause of death (14). According to conservative estimates, physical inactivity accounts for about 4% and obesity for about 7% of direct healthcare costs in the United States, figures that are comparable to those of smoking (15).

Diabetes is one of the most costly and burdensome chronic diseases and one of the fastest growing public health problems in the world (16). It has been estimated that the number of individuals with diabetes among adults 20 or more years of age will double from the current 171 million in 2000 to 366 million in 2030 (16). Recent data show that the lifetime risk of Type 2 diabetes is over 30% in Europe, Asia, and the United States (17–19). In addition, whereas Type 2 diabetes was previously considered to be a disease of middle and late adulthood, it is now increasingly prevalent also in children and adolescents (20). Cardiovascular disease (CVD) accounts for more than 70% of total mortality among patients with Type 2 diabetes (21). Some recent studies have shown that Type 2 diabetes and CVD share many common risk factors such as obesity, hypertension, dyslipidemia, and hyperglycemia. These clusters of metabolic abnormalities were named as the metabolic syndrome (22). The pathogenesis of the syndrome is complex (23). It has been proposed that the metabolic syndrome is a powerful determinant of Type 2 diabetes (24–29) and atherosclerotic CVD (30–35).

The development of Type 2 diabetes and the metabolic syndrome involves an interaction between genetics and lifestyle factors (36–38). Sedentary behaviors and obesity are independent risk factors for the metabolic syndrome and Type 2 diabetes (1,39–41). In this chapter, we summarize the current evidence about the management of obesity and the role of increased exercise and nutritional factors in the primary prevention of Type 2 diabetes and the metabolic syndrome.

PHYSICAL ACTIVITY AND ENERGY EXPENDITURE

Regular physical activity is a major determinant of total energy expenditure. Physical activity accounts for 20% to 30% of total daily energy expenditure in sedentary individuals, but it may represent up to 50% of all energy expended in persons who engage in heavy manual work or demanding exercise training (42). Physical activity accounts for most of the variation in total energy expenditure within and between individuals (43). The contribution of physical activity to total energy expenditure depends not only on the amount and intensity of physical activity, but also on many other factors such as body mass (42,43). Total physical activity can be divided into (*i*) spontaneous activity such as movement of arms, legs, and head, taking small steps, fidgeting, and even mastication; (*ii*) work-related activities such as office work; (*iii*) the activities of daily living such as climbing stairs, walking a few blocks instead of taking a car or bus, walking and cycling to and from work, household work, and yard work; and (*iv*) conditioning exercise such as walking, running, cycling, skiing, swimming, dancing, ball games, aerobics, and resistance training. In modern societies, the contribution of work-related activities to total energy expenditure is much smaller than it used to be. The activities of daily living account for most of the energy cost of physical activity in individuals who do not engage in regular exercise and who represent the majority of the populations in developed countries. In physically active individuals, however, purposeful conditioning exercise is the most important determinant of the energy expenditure of physical activity.

PHYSICAL ACTIVITY, OVERWEIGHT, AND OBESITY

Physical Activity in the Prevention of Weight Gain

Cross-sectional studies have shown that physically active adults and children are leaner and have less abdominal fat than sedentary individuals (44,45). The difference in body adiposity between physically active and inactive individuals appears to persist from early adulthood to old age (46). Total energy expenditure has been inversely associated with body weight and weight gain in adults and children (47–49). Prospective epidemiological studies have observed that regular physical activity prevents unhealthy weight gain and obesity, whereas sedentary behaviors such as watching TV, working at the computer, or playing video games promote them (50–53). It has been estimated that about 30% of new cases of obesity could be prevented by adopting a relatively active lifestyle, including more than 30 minutes of brisk walking and fewer than 10 hours of TV watching per week (53). There is some evidence that a sedentary lifestyle is a better population-level predictor of weight gain than increased caloric or fat intake (8). Regular physical activity, as estimated by cardiorespiratory fitness, may play a stronger role in attenuating age-related weight gain than in promoting long-term weight loss (54).

Epidemiological studies suggest that moderate-intensity physical activity 45 to 60 minutes per day is needed to prevent unhealthy weight gain and obesity (52). Brisk walking is effective in the prevention of obesity, but low-intensity activities of daily living also appear to be beneficial (53). Vigorous exercise may provide some additional benefit beyond low- and moderate-intensity physical activity in the prevention of weight gain (50). There are no randomized controlled trials that specifically address the questions of whether regular physical activity prevents long-term weight gain and fat accumulation, and what types, amount, and intensity of physical activity are needed to achieve such long-term benefits. Long-term energy balance will be easier to achieve if regular physical activity and a healthy diet are combined.

Physical Activity in the Promotion of Weight Loss

A number of randomized controlled trials have shown that regular physical activity can markedly reduce body weight and fat mass without dietary caloric restriction in overweight men and women (52,55–64). The effective exercise training programs have typically lasted for 3 to 12 months and have included three to five exercise sessions per week of 30 to 60 minutes each, and the total duration of physical activity has varied between three and five hours per week (52,55–64). Regular physical activity reduces body weight and adiposity within just three months (58), and further reductions can be seen at least until nine months (65). An increase in total energy expenditure appears to be the most important determinant of successful exercise-induced weight loss. The larger the reduction in body weight and fat, the greater has been the amount of physical activity (58,60–62,64), which suggests that regular exercise decreases body adiposity in a dose-dependent manner. The best long-term results may be achieved when physical activity produces an energy expenditure of at least 2500 kcal per week (62). Short-term studies have generally resulted in a greater weight and fat loss than long-term studies. The most likely explanation for this apparent discrepancy is that it is difficult to maintain high levels of energy expenditure for a long period of time (52,59). Indeed, adherence to the exercise-training program is a critical factor for a successful long-term weight loss. Adherence may be particularly problematic among obese subjects (66).

Most randomized controlled trials have included mainly aerobic exercise such as running, walking, and cycling (52,55–64). However, there is some evidence that resistance training also reduces body fat (67,68), and that the effect is independent of other physical activities and changes in energy intake (68). A combination of aerobic and weight training may be more effective in producing changes in body composition than aerobic exercise alone (67). Another advantage of resistance training is that it may increase skeletal muscle mass and perhaps resting metabolic rate if the program is sufficiently intense and demanding. Resistance exercise may also improve insulin sensitivity, an important benefit for overweight and obese individuals (55,56,69). The effects of regular physical activity on cardiovascular risk factors such as insulin resistance, glucose tolerance, Type 2 diabetes, dyslipidemia, and elevated blood pressure are stronger if associated with weight reduction (2). Yet, the optimal approach in weight-reduction programs appears to be a combination of regular physical activity and caloric restriction (52,55,56,58–61,64,70). It not only results in effective weight reduction, but also has the strongest effect on cardiovascular risk factors (2). Including physical activity, especially resistance training, in weight-reduction programs helps in maintaining skeletal muscle mass (55,56).

Physical Activity in the Prevention of Weight Regain After Weight Loss

Although several approaches, including dietary energy restriction and drugs, are available for weight reduction, weight maintenance after successful weight loss remains difficult. A large proportion of individuals will eventually regain weight up to their initial body weight (70), and new approaches to prevent weight regain are needed. Ninety percent of individuals, who have been able to maintain weight after a significant weight loss, report that regular physical activity is a critical component of their success (71). Randomized controlled trials have shown a modest and inconsistent effect of regular physical activity on weight maintenance (66). One explanation for the mild effect may be that the amount of physical activity has been inadequate to maintain reduced body weight in overweight and obese individuals who are prone to weight regain. Indeed, exercise programs have typically consisted of 1.5 to 3 hours per week of walking or cycling, which corresponds to an energy expenditure of 500 to 1000 kcal per week. It is likely that much larger amounts of physical activity are required to prevent weight gain after weight loss. People who have succeeded in avoiding weight regain have reported a mean exercise energy expenditure of about 2700 kcal per week, which equals to about four miles of walking per day (71). Recent reviews have concluded that a minimum of 60 minutes, but most likely 80 to 90 minutes of moderate-intensity physical activity per day, corresponding to about 2000 to 2500 kcal per week, may be needed to avoid or limit weight regain in formerly overweight or obese individuals (52,66).

Physical Activity and Fat Distribution

There is some evidence that abdominal obesity is an independent risk factor for CVD and may provide additional information beyond overall adiposity (72–81). Regular physical activity reduces abdominal visceral and subcutaneous fat independent of changes in dietary energy intake in healthy, overweight, and obese men and women (58,60,63,82,83). However, regular exercise does not appear to preferentially reduce total abdominal and visceral fat beyond the changes in total adiposity (58,60,64). Although most studies have not been able to demonstrate a dose–response relationship between regular physical activity and reduction in abdominal adiposity (59), a recent study in overweight postmenopausal women showed that larger amounts of regular exercise resulted in a greater reduction in abdominal fat (60).

OBESITY, DIABETES, AND THE METABOLIC SYNDROME

Obesity and Type 2 Diabetes: Data from Prospective Epidemiological Studies

Overweight, obesity, and weight gain have been shown to be important risk factors for the development of Type 2 diabetes regardless of age and sex. In the Nurses' Health Study involving 84,941 U.S. women, 34 to 59 years of age, free of diagnosed diabetes, CVD and cancer at baseline, a strong positive association between overall obesity as measured by BMI and the risk of incident diabetes was observed during 16 years follow-up (84). After adjustment for age, family history of diabetes, dietary score, physical activity, smoking, and alcohol consumption, the relative risks of incident diabetes were 2.7 for normal weight (BMI 23–24.9 kg/m^2), 7.6 for overweight (25–29.9 kg/m^2), 20.1 for obesity (30–34.9 kg/m^2), and 39 for severe obesity (greater than or equal to 35 kg/m^2) women compared with lean weight women (less than 23 kg/m^2) (84). In the Health Professionals' Follow-up Study of 22,171 U.S. men aged 40 to 84 years, the investigators found that the multivariate-adjusted relative risks of incident diabetes at different levels of BMI (less than 23, 23–24.9, 25–26.9, 27–29.9, and greater than or equal to 30 kg/m^2) were 1.0, 1.9, 2.7, 3.9, and 7.6, respectively (85). In the Women's Health Study including 37,878 U.S. women aged 45 years and older, the relative risks of developing Type 2 diabetes were 3.2 for overweight (BMI 25–29.9 kg/m^2), and 9.1 for obesity (greater than or equal to 30 kg/m^2) women compared with normal weight women (less than 25 kg/m^2) (86). In nondiabetic Finnish men and women confirmed by the standard oral glucose tolerance test at baseline, it is found that overweight and obesity participants had 1.7- and 5.6-fold increased risks of incident diabetes, respectively, compared with normal weight participants (87).

Abdominal obesity, measured by waist circumference or waist to hip ratio, predicts the risk of Type 2 diabetes independently of BMI. In the Nurses' Health Study, after controlling for BMI and other potentially confounding factors, the relative risk of incident diabetes for the 90th percentile of waist to hip ratio (≥0.86) versus the 10th percentile (waist to hip ratio <0.70) was 3.1, and the relative risk for the 90th percentile of waist circumference (≥92 cm) versus the 10th percentile (waist circumference <67 cm) was 5.1 (88). In the Physicians' Health Study, both overall and abdominal adiposity strongly and independently predicted the risk of Type 2 diabetes, and waist circumference was a better predictor than BMI or waist to hip ratio (89). The atherosclerosis risk in communities cohort reported that waist circumference, waist to hip ratio, and BMI were equivalent in their ability to predict Type 2 diabetes (90).

Weight gain during adulthood was also associated with an increased risk of diabetes independent of initial body weight. In a national cohort of 8545 U.S. adults from the National Health and Nutrition Examination Survey Epidemiologic Follow-up Study, participants with 5 to 7.9, 8 to 10.9, 11 to 19.9, and ≥20 kg weight gains were associated with a 2.1-, 1.1-, 2.6-, and 3.9-fold increased risk of incident diabetes, respectively, compared with participants whose weights remained relatively stable (those who gained or lost less than 5 kg weight) (91). In the Nurses' Health Study, the corresponding relative risks of diabetes for women were 1.9, 2.7, 5.5, and 12.3, respectively (92). In contrast, women who lost more than 5 kg weight reduced their risk of diabetes by 50% or more (92). In the Physicians' Health Study, an increase in every kilogram of weight was associated with a 7.3% increased risk of diabetes (85).

Obesity and the Metabolic Syndrome: Data from Prospective Epidemiological Studies

Because there are no studies regarding weight change and the development of the metabolic syndrome, abdominal obesity has been made as the key component of the metabolic syndrome in the International Diabetes Foundation (IDF) clinical definition for the metabolic syndrome (93), and as one important component of the metabolic syndrome in the definitions by the World Health Organization (WHO) Consultation (22), the European Group for Study of Insulin Resistance (EGIR) (94), and the National Cholesterol Education Program Expert Panel (NCEP) (95,96). Increases in body weight were, however, shown to predict the metabolic syndrome as assessed by the presence of hypertension, hyperinsulinemia, and dyslipidemia as well as worsening of individual features of the metabolic syndrome in nondiabetic middle-aged men from the Kuopio Ischemic Heart Disease Risk Factor Study (97).

PHYSICAL ACTIVITY, DIABETES, AND THE METABOLIC SYNDROME

Physical Activity and Type 2 Diabetes: Data from Prospective Epidemiological Studies

Physical inactivity is another important risk factor for the development of Type 2 diabetes. The first study confirming the association between physical activity and the risk of Type 2 diabetes was carried out in 5990 male alumni from the University of Pennsylvania (98). Increasing leisure time physical activity was associated with a lower risk of developing Type 2 diabetes. For each 500 kcal per week increment in leisure time physical activity, the risk of diabetes declined by 6% (98). Subsequently, two large studies confirmed these findings. The Nurses' Health Study involved 87,253 U.S. women, 34 to 59 years of age, free of diagnosed diabetes, CVD and cancer at baseline (99). During 1980 to 1988, 1303 cases of self-reported Type 2 diabetes developed (99). Women who were engaged in vigorous exercise at least once per week had a 33% reduced age- and multivariate-adjusted risk of Type 2 diabetes compared with women who did not exercise weekly. The Physicians' Health Study including 21,271 U.S. men aged 40 to 84 years indicated that those who exercised at least once a week had a multivariate-adjusted relative risk of Type 2 diabetes of 0.71 during five years from 1982 to 1988 (100). In subsequent analyses of these two large studies, extending the period of follow-up, the Nurses' Health Study from 1986 to 1994, and the Health Professionals' Follow-up Study from 1986 to 1996, the investigators found a progressive reduction in the multivariate-adjusted relative risk of Type 2 diabetes across increasing quintiles of leisure time physical activity (101,102).

Several other studies of men in different countries also confirmed the association between higher levels of physical activity and a lower risk of developing Type 2 diabetes. In the Honolulu Heart Program, the risk of Type 2 diabetes was inversely related to total physical activity during a follow-up of two to six years among 6815 Japanese American men 45 to 68 years of age (103). The results from the British Regional Heart Study indicated that men who were engaged in moderate levels of physical activity had a substantially reduced risk of Type 2 diabetes, compared with physically inactive men, after adjustment for age, BMI, systolic blood pressure, high-density lipoprotein (HDL) cholesterol, smoking, alcohol intake, and prevalent CAD (104). In Sweden, the Malmö Preventive Trial reported that men who developed Type 2 diabetes during a six-year follow-up had a 16% lower baseline mean value of physical activity score compared with men who did not develop diabetes (105). In middle-aged Finnish men, physical activity of moderate intensity ($\geq$5.5 metabolic units) for at least 40 minutes per week was associated with decreased rates of Type 2 diabetes after adjusting for age, baseline glucose levels, and known risk factors (106). In Japanese men aged 35 to 60 years free of diabetes, impaired fasting glycemia and hypertension (107) those who participated in regular physical exercise at least once a week, and vigorous activity only once a week on weekends were at a decreased risk of Type 2 diabetes. In another recent study of 2924 Japanese male office workers aged 35 to 59 years, physical activity in daily life expressed in terms of daily energy expenditure was inversely associated with the risk of developing impaired fasting glucose or Type 2 diabetes after adjustment for potential confounding factors (108).

The inverse relation between physical activity and Type 2 diabetes has also been observed in prospective studies that included women, as well as in studies of women alone, from several different countries. A Finnish prospective study that examined 891 men and 973 women 35 to 63 years of age reported that only women with a higher total amount of physical activity or weekly vigorous exercise had a reduced risk of developing Type 2 diabetes during 10 years of follow-up (109). An age-adjusted relative risk of 2.6 for Type 2 diabetes was found for the lowest third of physical activity, compared with the highest third. Among 6898 Finnish men and 7392 women aged 35 to 64 years (39), 373 incident cases of Type 2 diabetes were ascertained during a 12-year follow-up. Physically moderately active and very active work were associated with a 30% and 26% reduction in the risk of Type 2 diabetes compared with sedentary work (Table 1). For leisure time physical activity, corresponding risk reductions were 19% and 16%. Daily walking or cycling to and from work for more than 30 minutes was also significantly and inversely associated with the diabetes risk. These associations were independent of age, systolic blood pressure, smoking, education, the other two kinds of physical activity, and BMI. Simultaneous engagement in at least two kinds of physical activity (occupational, leisure time, or commuting) at a moderate or high level was associated with a lower risk of Type 2 diabetes than engagement in any one kind of activity at a moderate or high level. In a separate analysis, the independent and joint associations of physical activity, BMI, and plasma glucose levels with the risk of Type 2 diabetes among 2017 Finnish men and 2352 women were evaluated (87). We classified the subjects into three levels of physical activity (*i*) low levels of occupational, leisure time, and commuting (less than 30 minutes) physical activity, (*ii*) moderate to high physical activity in only one kind of activity, and (*iii*) moderate to high physical activity in at least two kinds of activity. Level 2 physical activity, compared with level 1, was associated with a 15% reduction in the risk of Type 2 diabetes; whereas level 3, with a 57% decrease. The inverse association was observed among individuals with BMI < 30 kg/m^2 and BMI $\geq$30 kg/m^2 (Fig. 1A), and among those with normal and impaired glucose homeostasis (Fig. 1B). We also examined the joint relations among physical

Table 1 Relative Risk of Type 2 Diabetes According to Different Levels of Occupational, Commuting, and Leisure Time Physical Activity Among Finns

Physical activity	No. of cases	Person-year	Relative risk[a] (95% confidence interval)		
			Model 1	Model 2	Model 3
Occupational physical activity					
Light	199	67250	1.00	1.00	1.00
Moderate	63	48184	0.57 (0.43–0.76)	0.66 (0.49–0.90)	0.70 (0.52–0.96)
Active	111	55695	0.76 (0.60–0.97)	0.73 (0.56–0.94)	0.74 (0.57–0.95)
P value for trend			<0.001	0.008	0.020
Walking or cycling to/from work					
0 min/day	242	81556	1.00	1.00	1.00
1–29 min/day	93	54576	0.75 (0.59–0.96)	0.88 (0.68–1.15)	0.96 (0.74–1.25)
≥30 min/day	38	34998	0.42 (0.30–0.59)	0.54 (0.38–0.77)	0.64 (0.45–0.92)
P value for trend			<0.001	0.003	0.048
Leisure time physical activity					
Low	173	56387	1.00	1.00	1.00
Moderate	166	88350	0.63 (0.50–0.78)	0.67 (0.53–0.84)	0.81 (0.64–1.02)
Active	34	26392	0.52 (0.36–0.75)	0.61 (0.41–0.90)	0.84 (0.57–1.25)
P value for trend			<0.001	0.001	0.186

[a]Model 1, adjusted for age, sex, and study year; Model 2, adjusted for the factors in Model 1, plus systolic blood pressure, smoking status, education, and the two other kinds of physical activity; Model 3, adjusted for the factors in Model 2, plus body mass index.
Source: From Ref. 39.

(**A**)

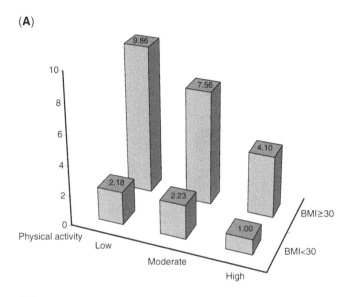

(**B**)

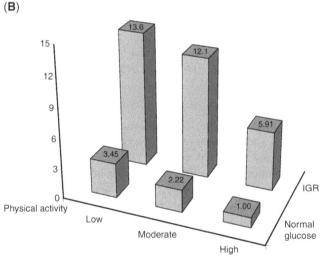

Figure 1   Relative risk of Type 2 diabetes according to different levels of (**A**) physical activity and BMI (<30 kg/m^2 and ≥30 kg/m^2) and (**B**) physical activity and glucose (normal glucose, IGR). Adjusted for age, sex, study year, systolic blood pressure, smoking status, education, and BMI. *Abbreviations*: BMI, body mass index; IGR, impaired glucose regulation. *Source*: From Ref. 87.

activity, BMI, plasma glucose, and the risk of Type 2 diabetes (Fig. 2). Obese subjects with low physical activity and impaired glucose regulation had a 30-fold increase in risk compared with nonobese persons with high physical activity and normal glucose homeostasis. The Iowa Women's Health Study

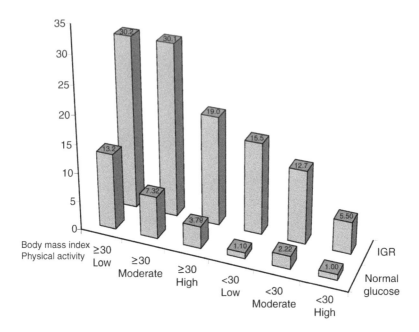

Figure 2 Relative risk of Type 2 diabetes according to joint levels of physical activity, body mass index, and glucose homeostasis. Adjusted for age, sex, study year, systolic blood pressure, smoking status, and education. *Abbreviation*: IGR, impaired glucose regulation. *Source*: From Ref. 87.

investigated 34,257 postmenopausal women 55 to 69 years of age without diabetes at baseline (110). In this study, women who participated in any leisure time physical activity had a 14% lower risk of Type 2 diabetes compared with sedentary women, after adjustment for age and other confounding factors. The Monitoring trends and determinants on cardiovascular diseases Kooperative Gesundheisforschung in der Region Augsburg (MONICA/KORA) Augsburg Cohort Study examined sex-specific associations between leisure time physical activity and incident Type 2 diabetes among 4069 German men and 4034 women 25 to 74 years of age, who were followed for 7.4 years (111,112). A significant inverse association between leisure time physical activity and incident Type 2 diabetes was found in both men and women, but more consistently in women. Among 2017 Swedish women in the Gothenburg BEDA Study, the investigators observed a significant inverse association between leisure time physical activity and the risk of Type 2 diabetes (113). The Women's Health Study examined the joint association of leisure time physical activity and BMI with the risk of Type 2 diabetes among 37,878 U.S. women free of CVD, cancer, and diabetes who were followed for 6.9 years (86). BMI and physical inactivity were independent predictors of incident diabetes when examined separately. However, when examined together, BMI was a far more important predictor, and the inverse relation between physical activity and the risk of Type 2 diabetes was attenuated once BMI was taken into account.

In the United States, African American men and women who were engaged in moderate physical activity had a 65% lower risk of developing Type 2 diabetes than their physically inactive counterparts (114). The Pima Indian Community Study also indicated that leisure time physical activity was associated with the lower risk of Type 2 diabetes (115). The Women's Health Initiative Observational Study evaluated whether physical activity independently predicted the risk of Type 2 diabetes in postmenopausal African American, Hispanic, Asian, and Caucasian women (116). After adjusting for age and multiple other risk factors, a significant inverse association between total physical activity and diabetes risk was apparent in Caucasian but not in African American, Hispanic, or Asian women (116). The lack of associations in the nonCaucasian women may have reflected the smaller sample sizes of these groups.

These prospective epidemiologic studies, conducted among different populations and assessing different domains of activity, indicate that regular physical activity during occupation, commuting, leisure time, or daily life reduces the risk of Type 2 diabetes by 15% to 60%, with most studies showing a 30% to 50% reduction in the risk. The benefit of physical activity is apparent in both men and women, and in younger and older individuals. These studies generally controlled for age, BMI, and several other important confounding factors. Nevertheless, residual confounding due to unmeasured factors may still be present. Another issue to consider is that questionnaires are imprecise measures of habitual physical activity. Misclassification may result in underestimation of the association between physical activity and the outcome. To provide additional information, studies assessing physical fitness (see below) are useful because maximal exercise testing to quantify cardiorespiratory fitness is an objective evaluation of an individual's recent physical activity pattern and accounts for up to 70% to 80% of variance in detailed recordings of physical activity (117). Residual confounding and misclassification of physical activity are unlikely to be major concerns, in view of the consistency of findings among these prospective studies, studies of physical fitness, and randomized clinical trials of behavior modification.

How much physical activity is required for a reduction in the risk of Type 2 diabetes? While the data are sparse, it appears that even moderate-intensity physical activity is sufficient to reduce risk. In the Nurses' Health Study (101), the Health Professionals' Follow-up Study (102), the Japanese Male Office Workers Survey (108), the Women's Health Study (86), and the Women's Health Initiative Observational Study (116), the magnitude of the inverse association between walking and the risk of Type 2 diabetes was similar to that between vigorous leisure activity and the risk. Perhaps some 30 minutes per day of brisk walking is sufficient. Additionally, decreasing the amount of time spent watching TV is helpful for reducing the risk (53,102). Each two-hour increment in TV watching per day was associated with a 14% to 20% increase in the risk of Type 2 diabetes in men and women. In the Finnish Diabetes Prevention Study (DPS), the increase in leisure time physical activity by three to four hours per week reduced the risk of diabetes more than 70% compared with no change in physical activity in high-risk subjects (118).

Physical Fitness and Type 2 Diabetes: Data from Prospective Epidemiological Studies

Only six prospective epidemiological studies have assessed the association of physical fitness with the risk of Type 2 diabetes (105,106,119–122). The Malmö Preventive Trial found that poor physical fitness, measured by vital capacity and maximal oxygen uptake, was inversely associated with the risk of Type 2 diabetes (105). Higher levels of cardiorespiratory fitness (maximal oxygen uptake of ≥ 31.0 mL per kilogram per minute) among men 42 to 60 years of age were associated with lower risks after adjusting for age, baseline glucose levels, and other risk factors (106). Another Norwegian study, the Oslo Healthy Men Study, comprising 2014 men without diabetes at baseline, reported that each unit increase in physical fitness was associated with a 54% decrease in the risk of Type 2 diabetes after adjustment for confounding factors (121). The Aerobic Center Longitudinal Study, conducted among 8633 U.S. men 30 to 79 years of age without diabetes at baseline, indicated that men with low cardiorespiratory fitness (the least fit 20%) had a 3.7-fold increase in the risk of developing Type 2 diabetes, compared with those with high fitness (the most fit 40%) (119). The Coronary Artery Risk Development in Young Adults Study among 4487 U.S. men and women 18 to 30 years of age assessed whether low fitness, estimated by short duration on a maximal treadmill test, predicted the development of Type 2 diabetes or the metabolic syndrome, and whether improving fitness (increase in treadmill test duration between examinations) was associated with the risk reduction (122). After multivariate adjustments, participants with low fitness (bottom 20%) were about two-fold more likely to develop Type 2 diabetes or the metabolic syndrome than those with high fitness (top 40%). Increasing fitness during the seven-year study was associated with a 60% reduction in the risk of Type 2 diabetes, and a 50% reduction in the risk of the metabolic syndrome (122). Low cardiorespiratory fitness, measured by a cycle ergometer test and maximal oxygen uptake was associated with an increased risk of incident Type 2 diabetes in nondiabetic Japanese men 20 to 40 years of age at baseline (120).

These studies of physical fitness—primarily but not only in men—show similar findings to the studies of physical activity, but also with somewhat larger magnitudes of the association. This may be due to fitness measurements being less prone to measurement error and misclassification. Additionally, factors other than physical activity may influence both physical fitness and health through related biological factors (123).

Physical Activity or Physical Fitness and the Metabolic Syndrome: Data from Prospective Epidemiological Studies

Regular physical activity prevents and also helps in the treatment of many cardiovascular risk factors, and most of these factors belong to the metabolic syndrome.

Regular exercise reduces body adiposity, increases insulin sensitivity, improves glucose tolerance, reduces postprandial hyperglycemia, decreases plasma triglyceride concentrations and increases plasma HDL cholesterol concentrations, decreases blood pressure, favorably affects hemostatic factors (2), improves endothelial function (124), and reduces the risk of developing the metabolic syndrome (125) and Type 2 diabetes. The effects of regular physical activity on cardiovascular risk factors such as insulin resistance, glucose tolerance, Type 2 diabetes, dyslipidemia, and elevated blood pressure are stronger if associated with weight reduction (2). Another advantage of including regular exercise in weight-reduction programs is that physical activity can decrease plasma low-density lipoprotein (LDL) cholesterol and limit the reduction in plasma HDL cholesterol that often occurs with a decrease in dietary saturated fat (126). The favorable effects of exercise on insulin sensitivity and the lipid profile tend to dissipate a few days after the last exercise session (127), which provides support for the recommendation that adults should participate in moderate-intensity physical activity on most days of the week (1,2).

It is important to recognize that regular physical activity favorably affects many cardiovascular risk factors, and the summation of these effects results in a marked reduction in the incidence of atherosclerotic CVD and premature mortality (128–136). There are also large individual differences in the magnitude of the effect of regular exercise on cardiovascular risk factors, and this variation in responses is influenced by age, sex, health status, body size, and genetic factors (137,138).

Several studies have assessed the association of physical activity or physical fitness with the risk of developing the metabolic syndrome. Finnish men who were engaged in moderate or vigorous leisure time physical activity greater than three hours per week had halved their risk to develop the metabolic syndrome compared with sedentary men after adjustment for major confounders (age, BMI, smoking, alcohol, and socioeconomic status) and potential mediating factors (insulin, glucose, lipids, and blood pressure) (125). The results of this study also suggested that poor cardiorespiratory fitness is not only associated with all components of the metabolic syndrome, but can also be considered as an underlying feature of the metabolic syndrome (139). In Japanese male office workers physical activity in daily life, expressed in terms of daily energy expenditure, was inversely associated with the risk of developing the metabolic syndrome in both nonobese and obese men (140). In a longitudinal Dutch study, from the age of 13 to 36 years, subjects with the metabolic syndrome at age 36, compared with those without the syndrome, had a more marked decrease in cardiopulmonary fitness levels, a more marked increase in light-to-moderate intensity physical activity, but a more marked decrease in hard physical activity (141). In a recent analysis from the Aerobic Center Longitudinal Study including 9007 U.S. men and 1491 women 20 to 80 years of age without the metabolic syndrome at baseline, the investigators found that cardiorespiratory fitness was inversely associated with the metabolic syndrome incidence in both men and women (142).

Change in Lifestyle and Type 2 Diabetes or the Metabolic Syndrome: Data from Clinical Trials

In recent years, five clinical trials have assessed whether regular physical activity, with or without dietary intervention, can reduce progression to Type 2 diabetes among adults with impaired glucose tolerance (IGT) (143–146), and among men with high cardiovascular risk (147). Two early reports from Sweden and China demonstrated that change in lifestyle can prevent Type 2 diabetes, but a major limitation of these two studies was that the individual subject was not randomly assigned to intervention and control groups (143,144). Subsequently, recently two well-designed randomized controlled trials in Finland and the United States confirmed these earlier findings (145,146).

The Malmö study from Sweden targeted increased physical exercise and weight loss as major intervention strategies to prevent and delay Type 2 diabetes (143). Subjects with IGT had less than half the risk of developing Type 2 diabetes during the five-year follow-up, compared with those who did not take part in the exercise program. In the Chinese study from Da Qing, 577 individuals with IGT were randomized, by clinic, into one of the four groups: exercise only, diet only, diet plus exercise, and a control group (144). The cumulative incidence of Type 2 diabetes during six years was significantly lower in the exercise group (41%), diet group (44%), and diet plus exercise group (46%), compared with the control group (68%), and remained significant even after adjusting for differences in baseline BMI and fasting glucose.

In the Finnish DPS, 522 middle-aged (mean age 55 years) men (33%) and women (67%), who were overweight (mean BMI 31 kg/m²) and had IGT, were randomized either to an intensive lifestyle intervention group or a control group (145,148). The subjects in the intervention group had frequent consultation visits with a nutritionist (seven times during the first year). They received individual advice about how to achieve the intervention goals, including (*i*) reduction in body weight of 5% or more, (*ii*) total fat intake less than 30% of energy consumed, (*iii*) saturated fat intake less than 10% of energy consumed, (*iv*) fiber intake of at least 15 g per 1000 kcal, and (*v*) moderate exercise for at least 30 minutes per day. After the intensive intervention period, there was a maintenance phase that included a counseling session every three months. At each of these counseling sessions, exercise habits were discussed, all kinds of physical activity were strongly recommended, and increased physical activity was considered an essential part of successful weight loss program (149). Endurance exercise, including walking, jogging, swimming, aerobic ball games, and skiing, was recommended to increase aerobic capacity and cardiorespiratory fitness. Participants were also offered an opportunity to attend supervised, progressive, individually tailored circuit-type resistance training sessions. The moderate intensity and medium to high volume programs were designed to improve the functional capacity and strength of the large muscle groups of the upper and lower body. The cumulative incidence of Type 2 diabetes after four years was 11% in the intervention group and 23% in the control group. During the entire trial, the risk of diabetes was reduced by 58% in the intervention group. The reduction in the incidence of diabetes was directly associated with changes in lifestyle, because majority of the people who reached four or five of the five-lifestyle targets developed diabetes. Improvements in both physical activity and diet were important; with a multifactorial study design it is not possible to point out a single factor that could be called the primary reason for the reduced risk of developing diabetes.

In additional analyses of data from the DPS, the role of leisure time physical activity in preventing Type 2 diabetes was evaluated by examining the association of changes in leisure time physical activity with the incidence of diabetes among participants in both the combined intervention and control groups (118). The change in total leisure time physical activity was more strongly associated with incident diabetes than changes in subcategories of leisure time physical activity (Table 2). After adjustment for confounding factors (including low-intensity leisure time physical activity and its change), participants in the upper third of the change in total leisure time physical activity were 66% less likely to develop diabetes than those in the lower third; those in the upper third of a change in moderate-to-vigorous leisure time physical activity were 49% to 65% less likely to develop diabetes than those who were in the lower third. Even changes in low-intensity leisure time physical activity also predicted a 59% to 64% reduction in the risk of incident diabetes.

In the U.S. Diabetes Prevention Program (DPP), 3234 nondiabetic persons with elevated fasting and postload plasma glucose concentrations were randomized to a placebo group, a group assigned metformin, or a group assigned a lifestyle-modification program with the goals of at least a 7% weight loss and at least 150 minutes of physical activity per week (146,150). The mean age of the participants was 51 years, the mean BMI was 34.0 kg/m^2, 68% of the participants were women, and 45% of them were members of nonCaucasian ethnic groups. The exercise intervention emphasized brisk walking, but other activities with equivalent intensity, including aerobic dance, bicycle riding, skating, and swimming, were also recommended. The participants were advised to distribute their physical activity throughout the week, with at least 10 minutes per session. Voluntary, supervised physical activity sessions were offered at least twice per week throughout the study, including group walks, aerobic classes, and one-to-one personal training. After an average follow-up of 2.8 years, the incidence of diabetes was 11.0, 7.8, and 4.8 cases per 100 person-years in the placebo, metformin, and lifestyle groups, respectively. The lifestyle intervention reduced the incidence by 58% and metformin by 31%, compared with placebo, and the lifestyle intervention was significantly more effective than metformin in the prevention of Type 2 diabetes.

Additional analyses of the U.S. DPP data examined the effect of intensive lifestyle intervention and metformin therapy on the incidence of the metabolic syndrome among adults without the syndrome at baseline (151). After a mean follow-up of 3.0 years, the cumulative incidence per 100 person-years of the

Table 2 Relative Risk[a] (95% Confidence Interval) of Developing Type 2 Diabetes, According to Tertiles of Change in Leisure Time Physical Activity Among Finns in the Diabetes Prevention Study

Change in total leisure time physical activity			
Tertiles[b] (hr/wk)	Model 1	Model 2	Model 3
-3.2 ((-35)–(-0.5))	1.00	1.00	1.00
0.5 (-0.5–1.7)	0.47 (0.28–0.79)	0.48 (0.28–0.82)	0.52 (0.31–0.89)
3.8 (1.8–19)	0.26 (0.15–0.47)	0.29 (0.16–0.53)	0.34 (0.19–0.62)
P for the trend	<0.001	<0.001	<0.001
Change in moderate-to-vigorous leisure time physical activity (≥3.5 METs)			
-1.5 ((-13.5)–(-0.1))	1.00	1.00	1.00
0.5 (-0.1–1.3)	0.78 (0.46–1.33)	0.86 (0.49–1.48)	0.95 (0.54–1.65)
2.6 (1.3–14.4)	0.35 (0.18–0.65)	0.40 (0.21–0.76)	0.51 (0.26–0.97)
P for the trend	0.001	0.004	0.037
Change in low-intensity leisure time physical activity (<3.5 METs)			
-3.2 ((-34)–(-1.0))	1.00	1.00	1.00
0.8 (-0.9–1.1)	0.83 (0.47–1.45)	0.85 (0.47–1.53)	0.63 (0.34–1.17)
3.1 (1.1–15.0)	0.38 (0.20–0.70)	0.41 (0.22–0.77)	0.36 (0.19–0.67)
P for the trend	0.001	0.003	0.001

[a]Model 1: adjusted for age, sex, group, baseline physical activity. Model 2: adjusted for variables in Model 1, plus baseline values and changes in dietary intake of energy, total fat, saturated fat, and fiber. Model 3: adjusted for variables in model 2, plus baseline values and change in body mass index. For moderate-to-vigorous activity, adjustment was also made for baseline low-intensity activity and change in low-intensity activity.
[b]The median (range) of the change in leisure time physical activity is shown.
Abbreviation: MET, midwest exercise trial.
Source: From Ref. 118.

metabolic syndrome was 61% in the placebo group, 50% in the metformin group, and 38% in the lifestyle group. Compared with placebo, the incidence of the metabolic syndrome was reduced by 41% in the lifestyle group and 17% in the metformin group.

In the 1970s, the Multiple Risk Factor Intervention Trial (MRFIT) enrolled 12,866 middle-aged men 35 to 57 years of age at high risk for CAD and delivered either special intervention or usual care over six to seven years (147). This trial, initiated in 1973, was originally designed to examine CAD as the outcome of interest. The special intervention group was counseled to change diet (reduce saturated fat, cholesterol, and calorie intake), to stop smoking, and to increase physical activity. Recently, the data from the MRFIT were used to investigate the role of the lifestyle intervention program in preventing Type 2 diabetes. In 11,827 men without diabetes and impaired fasting glycemia at baseline, a total of 666 men (11.5%) in the special intervention group and 616 men (10.8%) in the usual care group met the criteria for diabetes during six years of follow-up. Among nonsmokers, the intervention program resulted in a statistically significant 18% reduction in the incidence of diabetes compared with the usual care group. In smokers, however, the diabetes risk increased significantly by 26%.

The available data from these trials indicate that lifestyle intervention, including counseling for physical activity, nutrition, and body weight, can reduce the risk of Type 2 diabetes by 40% to 60% among adults with IGT, and by about 20% among general nonsmoking individuals. Smokers have an increased risk of Type 2 diabetes (104,152–155), but thus far it has remained unclear as to how to reduce their risk because in the MRFIT men who stopped smoking did not reduce their diabetes risk (147).

Biological Mechanisms

While physical activity reduces the risk of Type 2 diabetes certainly through favorable energy balance and weight control, it also has direct effects on insulin sensitivity and the components of the metabolic syndrome (156,157), in addition to reducing the risk of developing the metabolic syndrome and Type 2 diabetes (118,125). The lifestyle intervention in the DPS (145,149) and the DPP (158) resulted not only in a marked reduction in the risk of developing Type 2 diabetes but also in favorable changes in several cardiovascular risk factors, including a reduction in body weight, a decrease in blood pressure, an increase in plasma levels of HDL cholesterol, a decrease in plasma levels of triglycerides, and a reduction in fasting and two-hour glucose and hemoglobin A_{1c}. Data from the Insulin Resistance Atherosclerosis Study showed that both vigorous and nonvigorous activities were associated with higher insulin sensitivity among 1467 men and women 40 to 69 years of age (156). The British Regional Heart Study examined the role of serum insulin concentration and components of the insulin resistance syndrome in the relation between physical activity and the incidence of Type 2 diabetes among 5159 men 40 to 59 years of age (157). The study found that physical activity was significantly and inversely associated with serum insulin concentrations and many components of the metabolic syndrome, and these associations partly explained the relation between physical activity and the incidence of Type 2 diabetes.

Although the exact mechanisms underlying the association between a low cardiorespiratory fitness and increased risk of Type 2 diabetes is unknown, several putative mechanisms have been proposed. Individuals with a low cardiorespiratory fitness tend to have insulin resistance (159), as well as fewer glucose transporters compared with those who are more fit (160). The Kuopio Ischemic Heart Disease Risk Factor Study suggested that poor cardiorespiratory fitness is not only associated with all components of the metabolic syndrome, but might also be considered a feature of the syndrome (139). Finally, low cardiorespiratory fitness is an indication of a sedentary lifestyle, which results in an increased risk of the metabolic syndrome and Type 2 diabetes.

Combined Physical Activity and Dietary Approaches

Another critical factor in preventing Type 2 diabetes is the prevention and treatment of obesity through dietary energy restriction and increasing physical activity. Regular exercise can markedly reduce body weight and fat mass without dietary caloric restriction in overweight individuals. An increase in total energy expenditure appears to be the most important determinant of successful exercise-induced weight loss. The best long-term results may be achieved when physical activity produces an energy expenditure of at least 2500 kcal per week. The optimal approach in weight-reduction programs appears to be a combination of regular physical activity and caloric restriction. A minimum of 60 minutes, but most likely 80 to 90 minutes of moderate-intensity physical activity per day may be needed to avoid or limit weight regain in former overweight or obese individuals. Regular moderate-intensity physical activity, a healthy diet, and avoiding unhealthy weight gain are effective and safe ways to prevent and treat Type 2 diabetes, as well as CVD, and to reduce premature mortality in all population groups (1,123,161–168). Particular attention should be paid to individuals who are physically inactive, have unhealthy diets or are prone to weight gain. To combat the epidemic of overweight at a population level, it is important to develop strategies to increase habitual physical activity and to prevent overweight and obesity in collaboration with communities, families, schools, work sites, healthcare professionals, media, and policymakers (169).

NUTRITIONAL FACTORS AND APPROACHES IN THE METABOLIC SYNDROME

Nutritional Factors: Data from Prospective Epidemiological Studies

Amount and Quality of Dietary Fat

A high-fat diet has been associated with obesity, increased body fat for a given weight, and altered fat distribution, and each of these changes has been associated with change in glucose metabolism (170,171). Results from some earlier prospective studies have shown a positive association between total fat intake and the risk of Type 2 diabetes (172,173); however, most large studies indicated no association between total fat intake and the risk of Type 2 diabetes (174–176). The quality of dietary fat may be more important than the total fat intake. Generally, high saturated fat intake has been associated with a higher risk of IGT (173), and higher fasting plasma glucose (177) and fasting serum insulin (178). Higher proportion of saturated fatty acids in serum lipids/muscle phospholipids has been reported to link to higher fasting insulin (179), lower insulin sensitivity (180), and a higher risk of developing Type 2 diabetes (181). Higher vegetable fat and polyunsaturated fat intake have in turn been associated with lower risk of Type 2 diabetes (175,182,183). Furthermore, high dietary polyunsaturated:saturated fat ratio was inversely associated with the risk of diabetes in the European Prospective Investigation of Cancer-Norfolk study; however, the association was attenuated and no longer significant after adjustment for BMI (176). A report from the Nurses Health Study suggests a positive association between trans fatty acid intake and the risk of Type 2 diabetes (183), but this association was not observed in other studies (175,184).

Amount and Quality of Carbohydrates

Some controversies surround the optimal ratio of carbohydrate-to-fat in the diet with respect to the prevention of chronic diseases, including Type 2 diabetes. Low fat and high carbohydrate diets may increase postprandial glucose and insulin levels as well as triglycerides, and may decrease HDL cholesterol. However, results from prospective studies did not find an association between total carbohydrate and diabetes risk (182,185,186). Metabolic consequences of carbohydrate intake depend not only on their quantity but also on their quality. Similar to total fat, the various types of dietary carbohydrates are more important than the total carbohydrate intake.

Several large studies clearly showed that a relatively low intake of dietary fiber significantly increased the risk of Type 2 diabetes (182,185–187). The association was found to be strong for cereal fiber, a rich source of insoluble fiber, but weaker for sources of soluble fiber (182,185–187).

Because the glycemic response varies substantially between different foods and because this variability is not explainable by glucose chain length, the concept of glycemic index was developed to quantify the glycemic responses induced by carbohydrates in different foods (187,188). Some prospective studies examining the relation between glycemic index and the risk of Type 2 diabetes have reported varying findings, including direct association (182,185,187), or no association (186,189).

Micronutrients

Magnesium is an important component of whole grains and other unprocessed foods, such as nuts and green leafy vegetables. A significant inverse relationship between magnesium intake and the risk of diabetes has been found in several prospective studies (186,190,191). Recently, it has been found that high levels of sodium intake, measured by the highest quartile of the 24-hour sodium excretion, significantly increased the risk of Type 2 diabetes (192). Moreover, the Nurses' Health Study has found that both vitamin D and calcium intakes were inversely associated with the development of Type 2 diabetes, and the benefits of the two nutrients appear to be additive (193).

Individual Foods

The association between specific food intake and the risk of Type 2 diabetes has been evaluated in the recent years. Coffee, one of the most consumed beverages in the world, has been found to have an inverse association with the risk of Type 2 diabetes in some (194–199), but not all (200,201) prospective studies. The data from the Health Professionals' Follow-up Study (184) and the Nurses' Health Study (202) also found that high intake of processed meats could increase the risk for developing Type 2 diabetes. Recent results from prospective studies have indicated that high intakes of nut (203) and dairy products (204) are associated with a decreased risk of Type 2 diabetes; however, high consumptions of sugar-sweetened beverages (205) and French fry consumption (206) are associated with an increased risk for the development of Type 2 diabetes.

Alcohol

A recent review including 32 studies has indicated that moderate alcohol consumption appears to be associated with a reduced risk for diabetes, whereas some evidence suggests that heavy alcohol consumption may be associated with an increased risk (207).

Overall Dietary Patterns

Several studies have assessed the association between overall dietary patterns and the risk of diabetes. A pattern characterized by higher intake of fruits and vegetables (prudent pattern) was associated with a reduced risk of Type 2 diabetes, whereas a pattern characterized by higher intake of foods typical of Western diets (Western pattern) was associated with an increased risk of Type 2 diabetes (208–210).

Nutritional Approaches: Data from Clinical Trials

Two recent studies, DPS and DPP, where reductions in total fat intake and saturated fat have been a part of lifestyle intervention aim to prevent Type 2 diabetes in a high risk group (145,146), which together with increase in exercise, weight loss, and increase in dietary fiber intake was efficient in reducing the incidence of diabetes by 58% in both studies (145,146).

One clinical trial has also assessed the effect of a Mediterranean-style diet on endothelial function and vascular inflammatory markers in patients with the metabolic syndrome (211). A total of 180 patients (99 men and 81 women) with the metabolic syndrome were randomized either to an intensive lifestyle intervention group ($n = 90$) or a control group ($n = 90$). Patients in the intervention group were instructed to follow a Mediterranean-style diet and received detailed advice on how to increase daily consumption of whole grains, fruits, vegetables, nuts, and olive oil; patients in the control group followed a prudent diet (carbohydrates, 50–60%; proteins, 15–20%; total fat, less than 30%). After two years of follow-up, mean body weight decreased more in patients in the intervention group (–4.0 kg) than in those in the control group (–1.2 kg) ($P < 0.001$). Compared with patients consuming the control diet, patients consuming the intervention diet had significantly reduced serum concentrations of C-reactive protein ($P = 0.01$) and interleukins 6 ($P = 0.04$), as well as decreased insulin resistance ($P < 0.001$). Endothelial function score improved in the intervention group (mean change, +1.9; $P < 0.001$) but remained stable in the control group (+0.2; $P = 0.33$). After two years of follow-up, 40 patients in the intervention group still had features of the metabolic syndrome, compared with 78 patients in the control group ($P < 0.001$).

LIFESTYLE RECOMMENDATIONS IN THE METABOLIC SYNDROME

Recently, an American Heart Association/National Heart, Lung, and Blood Institute Scientific Statement have provided a summary of clinical management for the metabolic syndrome (96). The primary goal of clinical management in individuals with the metabolic syndrome is to reduce the risk for clinical atherosclerotic disease. In people with the metabolic syndrome, first-line therapy is directed toward the major risk factors: LDL-C above goal, hypertension, and diabetes (96). Prevention of Type 2 diabetes is another important goal when it is not present in a person with the metabolic syndrome. For individuals with established diabetes, risk factor management must be intensified to diminish their higher risk for CVD (96). The prime emphasis in the management of the metabolic syndrome per se is on mitigating the modifiable, underlying risk factors (obesity, physical inactivity, and atherogenic diet) through lifestyle changes. Effective lifestyle change will reduce all of the metabolic risk factors. Moreover, smoking patients should be encouraged to stop smoking in order to reduce the increased cardiovascular risk.

Table 3 summarizes the current goals and recommendations for management of patients with the metabolic syndrome, which have been suggested by the American Heart Association/National Heart, Lung, and Blood Institute Scientific Statement (96). Structured lifestyle intervention in the metabolic syndrome should include

- A regular exercise regimen to improve cardiorespiratory fitness and maintain weight loss
- Strict goals for calorie restriction to ensure a health diet and gradual weight loss
- Comprehensive patient education
- Regular follow-up and counseling to monitor

Table 3 Lifestyle Goals and Recommendations for Clinical Management of Metabolic Syndrome[a]

Goals	Recommendations
Abdominal obesity	
Reduce body weight by 7% to 10% during Year 1 of therapy. Continue weight loss thereafter to extent possible with goal to ultimately achieve desirable weight (body mass index <25 kg/m^2)	Consistently encourage weight maintenance/reduction through appropriate balance of physical activity, caloric intake, and formal behavior modification programs when indicated to maintain/achieve waist circumference of <40 in. in men and <35 in. in women. Aim initially at slow reduction of and 7% to 10% from baseline weight. Even small amounts of weight loss are associated with significant health benefits
Physical inactivity	
Regular moderate-intensity physical activity; at least 30 min of continuous or intermittent (and preferably ≥60 min) 5 day/wk, but preferably daily	In patients with established cardiovascular disease, assess risk with detailed physical activity history and/or an exercise test, to guide prescription. Encourage 30 to 60 min of moderate-intensity aerobic activity: brisk walking, preferably daily, supplemented by increase in daily lifestyle activities (e.g., pedometer step tracking, walking breaks at work, gardening, and housework). Longer exercise times can be achieved by accumulating exercise throughout the day. Encourage resistance training 2 day/wk. Advise medically supervised programs for high-risk patients (e.g., recent acute coronary syndrome or revascularization, and congestive heart failure)
Atherogenic diet	
Reduced intake of saturated fat, *trans* fat, cholesterol	Recommendations: saturated fat <7% of total calories; reduce *trans* fat; dietary cholesterol <200 mg/dL; total fat 25% to 35% of total calories. Most dietary fat should be unsaturated; simple sugars should be limited

[a]A recommendation from an American Heart Association/National Heart, Lung, and Blood Institute Scientific Statement.
Source: From Ref. 96.

FUTURE RESEARCH

The currently available epidemiological evidence from prospective studies and clinical trials confirms that obesity, sedentary lifestyles, and unhealthy diet are the major contributors to the diabetes epidemic. Overweight and obesity are the stronger risk factors for diabetes; and daily engaging in 30 minutes of moderate or high level of physical activity can reduce the risk of diabetes. Several important questions, however, need to be addressed. Lifestyle interventions, including physical activity and a healthy diet, have been indicated to have beneficial effect on the prevention of diabetes in high-risk groups, but we should know if the lifestyle interventions have the similar effect in the general population at large, especially in younger people. On the other hand, older populations seem to benefit from lifestyle changes because they are likely to have various diseases within a short time. Future prospective studies should be able to provide more evidence on biological mechanisms underlying physical activity, obesity, and diabetes association, and the effects of gene–physical activity interaction on the diabetes risk. The most important task is finding out the effective public health strategies to promote physical activity and prevent overweight and obesity at whole population level.

CONCLUSIONS

Diabetes is one of the fastest growing public health problems in the world, and it is an economic, social, and personal suffering burden. A variety of organizations, including Centers for Disease Control and Prevention and the American College of Sports Medicine (1), National Institutes of Health (212), and the WHO (213) have suggested that every U.S. adult should have at least 30 minutes moderate-intensity physical activity (such as brisk walking, cycling, swimming, home repair, and yard work) on most, preferably all, days of the week. Our review based on the scientific evidence is consistent with this recommendation, and confirms that 30 minutes per day of moderate or high level of physical activity, avoiding excessive weight gain, and a healthy diet are effective and safe ways to prevent Type 2 diabetes in all populations. Regular physical activity and maintaining healthy weight are important components of healthy lifestyle. Public health messages, healthcare professionals, and healthcare system should aggressively promote physical activity during occupation, commuting, leisure time and daily life, and prevent overweight and obesity. This is not only a task for health personnel, but they should also take a lead in process toward the primary prevention of Type 2 diabetes.

REFERENCES

1. Pate RR, Pratt M, Blair SN, et al. Physical activity and public health. A recommendation from the Centers for Disease Control and Prevention and the American College of Sports Medicine. JAMA 1995; 273:402–407.

2. Thompson PD, Buchner D, Pina IL, et al. Exercise and physical activity in the prevention and treatment of atherosclerotic cardiovascular disease: a statement from the Council on Clinical Cardiology (Subcommittee on Exercise, Rehabilitation, and Prevention) and the Council on Nutrition, Physical Activity, and Metabolism (Subcommittee on Physical Activity). Circulation 2003; 107:3109–3116.

3. Kuczmarski RJ, Flegal KM, Campbell SM, et al. Increasing prevalence of overweight among US adults. The National Health and Nutrition Examination Surveys, 1960 to 1991. JAMA 1994; 272:205–211.

4. Flegal KM, Carroll MD, Ogden CL, et al. Prevalence and trends in obesity among US adults, 1999–2000. JAMA 2002; 288:1723–1727.

5. World Health Organisation. Obesity: prevention and managing the global epidemic. WHO Technical Report Series 894. Geneva: World Health Organization; 2000.

6. Ogden CL, Flegal KM, Carroll MD, et al. Prevalence and trends in overweight among US children and adolescents, 1999–2000. JAMA 2002; 288:1728–1732.

7. Crespo CJ, Smit E, Troiano RP, et al. Television watching, energy intake, and obesity in US children: results from the third National Health and Nutrition Examination Survey, 1988–1994. Arch Pediatr Adolesc Med 2001; 155:360–365.

8. Prentice AM, Jebb SA. Obesity in Britain: gluttony or sloth? BMJ 1995; 311:437–439.

9. Grundy SM. Multifactorial causation of obesity: implications for prevention. Am J Clin Nutr 1998; 67:563S–572S.

10. Popkin BM, Nielsen SJ. The sweetening of the world's diet. Obes Res 2003; 11:1325–1332.

11. Clinical Guidelines on the Identification, Evaluation, and Treatment of Overweight and Obesity in Adults–The Evidence Report. National Institutes of Health. Obes Res 1998; 6(suppl 2):51S–209S.

12. Fontaine KR, Redden DT, Wang C, et al. Years of life lost due to obesity. JAMA 2003; 289:187–193.

13. McGinnis JM, Foege WH. Actual causes of death in the United States. JAMA 1993; 270:2207–2212.

14. Allison DB, Fontaine KR, Manson JE, et al. Annual deaths attributable to obesity in the United States. JAMA 1999; 282:1530–1538.

15. Colditz G, Mariani A. The costs of obesity and sedentarism in the United States. In: Bouchard C, ed. Physical Activity and Obesity. Champaign, IL: Human Kinetics, 2000:55–65.

16. Wild S, Roglic G, Green A, et al. Global prevalence of diabetes: estimates for the year 2000 and projections for 2030. Diabetes Care 2004; 27:1047–1053.

17. DECODE Study Group. Age- and sex-specific prevalences of diabetes and impaired glucose regulation in 13 European cohorts. Diabetes Care 2003; 26:61–69.

18. Qiao Q, Hu G, Tuomilehto J, et al. Age- and sex-specific prevalence of diabetes and impaired glucose regulation in 11 Asian cohorts. Diabetes Care 2003; 26:1770–1780.

19. Narayan KM, Boyle JP, Thompson TJ, et al. Lifetime risk for diabetes mellitus in the United States. JAMA 2003; 290:1884–1890.

20. Arslanian S. Type 2 diabetes in children: clinical aspects and risk factors. Horm Res 2002; 57(suppl 1):19–28.

21. Laakso M. Hyperglycemia and cardiovascular disease in Type 2 diabetes. Diabetes 1999; 48:937–942.

22. WHO Consultation. Definition, diagnosis, and classification of diabetes mellitus and its complications. Part 1: diagnosis and classification of diabetes mellitus. Geneva: World Health Organisation, 1999.

23. Reaven GM. Banting lecture. Role of insulin resistance in human disease. Diabetes 1988; 37:1595–1607.

24. Haffner SM, Valdez RA, Hazuda HP, et al. Prospective analysis of the insulin-resistance syndrome (syndrome X). Diabetes 1992; 41:715–722.

25. Hanson RL, Imperatore G, Bennett PH, et al. Components of the "metabolic syndrome" and incidence of Type 2 diabetes. Diabetes 2002; 51:3120–3127.

26. Laaksonen DE, Lakka HM, Niskanen LK, et al. Metabolic syndrome and development of diabetes mellitus: application and validation of recently suggested definitions of the metabolic syndrome in a prospective cohort study. Am J Epidemiol 2002; 156:1070–1077.

27. Lorenzo C, Okoloise M, Williams K, et al. The metabolic syndrome as predictor of Type 2 diabetes: the San Antonio Heart Study. Diabetes Care 2003; 26:3153–3159.

28. Wang JJ, Hu G, Miettinen ME, et al. The metabolic syndrome and incident diabetes: assessment of four suggested definitions of the metabolic syndrome in a Chinese population with high postprandial glucose. Horm Metab Res 2004; 36:708–715.

29. Wang JJ, Qiao Q, Miettinen ME, et al. The metabolic syndrome defined by factor analysis and incident Type 2 diabetes in a Chinese population with high postprandial glucose. Diabetes Care 2004; 27:2429–2437.

30. Isomaa B, Almgren P, Tuomi T, et al. Cardiovascular morbidity and mortality associated with the metabolic syndrome. Diabetes Care 2001; 24:683–689.

31. Lakka HM, Laaksonen DE, Lakka TA, et al. The metabolic syndrome and total and cardiovascular disease mortality in middle-aged men. JAMA 2002; 288:2709–2716.

32. Ford ES. The metabolic syndrome and mortality from cardiovascular disease and all-causes: findings from the National Health and Nutrition Examination Survey II Mortality Study. Atherosclerosis 2004; 173:309–314.

33. Hu G, Qiao Q, Tuomilehto J, et al. Prevalence of the metabolic syndrome and its relation to all-cause and cardiovascular mortality in nondiabetic European men and women. Arch Intern Med 2004; 164:1066–1076.

34. Malik S, Wong ND, Franklin SS, et al. Impact of the metabolic syndrome on mortality from coronary heart disease, cardiovascular disease, and all causes in United States adults. Circulation 2004; 110:1245–1250.

35. Hunt KJ, Resendez RG, Williams K, et al. National Cholesterol Education Program versus World Health Organization metabolic syndrome in relation to all-cause and cardiovascular mortality in the San Antonio Heart Study. Circulation 2004; 110:1251–1257.

36. Neel JV. Diabetes mellitus: a "thrifty" genotype rendered detrimental by "progress"? Am J Hum Genet 1962; 14:353–362.

37. Groop L, Orho-Melander M. The dysmetabolic syndrome. J Intern Med 2001; 250:105–120.

38. Tuomilehto J, Tuomilehto-Wolf E, Zimmet P, et al. Primary prevention of diabetes mellitus. London: John Wiley & Sons, 1997.

39. Hu G, Qiao Q, Silventoinen K, et al. Occupational, commuting, and leisure-time physical activity in relation to risk for Type 2 diabetes in middle-aged Finnish men and women. Diabetologia 2003; 46:322–329.

40. Laaksonen DE, Niskanen L, Lakka HM, et al. Epidemiology and treatment of the metabolic syndrome. Ann Med 2004; 36:332–346.

41. Wing RR, Goldstein MG, Acton KJ, et al. Behavioral science research in diabetes: lifestyle changes related to obesity, eating behavior, and physical activity. Diabetes Care 2001; 24:117–123.

42. Livingstone MB, Strain JJ, Prentice AM, et al. Potential contribution of leisure activity to the energy expenditure patterns of sedentary populations. Br J Nutr 1991; 65:145–155.

43. Ravussin E, Lillioja S, Anderson TE, et al. Determinants of 24-hour energy expenditure in man. Methods and results using a respiratory chamber. J Clin Invest 1986; 78:1568–1578.

44. Martinez-Gonzalez MA, Martinez JA, Hu FB, et al. Physical inactivity, sedentary lifestyle and obesity in the European Union. Int J Obes Relat Metab Disord 1999; 23:1192–1201.

45. Andersen RE, Crespo CJ, Bartlett SJ, et al. Relationship of physical activity and television watching with body weight and level of fatness among children: results from the Third National Health and Nutrition Examination Survey. JAMA 1998; 279:938–942.

46. Voorrips LE, Meijers JH, Sol P, et al. History of body weight and physical activity of elderly women differing in current physical activity. Int J Obes Relat Metab Disord 1992; 16:199–205.

47. Schulz LO, Schoeller DA. A compilation of total daily energy expenditures and body weights in healthy adults. Am J Clin Nutr 1994; 60:676–681.

48. Ravussin E, Lillioja S, Knowler WC, et al. Reduced rate of energy expenditure as a risk factor for body-weight gain. N Engl J Med 1988; 318:467–472.

49. Davies PS, Gregory J, White A. Physical activity and body fatness in preschool children. Int J Obes Relat Metab Disord 1995; 19:6–10.

50. Coakley EH, Rimm EB, Colditz G, et al. Predictors of weight change in men: results from the Health Professionals Follow-up Study. Int J Obes Relat Metab Disord 1998; 22:89–96.

51. Erlichman J, Kerbey AL, James WP. Physical activity and its impact on health outcomes. Paper 2: prevention of unhealthy weight gain and obesity by physical activity: an analysis of the evidence. Obes Rev 2002; 3:273–287.

52. Saris WH, Blair SN, van Baak MA, et al. How much physical activity is enough to prevent unhealthy weight gain? Outcome of the IASO 1st Stock Conference and consensus statement. Obes Rev 2003; 4:101–114.

53. Hu FB, Li TY, Colditz GA, et al. Television watching and other sedentary behaviors in relation to risk of obesity and Type 2 diabetes mellitus in women. JAMA 2003; 289:1785–1791.

54. DiPietro L, Kohl HW III, Barlow CE, et al. Improvements in cardiorespiratory fitness attenuate age-related weight gain in healthy men and women: the Aerobics Center Longitudinal Study. Int J Obes Relat Metab Disord 1998; 22:55–62.

55. Ballor DL, Keesey RE. A meta-analysis of the factors affecting exercise-induced changes in body mass, fat mass and fat-free mass in males and females. Int J Obes 1991; 15:717–726.

56. Garrow JS, Summerbell CD. Meta-analysis: effect of exercise, with or without dieting, on the body composition of overweight subjects. Eur J Clin Nutr 1995; 49:1–10.

57. Andersen RE, Wadden TA, Bartlett SJ, et al. Effects of lifestyle activity vs structured aerobic exercise in obese women: a randomized trial. JAMA 1999; 281:335–340.
58. Ross R, Dagnone D, Jones PJ, et al. Reduction in obesity and related comorbid conditions after diet-induced weight loss or exercise-induced weight loss in men. A randomized, controlled trial. Ann Intern Med 2000; 133:92–103.
59. Ross R, Janssen I. Physical activity, total and regional obesity: dose-response considerations. Med Sci Sports Exerc 2001; 33:S521–S527; discussion S528–S529.
60. Irwin ML, Yasui Y, Ulrich CM, et al. Effect of exercise on total and intra-abdominal body fat in postmenopausal women: a randomized controlled trial. JAMA 2003; 289:323–330.
61. Jakicic JM, Marcus BH, Gallagher KI, et al. Effect of exercise duration and intensity on weight loss in overweight, sedentary women: a randomized trial. JAMA 2003; 290:1323–1330.
62. Jeffery RW, Wing RR, Sherwood NE, et al. Physical activity and weight loss: does prescribing higher physical activity goals improve outcome? Am J Clin Nutr 2003; 78:684–689.
63. Donnelly JE, Hill JO, Jacobsen DJ, et al. Effects of a 16-month randomized controlled exercise trial on body weight and composition in young, overweight men and women: the Midwest Exercise Trial. Arch Intern Med 2003; 163:1343–1350.
64. Slentz CA, Duscha BD, Johnson JL, et al. Effects of the amount of exercise on body weight, body composition, and measures of central obesity: STRRIDE–a randomized controlled study. Arch Intern Med 2004; 164:31–39.
65. Kirk EP, Jacobsen DJ, Gibson C, et al. Time course for changes in aerobic capacity and body composition in overweight men and women in response to long-term exercise: the Midwest Exercise Trial (MET). Int J Obes Relat Metab Disord 2003; 27:912–919.
66. Fogelholm M, Kukkonen-Harjula K. Does physical activity prevent weight gain–a systematic review. Obes Rev 2000; 1:95–111.
67. Santa-Clara H, Fernhall B, Baptista F, et al. Effect of a one-year combined exercise training program on body composition in men with coronary artery disease. Metabolism 2003; 52:1413–1417.
68. Schmitz KH, Jensen MD, Kugler KC, et al. Strength training for obesity prevention in midlife women. Int J Obes Relat Metab Disord 2003; 27:326–333.
69. Cuff DJ, Meneilly GS, Martin A, et al. Effective exercise modality to reduce insulin resistance in women with Type 2 diabetes. Diabetes Care 2003; 26:2977–2982.
70. Jeffery RW, McGuire MT, French SA. Prevalence and correlates of large weight gains and losses. Int J Obes Relat Metab Disord 2002; 26:969–972.
71. Klem ML, Wing RR, McGuire MT, et al. A descriptive study of individuals successful at long-term maintenance of substantial weight loss. Am J Clin Nutr 1997; 66:239–246.
72. Welin L, Svardsudd K, Wilhelmsen L, et al. Analysis of risk factors for stroke in a cohort of men born in 1913. N Engl J Med 1987; 317:521–526.
73. Larsson B, Svardsudd K, Welin L, et al. Abdominal adipose tissue distribution, obesity, and risk of cardiovascular disease and death: 13 year follow up of participants in the study of men born in 1913. Br Med J (Clin Res Ed) 1984; 288:1401–1404.
74. Casassus P, Fontbonne A, Thibult N, et al. Upper-body fat distribution: a hyperinsulinemia-independent predictor of coronary heart disease mortality. The Paris Prospective Study. Arterioscler Thromb 1992; 12:1387–1392.

75. Fujimoto WY, Bergstrom RW, Boyko EJ, et al. Visceral adiposity and incident coronary heart disease in Japanese American men. The 10-year follow-up results of the Seattle Japanese American Community Diabetes Study. Diabetes Care 1999; 22:1808–1812.

76. Lakka HM, Lakka TA, Tuomilehto J, et al. Abdominal obesity is associated with increased risk of acute coronary events in men. Eur Heart J 2002; 23:706–713.

77. Rexrode KM, Buring JE, Manson JE. Abdominal and total adiposity and risk of coronary heart disease in men. Int J Obes Relat Metab Disord 2001; 25:1047–1056.

78. Folsom AR, Kaye SA, Sellers TA, et al. Body fat distribution and 5-year risk of death in older women. JAMA 1993; 269:483–487.

79. Rexrode KM, Carey VJ, Hennekens CH, et al. Abdominal adiposity and coronary heart disease in women. JAMA 1998; 280:1843–1848.

80. Folsom AR, Kushi LH, Anderson KE, et al. Associations of general and abdominal obesity with multiple health outcomes in older women: the Iowa Women's Health Study. Arch Intern Med 2000; 160:2117–2128.

81. Silventoinen K, Jousilahti P, Vartiainen E, et al. Appropriateness of anthropometric obesity indicators in assessment of coronary heart disease risk among Finnish men and women. Scand J Public Health 2003; 31:283–290.

82. Mourier A, Gautier JF, De Kerviler E, et al. Mobilization of visceral adipose tissue related to the improvement in insulin sensitivity in response to physical training in NIDDM. Effects of branched-chain amino acid supplements. Diabetes Care 1997; 20:385–391.

83. Wilmore JH, Despres JP, Stanforth PR, et al. Alterations in body weight and composition consequent to 20 wk of endurance training: the HERITAGE Family Study. Am J Clin Nutr 1999; 70:346–352.

84. Hu FB, Manson JE, Stampfer MJ, et al. Diet, lifestyle, and the risk of Type 2 diabetes mellitus in women. N Engl J Med 2001; 345:790–797.

85. Koh-Banerjee P, Wang Y, Hu FB, et al. Changes in body weight and body fat distribution as risk factors for clinical diabetes in US men. Am J Epidemiol 2004; 159:1150–1159.

86. Weinstein AR, Sesso HD, Lee IM, et al. Relationship of physical activity vs body mass index with Type 2 diabetes in women. JAMA 2004; 292:1188–1194.

87. Hu G, Lindstrom J, Valle TT, et al. Physical activity, body mass index, and risk of Type 2 diabetes in patients with normal or impaired glucose regulation. Arch Intern Med 2004; 164:892–896.

88. Carey VJ, Walters EE, Colditz GA, et al. Body fat distribution and risk of noninsulin-dependent diabetes mellitus in women. The Nurses' Health Study. Am J Epidemiol 1997; 145:614–619.

89. Wang Y, Rimm EB, Stampfer MJ, et al. Comparison of abdominal adiposity and overall obesity in predicting risk of Type 2 diabetes among men. Am J Clin Nutr 2005; 81:555–563.

90. Stevens J, Couper D, Pankow J, et al. Sensitivity and specificity of anthropometrics for the prediction of diabetes in a biracial cohort. Obes Res 2001; 9:696–705.

91. Ford ES, Williamson DF, Liu S. Weight change and diabetes incidence: findings from a national cohort of US adults. Am J Epidemiol 1997; 146:214–222.

92. Colditz GA, Willett WC, Rotnitzky A, et al. Weight gain as a risk factor for clinical diabetes mellitus in women. Ann Intern Med 1995; 122:481–486.

93. International Diabetes Federation. Worldwide definition of the metabolic syndrome. http://www.idf.org/webdata/docs/IDF_Metasyndrome_definition.pdf August 24, 2005.

94. Balkau B, Charles MA. Comment on the provisional report from the WHO consultation. European Group for the Study of Insulin Resistance (EGIR). Diabet Med 1999; 16:442–443.

95. National Institute of Health. Executive Summary of The Third Report of The National Cholesterol Education Program (NCEP) Expert Panel on Detection, Evaluation, And Treatment of High Blood Cholesterol In Adults (Adult Treatment Panel III). JAMA 2001; 285:2486–2497.

96. Grundy SM, Cleeman JI, Daniels SR, et al. Diagnosis and management of the metabolic syndrome: an American Heart Association/National Heart, Lung, and Blood Institute Scientific Statement. Circulation 2005; 112:2735–2752.

97. Everson SA, Goldberg DE, Helmrich SP, et al. Weight gain and the risk of developing insulin resistance syndrome. Diabetes Care 1998; 21:1637–1643.

98. Helmrich SP, Ragland DR, Leung RW, et al. Physical activity and reduced occurrence of noninsulin-dependent diabetes mellitus. N Engl J Med 1991; 325:147–152.

99. Manson JE, Rimm EB, Stampfer MJ, et al. Physical activity and incidence of noninsulin-dependent diabetes mellitus in women. Lancet 1991; 338:774–778.

100. Manson JE, Nathan DM, Krolewski AS, et al. A prospective study of exercise and incidence of diabetes among US male physicians. JAMA 1992; 268:63–67.

101. Hu FB, Sigal RJ, Rich-Edwards JW, et al. Walking compared with vigorous physical activity and risk of Type 2 diabetes in women: a prospective study. JAMA 1999; 282:1433–1439.

102. Hu FB, Leitzmann MF, Stampfer MJ, et al. Physical activity and television watching in relation to risk for Type 2 diabetes mellitus in men. Arch Intern Med 2001; 161:1542–1548.

103. Burchfiel CM, Sharp DS, Curb JD, et al. Physical activity and incidence of diabetes: the Honolulu Heart Program. Am J Epidemiol 1995; 141:360–368.

104. Perry IJ, Wannamethee SG, Walker MK, et al. Prospective study of risk factors for development of noninsulin dependent diabetes in middle aged British men. BMJ 1995; 310:560–564.

105. Eriksson KF, Lindgarde F. Poor physical fitness, and impaired early insulin response but late hyperinsulinaemia, as predictors of NIDDM in middle-aged Swedish men. Diabetologia 1996; 39:573–579.

106. Lynch J, Helmrich SP, Lakka TA, et al. Moderately intense physical activities and high levels of cardiorespiratory fitness reduce the risk of noninsulin-dependent diabetes mellitus in middle-aged men. Arch Intern Med 1996; 156:1307–1314.

107. Okada K, Hayashi T, Tsumura K, et al. Leisure-time physical activity at weekends and the risk of Type 2 diabetes mellitus in Japanese men: the Osaka Health Survey. Diabet Med 2000; 17:53–58.

108. Nakanishi N, Takatorige T, Suzuki K. Daily life activity and risk of developing impaired fasting glucose or Type 2 diabetes in middle-aged Japanese men. Diabetologia 2004; 47:1768–1775.

109. Haapanen N, Miilunpalo S, Vuori I, et al. Association of leisure time physical activity with the risk of coronary heart disease, hypertension and diabetes in middle-aged men and women. Int J Epidemiol 1997; 26:739–747.

110. Folsom AR, Kushi LH, Hong CP. Physical activity and incident diabetes mellitus in postmenopausal women. Am J Public Health 2000; 90:134–138.

111. Meisinger C, Thorand B, Schneider A, et al. Sex differences in risk factors for incident Type 2 diabetes mellitus: the MONICA Augsburg cohort study. Arch Intern Med 2002; 162:82–89.

112. Meisinger C, Lowel H, Thorand B, et al. Leisure time physical activity and the risk of Type 2 diabetes in men and women from the general population. The MONICA/KORA Augsburg Cohort Study. Diabetologia 2005; 48:27–34.

113. Dotevall A, Johansson S, Wilhelmsen L, et al. Increased levels of triglycerides, BMI and blood pressure and low physical activity increase the risk of diabetes in Swedish women. A prospective 18-year follow-up of the BEDA*study. Diabet Med 2004; 21:615–622.

114. James SA, Jamjoum L, Raghunathan TE, et al. Physical activity and NIDDM in African Americans. The Pitt County Study. Diabetes Care 1998; 21:555–562.

115. Kriska AM, Saremi A, Hanson RL, et al. Physical activity, obesity, and the incidence of Type 2 diabetes in a high-risk population. Am J Epidemiol 2003; 158:669–675.

116. Hsia J, Wu L, Allen C, et al. Physical activity and diabetes risk in postmenopausal women. Am J Prev Med 2005; 28:19–25.

117. Paffenbarger RS Jr, Blair SN, Lee IM, et al. Measurement of physical activity to assess health effects in free-living populations. Med Sci Sports Exerc 1993; 25:60–70.

118. Laaksonen DE, Lindstrom J, Lakka TA, et al. Physical activity in the prevention of Type 2 diabetes: the finnish diabetes prevention study. Diabetes 2005; 54:158–165.

119. Wei M, Gibbons LW, Mitchell TL, et al. The association between cardiorespiratory fitness and impaired fasting glucose and Type 2 diabetes mellitus in men. Ann Intern Med 1999; 130:89–96.

120. Sawada SS, Lee IM, Muto T, et al. Cardiorespiratory fitness and the incidence of Type 2 diabetes: prospective study of Japanese men. Diabetes Care 2003; 26:2918–2922.

121. Bjornholt JV, Erikssen G, Liestol K, et al. Prediction of Type 2 diabetes in healthy middle-aged men with special emphasis on glucose homeostasis. Results from 22.5 years' follow-up. Diabet Med 2001; 18:261–267.

122. Carnethon MR, Gidding SS, Nehgme R, et al. Cardiorespiratory fitness in young adulthood and the development of cardiovascular disease risk factors. JAMA 2003; 290:3092–3100.

123. Blair SN, Cheng Y, Holder JS. Is physical activity or physical fitness more important in defining health benefits? Med Sci Sports Exerc 2001; 33:S379–S399.

124. Hambrecht R, Wolf A, Gielen S, et al. Effect of exercise on coronary endothelial function in patients with coronary artery disease. N Engl J Med 2000; 342:454–460.

125. Laaksonen DE, Lakka HM, Salonen JT, et al. Low levels of leisure-time physical activity and cardiorespiratory fitness predict development of the metabolic syndrome. Diabetes Care 2002; 25:1612–1618.

126. Stefanick ML, Mackey S, Sheehan M, et al. Effects of diet and exercise in men and postmenopausal women with low levels of HDL cholesterol and high levels of LDL cholesterol. N Engl J Med 1998; 339:12–20.

127. Thompson PD, Crouse SF, Goodpaster B, et al. The acute versus the chronic response to exercise. Med Sci Sports Exerc 2001; 33:S438–S445; discussion S452–S433.

128. Paffenbarger RS Jr, Hyde RT, Wing AL, et al. Physical activity, all-cause mortality, and longevity of college alumni. N Engl J Med 1986; 314:605–613.

129. Blair SN, Kohl HW III, Paffenbarger RS Jr, et al. Physical fitness and all-cause mortality. A prospective study of healthy men and women. JAMA 1989; 262:2395–2401.

130. Blair SN, Kampert JB, Kohl HW III, et al. Influences of cardiorespiratory fitness and other precursors on cardiovascular disease and all-cause mortality in men and women. JAMA 1996; 276:205–210.

131. Sandvik L, Erikssen J, Thaulow E, et al. Physical fitness as a predictor of mortality among healthy, middle-aged Norwegian men. N Engl J Med 1993; 328:533–537.

132. Lakka TA, Venalainen JM, Rauramaa R, et al. Relation of leisure-time physical activity and cardiorespiratory fitness to the risk of acute myocardial infarction. N Engl J Med 1994; 330:1549–1554.

133. Manson JE, Hu FB, Rich-Edwards JW, et al. A prospective study of walking as compared with vigorous exercise in the prevention of coronary heart disease in women. N Engl J Med 1999; 341:650–658.

134. Sesso HD, Paffenbarger RS Jr, Lee IM. Physical activity and coronary heart disease in men: the Harvard Alumni Health Study. Circulation 2000; 102:975–980.

135. Tanasescu M, Leitzmann MF, Rimm EB, et al. Exercise Type and intensity in relation to coronary heart disease in men. JAMA 2002; 288:1994–2000.

136. Lakka TA, Laukkanen JA, Rauramaa R, et al. Cardiorespiratory fitness and the progression of carotid atherosclerosis in middle-aged men. Ann Intern Med 2001; 134:12–20.

137. Wilmore JH. Dose-response: variation with age, sex, and health status. Med Sci Sports Exerc 2001; 33:S622–S634; discussion S640–S621.

138. Bouchard C, Rankinen T. Individual differences in response to regular physical activity. Med Sci Sports Exerc 2001; 33:S446–S451; discussion S452–S443.

139. Lakka TA, Laaksonen DE, Lakka HM, et al. Sedentary lifestyle, poor cardiorespiratory fitness, and the metabolic syndrome. Med Sci Sports Exerc 2003; 35:1279–1286.

140. Nakanishi N, Takatorige T, Suzuki K. Daily life activity and risk of developing cardiovascular risk factors. Diabetes Care 2005; 28:1500–1502.

141. Ferreira I, Twisk JW, van Mechelen W, et al. Development of fatness, fitness, and lifestyle from adolescence to the age of 36 years: determinants of the metabolic syndrome in young adults: the Amsterdam growth and health longitudinal study. Arch Intern Med 2005; 165:42–48.

142. LaMonte MJ, Barlow CE, Jurca R, et al. Cardiorespiratory fitness is inversely associated with the incidence of metabolic syndrome: a prospective study of men and women. Circulation 2005; 112:505–512.

143. Eriksson KF, Lindgarde F. Prevention of Type 2 (noninsulin-dependent) diabetes mellitus by diet and physical exercise. The 6-year Malmo feasibility study. Diabetologia 1991; 34:891–898.

144. Pan X, Li G, Hu Y, et al. Effects of diet and exercise in preventing NIDDM in people with impaired glucose tolerance. The Da Qing IGT and Diabetes Study. Diabetes Care 1997; 20:537–544.

145. Tuomilehto J, Lindstrom J, Eriksson JG, et al. Prevention of Type 2 diabetes mellitus by changes in lifestyle among subjects with impaired glucose tolerance. N Engl J Med 2001; 344:1343–1350.

146. Knowler WC, Barrett-Connor E, Fowler SE, et al. Reduction in the incidence of Type 2 diabetes with lifestyle intervention or metformin. N Engl J Med 2002; 346:393–403.

147. Davey Smith G, Bracha Y, Svendsen KH, et al. Incidence of Type 2 diabetes in the randomized multiple risk factor intervention trial. Ann Intern Med 2005; 142:313–322.

148. Eriksson J, Lindstrom J, Valle T, et al. Prevention of Type II diabetes in subjects with impaired glucose tolerance: the Diabetes Prevention Study (DPS) in Finland. Study design and 1-year interim report on the feasibility of the lifestyle intervention programme. Diabetologia 1999; 42:793–801.

149. Lindstrom J, Louheranta A, Mannelin M, et al. The Finnish Diabetes Prevention Study (DPS): lifestyle intervention and 3-year results on diet and physical activity. Diabetes Care 2003; 26:3230–3236.

150. The Diabetes Prevention Program Research Group. The Diabetes Prevention Program (DPP): description of lifestyle intervention. Diabetes Care 2002; 25: 2165–2171.

151. Orchard TJ, Temprosa M, Goldberg R, et al. The effect of metformin and intensive lifestyle intervention on the metabolic syndrome: the Diabetes Prevention Program randomized trial. Ann Intern Med 2005; 142:611–619.

152. Patja K, Jousilahti P, Hu G, et al. Effects of smoking, obesity and physical activity on the risk of Type 2 diabetes in middle-aged Finnish men and women. J Intern Med 2005; 258:356–362.

153. Persson PG, Carlsson S, Svanstrom L, et al. Cigarette smoking, oral moist snuff use and glucose intolerance. J Intern Med 2000; 248:103–110.

154. Wannamethee SG, Shaper AG, Perry IJ. Smoking as a modifiable risk factor for Type 2 diabetes in middle-aged men. Diabetes Care 2001; 24:1590–1595.

155. Rimm EB, Manson JE, Stampfer MJ, et al. Cigarette smoking and the risk of diabetes in women. Am J Public Health 1993; 83:211–214.

156. Mayer-Davis EJ, D'Agostino R Jr, Karter AJ, et al. Intensity and amount of physical activity in relation to insulin sensitivity: the Insulin Resistance Atherosclerosis Study. JAMA 1998; 279:669–674.

157. Wannamethee SG, Shaper AG, Alberti KG. Physical activity, metabolic factors, and the incidence of coronary heart disease and Type 2 diabetes. Arch Intern Med 2000; 160:2108–2116.

158. The Diabetes Prevention Program Research Group. Impact of Intensive Lifestyle and Metformin Therapy on Cardiovascular Disease Risk Factors in the Diabetes Prevention Program. Diabetes Care 2005; 28:888–894.

159. Sato Y, Iguchi A, Sakamoto N. Biochemical determination of training effects using insulin clamp technique. Horm Metab Res 1984; 16:483–486.

160. Ivy JL, Kuo CH. Regulation of GLUT4 protein and glycogen synthase during muscle glycogen synthesis after exercise. Acta Physiol Scand 1998; 162:295–304.

161. Willett WC, Dietz WH, Colditz GA. Guidelines for healthy weight. N Engl J Med 1999; 341:427–434.

162. Wannamethee SG, Shaper AG. Physical activity in the prevention of cardiovascular disease: an epidemiological perspective. Sports Med 2001; 31:101–114.

163. Dubbert PM, Carithers T, Sumner AE, et al. Obesity, physical inactivity, and risk for cardiovascular disease. Am J Med Sci 2002; 324:116–126.

164. Erlichman J, Kerbey AL, James WP. Physical activity and its impact on health outcomes. Paper 1: the impact of physical activity on cardiovascular disease and all-cause mortality: an historical perspective. Obes Rev 2002; 3:257–271.

165. Katzmarzyk PT, Janssen I, Ardern CI. Physical inactivity, excess adiposity and premature mortality. Obes Rev 2003; 4:257–290.

166. Hu FB, Willett WC, Li T, et al. Adiposity as compared with physical activity in predicting mortality among women. N Engl J Med 2004; 351:2694–2703.

167. Hu G, Tuomilehto J, Silventoinen K, et al. Joint effects of physical activity, body mass index, waist circumference and waist-to-hip ratio with the risk of cardiovascular disease among middle-aged Finnish men and women. Eur Heart J 2004; 25:2212–2219.

168. Hu G, Tuomilehto J, Silventoinen K, et al. The effects of physical activity and body mass index on cardiovascular, cancer and all-cause mortality among 47,212 middle-aged Finnish men and women. Int J Obes Relat Metab Disord 2005; 29:894–902.

169. Lakka TA, Bouchard C. Physical activity, obesity and cardiovascular diseases. Hand b Exp Pharmacol. 2005; 170:137–163.

170. Hu FB, van Dam RM, Liu S. Diet and risk of Type II diabetes: the role of types of fat and carbohydrate. Diabetologia 2001; 44:805–817.

171. Steyn NP, Mann J, Bennett PH, et al. Diet, nutrition and the prevention of Type 2 diabetes. Public Health Nutr 2004; 7:147–165.

172. Marshall JA, Hoag S, Shetterly S, et al. Dietary fat predicts conversion from impaired glucose tolerance to NIDDM. The San Luis Valley Diabetes Study. Diabetes Care 1994; 17:50–56.

173. Feskens EJ, Virtanen SM, Rasanen L, et al. Dietary factors determining diabetes and impaired glucose tolerance. A 20-year follow-up of the Finnish and Dutch cohorts of the Seven Countries Study. Diabetes Care 1995; 18:1104–1112.

174. Colditz GA, Manson JE, Stampfer MJ, et al. Diet and risk of clinical diabetes in women. Am J Clin Nutr 1992; 55:1018–1023.

175. Meyer KA, Kushi LH, Jacobs DR Jr, et al. Dietary fat and incidence of Type 2 diabetes in older Iowa women. Diabetes Care 2001; 24:1528–1535.

176. Harding AH, Day NE, Khaw KT, et al. Dietary fat and the risk of clinical Type 2 diabetes: the European prospective investigation of Cancer-Norfolk study. Am J Epidemiol 2004; 159:73–82.

177. Feskens EJ, Kromhout D. Habitual dietary intake and glucose tolerance in euglycaemic men: the Zutphen Study. Int J Epidemiol 1990; 19:953–959.

178. Marshall JA, Bessesen DH, Hamman RF. High saturated fat and low starch and fibre are associated with hyperinsulinaemia in a nondiabetic population: the San Luis Valley Diabetes Study. Diabetologia 1997; 40:430–438.

179. Folsom AR, Ma J, McGovern PG, et al. Relation between plasma phospholipid saturated fatty acids and hyperinsulinemia. Metabolism 1996; 45:223–228.

180. Vessby B, Tengblad S, Lithell H. Insulin sensitivity is related to the fatty acid composition of serum lipids and skeletal muscle phospholipids in 70-year-old men. Diabetologia 1994; 37:1044–1050.

181. Vessby B, Aro A, Skarfors E, et al. The risk to develop NIDDM is related to the fatty acid composition of the serum cholesterol esters. Diabetes 1994; 43:1353–1357.

182. Salmeron J, Ascherio A, Rimm EB, et al. Dietary fiber, glycemic load, and risk of NIDDM in men. Diabetes Care 1997; 20:545–550.

183. Salmeron J, Hu FB, Manson JE, et al. Dietary fat intake and risk of Type 2 diabetes in women. Am J Clin Nutr 2001; 73:1019–1026.

184. van Dam RM, Willett WC, Rimm EB, et al. Dietary fat and meat intake in relation to risk of Type 2 diabetes in men. Diabetes Care 2002; 25:417–424.

185. Salmeron J, Manson JE, Stampfer MJ, et al. Dietary fiber, glycemic load, and risk of noninsulin-dependent diabetes mellitus in women. JAMA 1997; 277:472–477.

186. Meyer KA, Kushi LH, Jacobs DR Jr, et al. Carbohydrates, dietary fiber, and incident Type 2 diabetes in older women. Am J Clin Nutr 2000; 71:921–930.

187. Schulze MB, Liu S, Rimm EB, et al. Glycemic index, glycemic load, and dietary fiber intake and incidence of Type 2 diabetes in younger and middle-aged women. Am J Clin Nutr 2004; 80:348–356.

188. Jenkins DJ, Wolever TM, Taylor RH, et al. Glycemic index of foods: a physiological basis for carbohydrate exchange. Am J Clin Nutr 1981; 34:362–366.

189. Stevens J, Ahn K, Juhaeri, et al. Dietary fiber intake and glycemic index and incidence of diabetes in African American and white adults: the ARIC study. Diabetes Care 2002; 25:1715–1721.

190. Lopez-Ridaura R, Willett WC, Rimm EB, et al. Magnesium intake and risk of Type 2 diabetes in men and women. Diabetes Care 2004; 27:134–140.

191. Song Y, Manson JE, Buring JE, et al. Dietary magnesium intake in relation to plasma insulin levels and risk of Type 2 diabetes in women. Diabetes Care 2004; 27:59–65.

192. Hu G, Jousilahti P, Peltonen M, et al. Urinary sodium and potassium excretion and the risk of Type 2 diabetes: a prospective study in Finland. Diabetologia 2005; 48:1477–1483.

193. Pittas AG, Dawson-Hughes B, Li T, et al. Vitamin D and calcium intake in relation to Type 2 diabetes in women. Diabetes Care 2006; 29:650–656.

194. van Dam RM, Feskens EJ. Coffee consumption and risk of Type 2 diabetes mellitus. Lancet 2002; 360:1477–1478.

195. Rosengren A, Dotevall A, Wilhelmsen L, et al. Coffee and incidence of diabetes in Swedish women: a prospective 18-year follow-up study. J Intern Med 2004; 255:89–95.

196. Salazar-Martinez E, Willett WC, Ascherio A, et al. Coffee consumption and risk for Type 2 diabetes mellitus. Ann Intern Med 2004; 140:1–8.

197. Tuomilehto J, Hu G, Bidel S, et al. Coffee consumption and risk of Type 2 diabetes mellitus among middle-aged Finnish men and women. JAMA 2004; 291:1213–1219.

198. Carlsson S, Hammar N, Grill V, et al. Coffee consumption and risk of Type 2 diabetes in Finnish twins. Int J Epidemiol 2004; 33:616–617.

199. van Dam RM, Hu FB. Coffee consumption and risk of Type 2 diabetes: a systematic review. JAMA 2005; 294:97–104.

200. Reunanen A, Heliovaara M, Aho K. Coffee consumption and risk of Type 2 diabetes mellitus. Lancet 2003; 361:702–703.

201. Saremi A, Tulloch-Reid M, Knowler WC. Coffee consumption and the incidence of Type 2 diabetes. Diabetes Care 2003; 26:2211–2212.

202. Schulze MB, Manson JE, Willett WC, et al. Processed meat intake and incidence of Type 2 diabetes in younger and middle-aged women. Diabetologia 2003; 46:1465–1473.

203. Jiang R, Manson JE, Stampfer MJ, et al. Nut and peanut butter consumption and risk of Type 2 diabetes in women. JAMA 2002; 288:2554–2560.

204. Pereira MA, Jacobs DR Jr, Van Horn L, et al. Dairy consumption, obesity, and the insulin resistance syndrome in young adults: the CARDIA Study. JAMA 2002; 287:2081–2089.

205. Schulze MB, Manson JE, Ludwig DS, et al. Sugar-sweetened beverages, weight gain, and incidence of Type 2 diabetes in young and middle-aged women. JAMA 2004; 292:927–934.

206. Halton TL, Willett WC, Liu S, et al. Potato and French fry consumption and risk of Type 2 diabetes in women. Am J Clin Nutr 2006; 83:284–290.
207. Howard AA, Arnsten JH, Gourevitch MN. Effect of alcohol consumption on diabetes mellitus: a systematic review. Ann Intern Med 2004; 140:211–219.
208. Fung TT, Schulze M, Manson JE, et al. Dietary patterns, meat intake, and the risk of Type 2 diabetes in women. Arch Intern Med 2004; 164:2235–2240.
209. van Dam RM, Rimm EB, Willett WC, et al. Dietary patterns and risk for Type 2 diabetes mellitus in U.S. men. Ann Intern Med 2002; 136:201–209.
210. Montonen J, Knekt P, Harkanen T, et al. Dietary patterns and the incidence of Type 2 diabetes. Am J Epidemiol 2005; 161:219–227.
211. Esposito K, Marfella R, Ciotola M, et al. Effect of a mediterranean-style diet on endothelial dysfunction and markers of vascular inflammation in the metabolic syndrome: a randomized trial. JAMA 2004; 292:1440–1446.
212. NIH Consensus Development Panel on Physical Activity and Cardiovascular Health. Physical activity and cardiovascular health. NIH Consensus Development Panel on Physical Activity and Cardiovascular Health. JAMA 1996; 276:241–246.
213. World Health Organisation. Global strategy on diet, physical activity, and health. Geneva 2004. WHA27.17, Agenda Item 12.6.

10

Management of Patients with the Metabolic Syndrome: Compliance with or Adherence to Treatment?

C. Tissa Kappagoda and Ezra A. Amsterdam
Department of Medicine, Division of Cardiology, University of California, Davis, California, U.S.A.

SUMMARY

■ The metabolic syndrome is a condition that affects nearly 40% of Americans and presents a significant public health problem.

■ Effective management of the metabolic syndrome is complicated by its multifaceted nature and by the fact that there is a strong behavioral element in its development.

■ In general, the current health-care systems in developed countries are not readily adaptable to managing chronic diseases of this nature.

■ Thus, agencies entrusted with the task of guiding health policy in this field have tended to advocate an approach that is centered upon pharmacologic interventions with a modest exhortation to promote lifestyle changes.

■ The latter which is probably the more cost-effective approach to the problem requires a regrouping of forces among health-care providers emphasizing a multidisciplinary team approach that blends the skills of physicians, nurses, dieticians, exercise physiologists, and behaviorists.

INTRODUCTION

The metabolic syndrome has been recognized as a clinical entity in one form or another for more than 80 years. Kylin described a clinical syndrome composed of hypertension, hyperglycemia, and hyperuricemia in 1923 (1). Since then, the combination of obesity, hypertension, diabetes, and serum lipid abnormalities has been described variously as the deadly quartet (Kaplan, 1989), syndrome "X" (2), plurimetabolic syndrome (3), the insulin resistance syndrome (4), and the dysmetabolic syndrome (5). The phenomenon is currently designated the metabolic syndrome (6).

The National Cholesterol Education Program Adult Treatment Panel (NCEP III) defines the condition based on the presence of three of the following factors: abdominal obesity, elevated serum triglycerides, low serum high-density lipoprotein concentration, elevated blood pressure, and an elevated blood glucose (7). These factors when viewed as individual entities do not usually engage the attention of physicians in a manner that would lead to effective therapy (8,9). It is their clustering that is even more demanding of consideration as an illness. The definitions of the syndrome by the World Health Organization and the European Group for the Study of Insulin Resistance differ slightly from the foregoing, but do not appear to influence the indications for treatment required for these patients (Table 1).

Recently, the American Diabetes Association (ADA) and the European Association for the Study of Diabetes (EASD) issued a joint statement urging caution on accepting a universal definition of the metabolic syndrome (10). Their thesis is based principally on the perceived lack of precision in the cut points of the various components of the syndrome. While there is a certain superficial validity in this claim, one has to temper these apparent shortcomings with the findings of other studies such as the Interheart study, which established the universality of the conventional cardiovascular risk factors in identifying those likely to develop a myocardial infarction (MI) (11). In this study, although the cut points were not defined with the level of precision demanded by the ADA and the EASD, the risks attached to some of the variables, which constitute the metabolic syndrome, were identified clearly. While scientific rigor requires that definitions of diseases should be as precise as possible, demands for an impossible level of precision in identifying the metabolic syndrome carry the risk of relegating what is an important public health issue to the status of the 800-lb somnolent simian in the room, whose lethality becomes apparent only when it awakes.

COMPLIANCE OR ADHERENCE?

Physicians tend to regard treatment and compliance as two sides of the same therapeutic coin in most diseases. Compliance, which is usually defined as obedience to a request or command, also carries all the connotations of the authoritarian physician who "knows best." Several recent societal developments have undermined this proposition. For instance, the relentless exposure of the public to health issues in the mass media has led many people to assume a greater role in decisions

Table 1 Three Definitions of the Metabolic Syndrome

WHO criteria (1999)	European Group for the Study of Insulin Resistance (1999)	NCEP III 2001
Diabetes, impaired fasting glycemia, impaired glucose tolerance, or insulin resistance, plus two of the following	Insulin resistance plus two of the following	Three occurrences of the following[a]:
Obesity: BMI >30 kg/m^2 or waist-to-hip ratio >0.9 (male) and >0.85 (female)	Central obesity: Waist circumference ≥37 in. (male) or 31.5 in. (female)	Central obesity: Waist circumference ≥40 in. (male) or 35 in. (female)
Dyslipidemia: Triglycerides >150 mg% or HDL <35 mg % (male) and <40 mg% (female)	Dyslipidemia: Triglycerides >175 mg% or HDL < 40 mg%	Dyslipidemia: Triglycerides ≥150 mg/dL or HDL <40 mg/dL (or medication for either)[b]
Hypertension: Blood pressure >140/90 mmHg	Hypertension: Blood pressure ≥140/90 mmHg with or without medications	Hypertension: Blood pressure ≥135/85 mmHg (or medication)[b]
Microalbuminuria: Excretion >20 µg/min	Fasting plasma glucose: >100 mg%	Fasting plasma glucose: >110 mg/dL (≥100 mg/dL or on hypoglycemic medication)[b]

[a]Elevated triglycerides and low HDL-C count as separate criteria.
[b]Revisions from AHA/NHLBI statement 2005 (24).
Abbreviations: WHO, world health organization; HDL, high-density lipoprotein; BMI, body mass index; NCEP, National Cholesterol Education Program; HDL-C, high-density lipoprotein-cholesterol; AHA/NHLBI.

concerning their health and fostered a belief that physicians require their guidance to make appropriate therapeutic decisions. The sale of untested nutraceuticals through the internet, the availability of over-the-counter ethical preparations, and direct media advertising to the public have all contributed to this trend.

Operating in such a climate of opinion, physicians have had to switch to a more collegial approach and embrace the idea of adherence instead of compliance. Implicit in adherence is the idea of behaving according to a plan, which ideally is developed jointly by the patient and the caregiver.

Treatment protocols for the management of the metabolic syndrome are made particularly difficult by two aspects of the condition, which are not evident in most other chronic diseases. The first is the sheer magnitude of the problem and the second is the nature of the condition.

Table 2 Prevalence of the Metabolic
Syndrome (%) in the United States
Based on NCEP III Criteria

Overall prevalence	37.9
Based on Race/Ethnicity	
NonHispanic White	39.2
NonHispanic Black	34.6
Mexican American	43.5
Other	35.9
Based on age (yr)	
50–59	30.6
60–69	41.5
70–79	42.6
>80	43.3

Source: From Ref. 12.

IMPACT OF PREVALENCE

The overall prevalence of the metabolic syndrome as defined by the NCEP III is
approximately 38% of the adult population in the United States. In certain seg-
ments of the population, the incidence is even higher (Table 2) (12). Given these
large numbers, the metabolic syndrome presents a public health hazard of
unprecedented proportions.

IMPACT OF THE MULTIFACETED NATURE OF THE SYNDROME

It is widely accepted that the metabolic syndrome is associated with a substantially
increased risk of developing diabetes mellitus. Regardless of which definition of the
syndrome is used, the odds ratio of developing diabetes varies between 5.0 and 8.8
(13). Apart from the impact of diabetes on cardiovascular risk (7), persons with the
metabolic syndrome alone, without evidence of diabetes, also have an enhanced
risk of developing coronary artery disease (CAD) and cardiovascular disease
(CVD) (14). Data derived from the second National Health and Nutrition
Examination Survey showed that over an average follow-up of 13.3 years, the hazard ratios for developing CAD and dying from CVD were 2.02 (95% CI, 1.42–2.89)
and 1.82 (95% CI, 1.40–2.37), respectively, in individuals with no preexisting
CVD. The hazard ratios were even higher in those with preexisting disease (14).

It should be appreciated that several features of the metabolic syndrome
have an independent association with the development of CVD. For instance
abdominal obesity, dyslipidemias, elevated blood pressure, insulin resistance,
and/or glucose intolerance, proinflammatory state, and prothrombotic mediators
are widely recognized as independent cardiovascular risk factors (15). Thus, the
metabolic syndrome presents a significant challenge to health-care professionals
involved in preventive cardiology.

INTERVENTIONS FOR PATIENTS WITH THE METABOLIC SYNDROME

From the perspective of preventive cardiology, there are certain specific issues that need to be addressed systematically. These are summarized in Table 3. In addition to the areas listed in the Table, recent evidence suggests that certain psychological variables such as hostility enhance the propensity of patients with the metabolic syndrome to sustain an MI (18).

Several surveys have repeatedly confirmed that these targets, though widely publicized, are often not adhered to in practice (8,9). It is likely that the reasons for this poor record of implementation reside in factors that could be laid at the feet of both physicians and patients.

It is evident that the management of the metabolic syndrome has to proceed along two parallel tracks, one based on the use of medications (Fig. 1) and the other based on therapeutic lifestyle change (see below). However, implementation of such a dual approach, though logical and evidence based, presents unique problems.

Pharmacologic Interventions for the Metabolic Syndrome

Several advisory bodies such as the American Heart Association, NCEP III, European Heart Association, and Joint National Committee for the management of hypertension have provided detailed recommendations for the management of blood pressure (17), lipid abnormalities (7,19), insulin resistance and hyperglycemia, and potential thrombotic complications associated with the metabolic

Table 3 Summary of Interventions to Prevent Cardiovascular Disease in Patients with the Metabolic Syndrome

Clinical problem	Action required
Abdominal obesity	Weight management consistent with FNB guidelines for diet and exercise (16)
Atherogenic dyslipidemia	Achieve (NCEP III) targets for HDL, LDL and triglycerides (7)
Raised blood pressure	Adherence to JNC 7 guidelines (17)
Insulin resistance ± glucose intolerance	Exercise, dietary management and medications to reduce insulin resistance
Proinflammatory state	No specific treatment
Prothrombotic state	Antiplatelet therapy
Physical inactivity	Regular moderate exercise (see text)
Dietary changes	Reduce intake of saturated fat and trans fat. Saturated fat: 7% of total calories and fat: approximately 25–30% of total calories
Cigarette smoking	Smoking cessation

Abbreviations: NCEP: National Cholesterol Education Program, FNB: Food Nutrition Board, JNC: Joint National Committee, HDL-C: high-density lipoprotein cholesterol, LDL-C: low-density lipoprotein cholesterol.

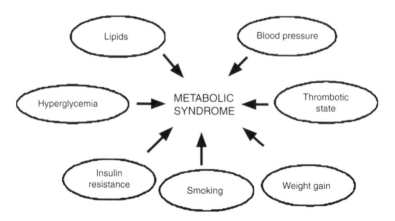

Figure 1   Potential areas for interventions in persons with the metabolic syndrome.

syndrome. These interventions are described in detail in other chapters in this book and summarized in Figure 1 and Table 4.

Among the recent developments in the area of pharmacologic approaches to the management of the metabolic syndrome is the use of selective cannabinoid 1 receptor blockers in the endocannabinoid system. In a randomized trial of such a drug (rimonabant) recently completed (21) in obese subjects with a body mass index (BMI) $\geq$ 30 kg/m^2 (or $\geq$ 27 kg/m^2 with treated or untreated dyslipidemias, hypertension, or both), subjects were randomized to receive double-blind treatment with placebo, 5 mg rimonabant, or 20 mg rimonabant once daily, in addition to a "mild" hypocaloric diet (600 kcal/day deficit). After one year of treatment, subjects receiving both dose levels of rimonabant had lost significantly more weight than those on the placebo. The 5-mg and 20-mg groups lost 3.4 kg and 6.6 kg, respectively, whereas the placebo group lost 1.8 kg during the period of the study. These results are interesting, but two notes of caution have to be

Table 4   Specific Therapeutic Targets for Patients with the Metabolic Syndrome

Parameters	Specific therapeutic targets	References
Serum lipids	LDL-C <100 mg/dL	
	HDL-C $\geq$45 mg/dL for men and	(7)
	>55 mg/dL for women	
Blood pressure	<120/80 mmHg	(17)
Fasting blood glucose	<100 mg/dL (hemoglobin A$_{1c}$<7.0%)	(20)
Weight loss	Aim to lose 3–4 lb/mo	
Exercise	Daily exercise (45 min/day)	

Note: Exercise should be an integral part of a weight loss program.
Abbreviations: HDL-C, high-density lipoprotein cholesterol; LDL-C, low-density lipoprotein cholesterol.

sounded. First the data was analyzed on the "last observation carried forward" principle, which means that adherence to the treatment program is questionable. Secondly, if the subjects had reduced their calorie intake by 600 cal/day, they should have lost in excess of 25 kg in weight over one year. For these reasons, the findings of the Rimonabant In Obesity (RIO-Europe) trial should be viewed with caution and emphasize the need to incorporate a strong behavioral element to the management of patients with the metabolic syndrome (see below).

Failure of Pharmacologic Interventions—The Efficacy Gap

Judging from the epidemiologic studies reported from the United States and Europe, it is apparent that these recommendations, despite their wealth of detail, have failed to provide a road map for physicians to combat the related "epidemics" of obesity, the metabolic syndrome, and Type 2 diabetes (Fig. 2).

Projections for the next two decades also suggest that the current system of healthcare in the United States is unlikely to deal effectively with these concerns in a meaningful fashion (Fig. 3). In addition, upon reviewing the latest recommendation of the American Heart Association and the National Institutes of Health for the management of the metabolic syndrome, one feels less than optimistic about the immediate future, because much of the emphasis is placed upon the therapeutic goals, and little attention is paid to the manner in which these goals are to be achieved (24). The absence of practical help in this area from policy makers compounds the problems experienced by those responsible for delivering care to these patients.

In general, physicians are ill-equipped to deal with chronic diseases such as the metabolic syndrome both by their training and the circumstances of their

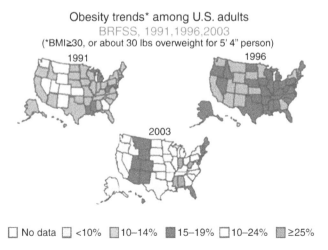

Figure 2 Trends in obesity in the United States for the period 1991 to 2003. *Source*: From Ref. 22.

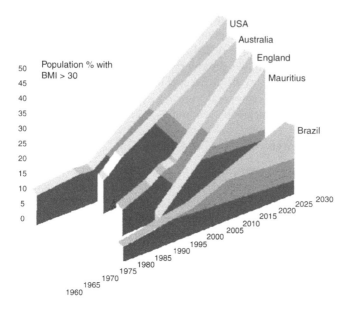

Figure 3 Projections for obesity in the next two decades. Data from the International Taskforce on Obesity. *Source*: From Ref. 23.

practice. The traditional medical curriculum places a premium on crisis management. This model is precise and well defined by established procedures and evidence-based algorithms that demand specific interventions in acute and subacute clinical settings. The conventional criteria for judging professional competence of young physicians is their ability to diagnose an acute condition rapidly, initiate appropriate therapy, and minimize the hospital stay. This type of training places little or no emphasis on the management of patients with chronic diseases. Ironically, nearly 90% of individuals requiring treatment need care for chronic disease, and they are found in an outpatient setting.

Lifestyle-Based Interventions for Patients with the Metabolic Syndrome

The nature of lifestyle interventions is a multimodal interaction between the patient and caregivers (Fig. 4). Patients with the metabolic syndrome need several modalities of care, which busy primary-care physicians, harried by the conveyor belt mind-set of payer agencies and hampered by inadequate training, are not in a position to provide. The situation is not significantly better in tertiary-care hospitals in which specialized services such as nutritional counseling, exercise training, and clinical psychological care are available. Even in this environment, there is an incessant need for physicians to balance the requirements of academic activity with the mundane but essential business of earning one's financial keep.

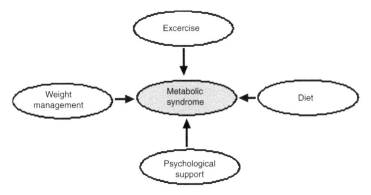

Figure 4   Lifestyle-based interventions in the metabolic syndrome.

The challenges presented by this combination of ill-prepared physicians working within a system that does not recognize the special needs of patients with chronic illnesses need to be addressed now. It calls for a significant regrouping of forces in order to create a team concept, where the patient is the driver and caregivers, the pit crew (Fig. 5).

AN ALTERNATIVE MEDICAL PARADIGM FOR MANAGING THE METABOLIC SYNDROME

The nature of the interaction in the model, depicted in Figure 5, moves a significant portion of the execution of the care plan away from the caregivers to the

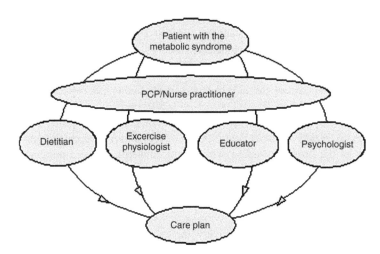

Figure 5   Care plan for patients with the metabolic syndrome.

patient, i.e., guides and empowers patients to undertake self-care. This model utilizes three related ideas that promote a lifestyle change: 1) Attitudes toward change—The Health Belief Model (HBM), 2) Stages of change, and 3) Motivational interviewing.

Health Belief Model

The central concept in this approach to care is the proposition that success or failure of management of a disease depends on the patient's attitude and beliefs regarding health-related matters. The HBM was probably the first formal attempt at providing a psychological framework for explaining and predicting health behaviors. The HBM was first developed in the 1950s by Hochbaum, Rosenstock, and Kegels working in the U.S. Public Health Service. The model was developed in response to the failure of a free tuberculosis health-screening program. Since then, the HBM has been applied to a variety of clinical situations that are relevant to patients diagnosed with the metabolic syndrome such as dietary management (25), exercise (26), adherence to medical regimens (27), and smoking cessation (28).

Core Issues in the Health Belief Model

The HBM (29) is based on the understanding that a person will take positive health-related actions under three circumstances. When viewed from the perspective of an overweight patient with the metabolic syndrome, these conditions could be adapted as follows:

1. Patient feels that a negative health condition such as CAD or the onset of Type 2 diabetes could be avoided.
2. Patient has a positive expectation that taking a recommended action would enable him/her to avoid a negative health condition (e.g., successful weight control to prevent the onset of Type 2 diabetes).
3. Patient believes that he/she can successfully change a behavior to promote weight loss (e.g., adopt a low-fat, hypocaloric diet).

The HBM was spelled out initially in terms of four concepts representing the perceived threat and net benefits: (i) perceived susceptibility of the individual to the adverse outcome, (ii) perceived severity of the current situation, (iii) perceived benefits to be derived from the proposed action, and (iv) perceived barriers to execution of the proposed action. These four concepts define a person's "readiness to act" with respect to their health problem (Table 5).

The original model has been modified to include a "cue to action," to translate intent into overt behavior. Later the concept of self-efficacy was added to the model to define one's confidence and ability to successfully perform an action to help the HBM better fit the challenges of changing habitually unhealthy behaviors that are common in patients with the metabolic syndrome, such as being sedentary, smoking, or overeating (29).

Table 5 Summary of Health Belief Model as Applied to the Metabolic Syndrome

Concept	Definition	Response of care giver
Perceived susceptibility	Patient's opinion of the chances of developing a complication of the metabolic syndrome	Define population risk Individualize risk based on patient characteristics Raise perceived susceptibility if patient's perception is too low
Perceived severity	Patient's opinion of his/her own chances of developing a complication of the metabolic syndrome	Specify individual consequences of developing the complication
Perceived benefit	Patient's belief in the efficacy of the advised action to reduce risk or seriousness of impact of complication	Define action to be taken in detail (how, when, where?) and positive effects to be expected
Perceived barriers	Patient's belief in the efficacy of the advised action to reduce risk or seriousness of impact of complication	Identify and reduce barriers through reassurance, incentives and assistance
Efficacy	Patient's confidence in his/her ability to take action	Provide education, guidance in performing action, i.e., cues to action

Source: Adapted from Ref. 29.

Stages of Change

Cues for change have to be based on an understanding of the processes of change experienced by those who wish to alter their lifestyle. This process is usually depicted as a five-stage model (30), and is widely used in the management of addictive behaviors. It is suggested that people move through five stages in making changes in lifestyle, but the progression is not always an orderly process and is often associated with relapses before attainment of a goal. These stages are as follows:

1. Precontemplation stage in which patients do not believe they have a disease or do not want to change (Many patients with the metabolic syndrome remain at this stage and need motivation to advance to another stage),
2. Contemplation stage in which patients begin to perceive their clinical problems and evaluate cost benefits.
3. Determination stage in which the patients have made a decision to change, and the caregiver is beginning to have a positive impact on them.

4. Action stage in which the patients have received the cues to action from the caregiver.
5. Maintenance stage in which the patients need reinforcement about the value of the changes they have made.

Recently, these concepts have been recommended as a means of addressing the problems of patients with chronic diseases. There are several studies in which the "stages of change" have played an integral part in the development of a care plan for patients in weight-management programs (31,32) and in exercise programs (33). However, other investigators have not been able to establish a definitive relationship between stages of change and success in weight management (34).

It is important to recognize also that in reality, relapses into a sedentary lifestyle or poor eating habits are common and often precipitated by general life stresses.

Motivational Interviewing

Motivation is the act of providing a reason for a person to undertake a particular course of action. Motivational interviewing is a counseling approach based on the principle that all human behavior is motivated (35). It acknowledges that many patients experience ambivalence when deciding to make lifestyle changes because they perceive both the advantages and the disadvantages of changing or continuing with their current behavior. The aim of motivational interviewing is to enhance motivation to change while not focusing on the change itself. The advantage in the technique is that patient maneuvers him/herself into a situation where a change is both logical and likely to be beneficial. The technique, which was first developed for the treatment of addictive behaviors, focuses on two specific areas. For instance, in the case of a patient with the metabolic syndrome aiming to lose weight, the interview will address the importance of the patient's current dietary habits and sedentary behavior and the level of confidence he/she has in affecting a change. The interviewer approaches the patients in a nonconfrontational, nonjudgmental fashion.

There are the five counseling techniques that are generally found to be effective:

1) Express empathy—acceptance facilitates change
2) Avoid arguments—resistance is a signal to change strategies
3) Look for inconsistency—consequences that conflict with important goals will favor change
4) Yield to resistance—use it to look for solutions with the patient
5) Support self responsibility—the client is responsible for choosing and carrying out change.

This approach has been used in clinical trials relating to hypertension (36) weight loss (37) and diabetes mellitus (31). Effects on smoking cessation have been explored in several small pilot studies (38). The findings of larger trials are not yet available. Although there have been no trials on patients with the metabolic syndrome per se, a recent meta-analysis of several clinical trials, which address various components of the metabolic syndrome, suggests that the technique is superior to conventional methods of proffering advice to patients.

HEALTH BELIEF MODEL AND THE METABOLIC SYNDROME

There are no studies that have examined the efficacy of the HBM in the management of patients with the metabolic syndrome. There are, however, studies that have examined the effects of treatment plans based on this model upon various components of the syndrome. These studies address the effects on exercise training, dietary management, and control of high blood pressure, and ability to consistently take prescribed medications. In addition, modifications of the HBM have been used in developing smoking cessation programs.

An example of such a study is that reported by Wdowik et al. (28) who examined the effect of a management program based on the HBM in college students suffering from Type 1 diabetes—a group that is traditionally considered to be relatively noncompliant. The study was undertaken to develop and test an intervention designed to enhance knowledge regarding Type 1 diabetes and positively alter attitudes and behaviors. These aspects were assessed before the start of the program, immediately after conclusion of the program and at follow-up in intervention cohorts and a control group. Reporting of glycated hemoglobin (HbA$_{1c}$) values and diabetes knowledge improved significantly as a result of the intervention compared with no increase in the control group. Furthermore, participants reported feeling more support on campus after the intervention, appeared to have overcome their fears associated with testing their blood glucose, reported an increased frequency of blood glucose testing, and were more likely to test when they felt their blood glucose level was low. The frequency of measurements of these parameters was in excess of the minimum standards of care defined by the ADA (20).

Similar studies have established the efficacy of using a patient-centered approach based on the HBM in adherence to dietary management (25), exercise (26), medical regimens (27), and smoking cessation (28). Additionally, the efficacy of this approach appears to transcend different cultures and ethnicities (26,27,30).

A REALITY CHECK

Most patients with the metabolic syndrome are seen by their health-care professionals in a nonresidential outpatient setting. In the majority of instances, such encounters are usually limited to 15 to 20 minutes. It is futile to attempt implementation of even the minimal requirements delineated by the clinical trials. For instance, in the Diabetes Prevention Program (DPP) (39), each patient received a

Table 6   The Interventions in a Multicenter Clinical Trial (Diabetes Prevention Program—DPP) Compared to What Could Be Offered in a Routine Clinic Visit

Intervention	DPP	Average PCP visit
Funding	+	??
Goals	+	+/-
Trained staff	+	-
Team	+	-
Supervised exercise	+	-
Frequent study visits	+	-
Group	+	-
Ethnic/cultural issues	+	-
Motivational component	+	-
Phone surveillance	+	-
Network feedback	+	-

Abbreviation: PCP, primary care physician.

series of interventions. Table 6 depicts the requirements delineated by this funded trial and the reality of conventional outpatient care.

In the DPP, lifestyle change was even more effective than pharmacologic therapy in averting the onset of Type 2 diabetes in patients with the metabolic syndrome (Fig. 6) and it was significantly less expensive, confirming the rationale of this approach. However, as seen in Table 6, the resources and expertise applied in the DPP exceed anything available to the average physician. The DPP is an example of a funded program and raises the obvious issue of the role of public (i.e. government) support to meet the threat of the metabolic syndrome to the health of our population. The demands of patients with the metabolic syndrome are no less exacting than those with Type 2 diabetes. Clearly, there are no means of providing this type of care outside the context of a clinical trial.

PROGRAMS BASED ON MULTIPLE INTERVENTIONS

It has been recognized for many years that patients with established CAD are significantly benefited by multiple interventions involving exercise training, dietary management, stress management, and pharmacologic therapy (40). Further, these programs are effective outside the context of strictly regulated clinical trials (41). However, one of the problems with such an approach is an attrition rate of almost 40%.

The NCEP III has defined the metabolic syndrome as a significant risk factor for CAD with greater than 20% risk of a fatal or nonfatal MI over 10 years. The elements of multiple intervention programs for CAD have features that are essential for the management of patients with the metabolic syndrome. Because such activities

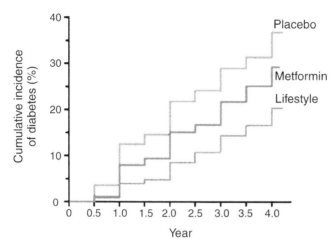

Figure 6 Results of the Diabetes Prevention Program Trial of the effects of lifestyle change, metformin, and placebo on the incidence of Type 2 diabetes in patients with impaired glucose tolerance. Lifestyle change resulted in a 58% reduction in the incidence of diabetes over 4.5 years. *Source*: From Ref. 39.

are available within cardiac rehabilitation programs, it seems reasonable to offer the services of cardiac rehabilitation programs to patients with the metabolic syndrome, especially if such programs also incorporate a version of the HBM and motivational interviewing. A scheme for such a program is depicted in Figure 7. This approach will reduce the frustrating experience of successive outpatient clinic visits, which accomplish little of clinical value besides renewing prescriptions and often place the physician and the patients in an adversarial situation.

The action plan identified above should encompass all elements of the multiple intervention programs with the provision that the patient adopts those portions, depending upon his/her perception of their importance and potential benefit. The role of the caregivers is to identify these elements and assist the patient to broaden the scope of these interventions during the course of treatment. This approach to the management of patients with the metabolic syndrome implies that the patients take an active role in their healthcare, which is tantamount to a partnership with the caregivers. This Utopian ideal has to be tempered with the reality that in a societal melting pot, (e.g., the United States) caregivers would be dealing with a wide spectrum of individuals, all requiring personalized care plans. The current mechanisms for the provision of healthcare for the majority of individuals are not capable of meeting such a challenge. However, before advocating such far ranging changes to the health-care system, it would be important to examine the evidence available for the efficacy of such an approach in the context of both a clinical trial and in free-living individuals.

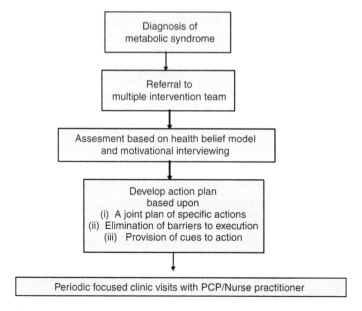

Figure 7   Scheme for developing a care plan for patients with the metabolic syndrome.

PRACTICAL CONSIDERATIONS

For the past 15 years, the University of California Davis Medical Center has offered multiple intervention programs to patients with cardiovascular risk factors (41) and, more recently, for patients with Type 2 diabetes. These programs have incorporated multiple modalities of care such as exercise training, dietary management, therapeutic education, and psychological support. More recently, increasing numbers of patients have been encouraged to undertake their programs at home in order to circumvent the logistic difficulties associated with attending the hospital several times each week. Hospital-based outreach operations of this type are ideally suited for patients with the metabolic syndrome.

Initiation into the Program

Patients are initially evaluated in a clinic, and their overall cardiovascular risk status is assessed. As a part of this assessment, their cardiovascular risk factors (previous cardiac events, serum lipids, blood pressure, smoking status, glycemic control, and criteria for the metabolic syndrome) are evaluated. Smokers are offered the services of a smoking cessation program. Individual care plans are then developed for those interested in making lifestyle changes. In order to avoid duplication of services, the care plans of individual patients are coordinated by a staff member who reports to the caregiver group at periodic intervals. Brief summaries of the various modalities of care offered to these patients are given below.

Exercise Programs

Exercise programs serve several purposes for patients with the metabolic syndrome. Those wishing to undertake an exercise program to improve physical fitness are given guidelines that define target heart rates and rates of perceived exertion, based on an initial treadmill test. In the absence of symptoms and electrocardiographic abnormalities, patients are encouraged to undertake aerobic training at a local gym of their choice. The patients are also given an exercise log to record their workouts, and these are reviewed periodically.

However, aerobic training, which is traditionally undertaken in a gym, has little value as a tool for weight loss. For instance, to lose weight at the rate of 1 lb (of fat) per week, it is necessary to be in a weekly negative energy balance of 3500 cal. This would be equivalent to a daily calorie deficit of 500 cal. A heavy workout of one hour in a gym could potentially result in a calorie expenditure of this magnitude (Table 7). When one adds the travel time to and from an exercise facility, the time commitment is likely to be unacceptably high.

An alternative approach is to increase the calorie expenditure by enhancing the daily activity level. A very useful device for this purpose is a pedometer.

Table 7 Calorie Expenditures of Activities Commonly Perceived as Workout

Activity and calories/min	120 lbs	140 lbs	160 lbs	180 lbs
Aerobics (traditional)	7.4	8.6	9.8	11.1
Basketball	7.5	8.8	10.0	11.3
Bowling	1.2	1.4	1.6	1.9
Cycling (10 mph)	5.5	6.4	7.3	8.2
Golf (pull/carry clubs)	4.6	5.4	6.2	7.0
Golf (power cart)	2.1	2.5	2.8	3.2
Hiking	4.5	5.2	6.0	6.7
Jogging	9.3	10.8	12.4	13.9
Running	11.4	13.2	15.1	17.0
Sitting quietly	1.2	1.3	1.5	1.7
Skating (ice and roller)	5.9	6.9	7.9	8.8
Skiing (cross country)	7.5	8.8	10.0	11.3
Skiing (downhill and water)	5.7	6.6	7.6	8.5
Swimming (crawl and moderate pace)	7.8	9.0	10.3	11.6
Tennis	6.0	6.9	7.9	8.9
Walking	6.5	7.6	8.7	9.7
Weight training	6.6	7.6	8.7	9.8

Note: The values are the calorie expenditures per minute. For instance, an individual weighing 180 lb wishing to spend 300 calories/day will have to jog for 21 minutes. Weights refer to body weight.
Source: From Ref. 42.

Table 8 The Pedometer Log

Week	Instructions		Record steps taken daily							
			Day 1	Day 2	Day 3	Day 4	Day 5	Day 6	Day 7	Total
Week 1 Dates:	If daily steps were: Aim for:									
	<2500 steps	3000 steps on at least 3 days								
	2500–5000 steps	3000–5500 steps on 3 days								
	5000–7500 steps	5500–8000 steps on 3 days								
	>7500 steps	8000–10,000 steps on 3 days								
Week 2 Dates:										
	<2500 steps	3000 steps on at least 3 days								
	2500–5000 steps	3000–5500 steps on 3 days								
	5000–7500 steps	5500–8000 steps on 3 days								
	>7500 steps	8000–10,000 steps on 3 days								
Week 3 Dates:										
	<2500 steps	3000 steps on at least 3 days								
	2500–5000 steps	3000–5500 steps on 3 days								
	5000–7500 steps	5500–8000 steps on 3 days								
	>7500 steps	8000–10,000 steps on 3 days								
Week 4 Dates:										
	<2500 steps	3000 steps on at least 3 days								
	2500–5000 steps	3000–5500 steps on 3 days								
	5000–7500 steps	5500–8000 steps on 3 days								
	>7500 steps	8000–10,000 steps on 3 days								

These devices, which record the number of steps taken during waking hours, provide a simple means of increasing a person's level of activity in a manner that could be documented. Such a record (Table 8) is used to motivate individuals to incorporate physical activity into their daily life, without committing a significant portion of the day to "exercise training."

Taking an average stride length of 2 ft, a little over 2000 steps would constitute a one-mile walk that results in the expenditure of approximately 100 cal. Patients are encouraged to increase their daily step rate at regular intervals in order to promote weight loss. Individual goals can be set depending on a person's lifestyle and weight. In patients with the metabolic syndrome, daily exercise is important, as a means of both reducing insulin resistance (43,44) and promoting weight loss.

Dietary Management

With certain notable exceptions (16), the training in nutrition provided to medical students is heavily tilted toward the biochemistry of nutrition. While this information is important, it does not equip the average physician to discuss the dietary management such as recipes, meal planning, and food preparation with patients. Thus, the advice provided tends to be of the broad-brush variety with exhortations to "avoid fatty foods," "lay off the French fries," "less pizza and more salads," etc. yet, ironically, dietary advice offered by physicians carries more gravitas than when it is provided by a registered dietitian. For this reason, physicians need to work closely with dietitians and be seen to endorse their professional activities.

In our program, patients have an initial interview with a registered dietitian who encourages patients to complete a five-day food diary. This is an important initial step as it provides the dietitian (and the physician) with a good "snapshot" of how the patient approaches meal planning and also to gauge knowledge about nutritional matters (Fig. 8).

Once this information is available, it is possible to begin a meaningful dialog regarding making changes, if the patient is willing to do so.

Patients also need detailed information about how to read food labels and select and prepare food. Many food labels are an exercise in obfuscation. For instance, many labels provide the fat content in bold letters as a percentage of the daily calorie intake, while the relevant number, which is the percentage of calories provided as fat in a serving, is often presented in small print (Fig. 9).

Patients also need information about portion control and appropriate substitutions for family recipes. To assist in this process, the dietitians accompany patients on shopping expeditions, give cooking demonstrations, and sponsor dinners to encourage patients to try new recipes. Food models are a useful method of teaching patients about serving portions. Although the fat content (%) of the U.S. diet has varied little over that last century, the average portion sizes have increased significantly as judged by the size of the dinner plates (Fig. 10).

Another major issue is the effect of aging on the daily calorie requirement. The recent report of the Food and Nutrition Board has shown that, as individuals get older, their daily calorie requirements diminish. Thus if a person continues to eat in

Cornary heart disease reversal program
food record

Name: _____   Date: __07-09-03__

Height: __52__ Weight: __279__ Age: __49__   Day of Work: __WED__

Food eaten (Detailed description)	How prepared (If applicable)	Amount	When (Approximate time)	Where	Blood sugars
Spaget	Pasta, meat, tomatoes	About L	5:30 pn	Home	600cal
2 slices B. PB.	toast		6:00	Home	350cal
Soda coffee	—	1 liter 1 cup	5:00 am	Work	800cal
Bag of corn chips	—	5 oz	7:30 am	work	400cal
Top Ramen Noodles	Boil	whole package	9:30	work	800cal
Potato chips bag	—	5 oz	11:30	work	
2 liters water					
Total calories = 2950/day					
Calorie needs = 1900/day					

Figure 8 An example of a daily food diary submitted by a 48-year-old woman with diabetes and coronary artery disease. There is little evidence of meal planning. Dietary advice is of little value without an appreciation of this patient's approach to food. The calorie content of the individual items are in bold, and the calorie needs are calculated on the basis of height, weight, age, and activity level. *Source*: From Ref. 45.

the same way as he/she did in the second decade of life, an increase in weight is inevitable in the ensuing decades unless there is an increase in physical activity (45).

Finally the method of preparation must also be taken into consideration. For instance, a vegetable salad, which usually contains few calories, is transformed by adding a French dressing into a menu item containing more than half the calories derived from fat. Patients, often unaware of this transformation, insist that they eat "healthy salads for lunch."

Psychological Support

Recent evidence from the Interheart study suggests that psychosocial stress is likely to enhance the odds ratio of developing an MI to a significant extent in people who have the features of the metabolic syndrome. In addition, in patients with the metabolic syndrome, the presence of "hostility" as defined by the Minnesota Multipurpose Personality Inventory (MMPI) is an important amplifier of the risk of MI (18). The Normative Aging Study examined prospectively the impact of the metabolic syndrome and hostility as defined by the MMPI on the incidence of MI in healthy, older men (mean ± SD, 59.7 ± 7.2 years). Seven hundred fifty-four men who were diagnosed as not having CAD or diabetes mellitus were recruited into the study. Men were assigned to one of four risk factor groups based on the presence or absence of the metabolic syndrome and low or

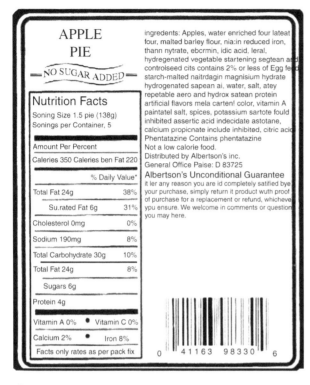

APPLE
PIE
═ NO SUGAR ADDED ═

Nutrition Facts

Soning Size 1.5 pie (138g)
Sonings per Container, 5

Amount Per Percent

Caleries 350 Caleries ben Fat 220

	% Daily Value*
Total Fat 24g	38%
Su.rated Fat 6g	31%
Cholesterol 0mg	0%
Sodium 190mg	8%
Total Carbohydrate 30g	10%
Total Fat 24g	8%
Sugars 6g	
Protein 4g	

Vitamin A 0%	•	Vitamin C 0%
Calcium 2%	•	Iron 8%

Facts only rates as per pack fix

ingredients: Apples, water enriched four lateat four, malted barley flour, nia:in reduced iron, thann nytrate, ebcrmin, idic acid, leral, hydregenated vegetable startening segtean and controlsed cits contains 2% or less of Egg feed starch-malted naitrdagin magnisium hydrate hydrogenated sapean ai, water, salt, atey repetable aero and hydrox satean protein artificial flavors mela carten! color, vitamin A paintatel salt, spices, potassium sartote fould inhibited assertic acid indecidate astotane, calcium propicnate include inhibited, citric acid Phentatazine Contains phentatazine
Not a low calorie food.
Distributed by Albertson's inc.
General Office Paise: D 83725

Albertson's Unconditional Guarantee
it ler any reason you are id completely satified bye your purchase, simply return it product wuth proof of purchase for a replacement or refund, whicheve ypu ensure. We welcome in comments or question you may here.

0 41163 98330 6

Figure 9 The labeling minefield. This common item is stated to contain 38% fat. This value refers to the percentage of fat based on the daily recommendation for fat and is presented in bold letters. The biologically relevant value for weight management is the percentage of calories derived from fat in a portion, which is $(220/350) \times 100 = 63\%$.

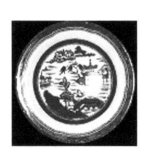

Ashworth Bros. dinner plate
circa 1910
9 inch diameter

Wedgewood dinner plate
by Jasper Conran, 2004
diameter 13.63 in

Figure 10 The changing face of the American dinner plate.

high hostility. Hierarchical logistic regression was used to assess the multivariate risk of MI over an average follow-up period of 13.8 years. It was found that the presence of hostility enhanced the probability of patients with the metabolic syndrome sustaining an MI (Fig. 11).

The definition of "Hostility" is interesting and refers to how an individual reacts with others he or she encounters, i.e. the anger is directed toward others. A corollary of this state would be hostility in the work place.

In addition, there is a significant body of evidence, which suggests that people who are overtly diabetic (46,47) or have some of the features of the metabolic syndrome such as obesity and hypertension (48) have cognitive deficits that could interfere with their ability to comprehend the nature of their own medical problems. The nature of this difficulty has been identified in some studies as their inability to make logical connections in their thinking. Such problems are very likely to have an adverse impact on the ability of patients to progress through the stages of change and make meaningful decisions regarding self-care.

For these reasons, the nature of the psychological support should be varied to suit the individuals. In the University of California, Davis program, the psychologists provide individual counseling as needed, conduct support groups, and engage in a variety of therapeutic teaching activities. The support groups usually focus on several topics such as anger management, eating disorders, depression, etc. Patients are encouraged to participate in these groups depending on their specific needs (49–51).

One of the practical problems encountered in offering these services to patients is the necessity for them to attend the outpatient facility, where these activities are undertaken. For patients unable to attend the programs, some support could be provided via telephones and e-mails.

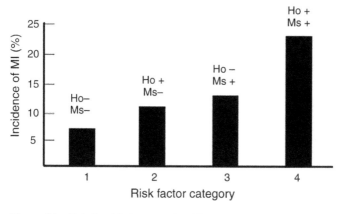

Figure 11 Relationship between hostility and the incidence of MI. Hostility amplifies the risk of developing a MI in men. Data obtained from the healthy aging study. *Abbreviations*: MS, metabolic syndrome; Ho, hostility; MI, myocardial infarction. *Source*: From Ref. 18.

Therapeutic Education

Central to all the activities described above is the role of therapeutic education (52). It is important to recognize that therapeutic education differs from health education. The latter is directed at healthy individuals and does not usually involve specific matters pertaining to people with medical problems. Therapeutic education is directed principally at enhancing self-care. It is important that every member of the care team utilizes every patient contact as an opportunity to further the aims of therapeutic education.

WHO PAYS THE PIPER?

Recent randomized clinical trials have shown that diabetes can be prevented in patients who have many of the features of the metabolic syndrome (39,53). The findings of the trial reported by the DPP (39) indicate that an intensive lifestyle intervention program resulted in a relative reduction in the incidence of diabetes (58%) (Fig. 6). The corresponding reduction in incidence in a group treated with metformin was 31% (95% CI, 48–66%). Findings such as these appear to present a compelling case for a national program to manage patients with the metabolic syndrome. Yet, two recent studies (54,55) present very divergent views on the cost-effectiveness of such an initiative.

Much of the controversy appears to reside in the type of statistical modeling used to estimate costs (56). Both groups working with virtually similar data appear to agree on several critical issues with respect to the effects of a lifestyle modification program in patients at risk of developing diabetes: (i) reduction in the incidence of diabetes, (ii) delaying onset of diabetes, (iii) reduction in complications of diabetes, (iv) extension of life expectancy, and (v) improvement in the quality of life. Both analyses also show that that the cost of the lifestyle interventions exceeds savings from lower rates of complications attributable to diabetes, suggesting that the treatment of the metabolic syndrome is unlikely to be cost neutral.

Thus, the issue resolves itself into what is deemed an acceptable cost to society. There is a consensus that an intervention that costs less than $50,000 per quality-adjusted life year (QALY) is a reasonable investment. By this yardstick, Eddy et al. (54) estimated that the cost/QALY of starting a lifestyle intervention program was $62,600 over 30 years. The corresponding cost for starting therapy with metfomin was $34,400. However, the cost of starting an intensive lifestyle intervention after the onset of diabetes was $24,000! A cynical interpretation of this projection is that the overall cost is lower because the duration of treatment (i.e., life expectancy) is reduced. In contrast, the analysis provided by Herman et al. (55) suggests that the cost/QALY was $8800 for the lifestyle intervention and $29,000 for metformin, both of which would be deemed acceptable.

Eddy et al. used a novel technique, called the Archimedes model, which takes into consideration a variety of physiological variables together with the costs of patients' health-care seeking behavior (57,58). It also takes into consideration an infinite number of patient states as continuous variables. In contrast, the model used by Herman et al. (55) applied the alternative, more widely used, Markov model, which takes into account the transitions experienced by patients as they move from one condition to another. A relevant example is a patient with the metabolic syndrome, who develops angina or an MI. The analyst enters the condition and the probability of its occurrence and outcome for each patient into a computer program that simulates the time course and outcomes. This analysis yields average values for various clinical events. It is beyond the scope of this chapter to assess the relative merits of each type of analysis.

However, there may be other more mundane reasons for this difference in calculated costs. The analysis performed by Eddy et al. (54) was based on a 30-year time horizon, which was shorter than the time span of the analysis by Herman et al. (55), which extended from time of diagnosis of impaired glucose tolerance to death. A shorter time span is likely to generate higher calculated costs, if the intervention takes several decades to show benefit (56). Another issue of interest is the projected rate of microvascular complications in the analysis by Herman et al. (55). It appears that the analysis used by Eddy et al. (54) assumed a slower rate of progression of fasting plasma glucose, which, in turn, would point to a lower rate of microvascular complications. In circumstances where the complication rate is high, the benefit from a lifestyle intervention would be greater as in the analysis by Herman et al. (55).

CONCLUSION

The metabolic syndrome presents a major challenge for both health-care professionals and policymakers alike. While it is tempting to seek cost-effective strategies for managing what has euphemistically come to be termed a disease of lifestyle, it is self-evident that the condition carries an enormous human cost as well. Ironically, this disease of lifestyle may well be a disease of life choice, albeit an ill-informed one resulting from a relentless media assault designed to alter the eating habits of the public. Neither health-care dollars alone nor an exclusively pharmacologic approach is likely to solve this problem.

REFERENCES

1. Kylin E. Studien ueber das Hypertonie-Hyperglykamie-Hyperurikamisyndrom. Zentrablatt fuer Innere Medizin 1923; 105–127.
2. Reaven GM. Banting lecture 1988. Role of insulin resistance in human disease. Diabetes 1988; 37(12):1595–1607
3. Descovich DC, Bennasi B, Canneli V et al. D'Addato S De Simone G Dormi A. An epidemic view of the plurimetabolic syndrome. In: Crepaldi G, Tiengo A, Manzato E, eds. Diabetes, Obesity and Hyperlipidemia. Amsterdam: Elsevier Science, 1993: 67–74
4. DeFronzo RA, Ferrannini E. Insulin resistance. A multifaceted syndrome responsible for NIDDM, obesity, hypertension, dyslipidemia, and atherosclerotic cardiovascular disease. Diabetes Care 2005; 14(3):173–194.
5. Groop L, Orho-Melander M. The dysmetabolic syndrome. J Intern Med 2001; 250(2):105–120.

6. Hanefeld M, Leonhardt W. Das Metabolische Syndrom. Dt Gdewsundh-Wesen 1981; 36:545–551.
7. Executive Summary of The Third Report of The National Cholesterol Education Program (NCEP) Expert Panel on Detection, Evaluation, and Treatment of High Blood Cholesterol In Adults (Adult Treatment Panel III). JAMA 2001; 285:2486–2497.
8. Pasternak RC, McKenney JM, Brown WV, et al. Understanding physician and consumer attitudes concerning cholesterol management: results from the National Lipid Association surveys. Am J Cardiol 2004; 94:9F–15F.
9. Echlin PS, Upshur RE, Markova TP. Lack of chart reminder effectiveness on family medicine resident JNC-VI and NCEP III guideline knowledge and attitudes. BMC Fam Pract 2004; 5:14–21.
10. Kahn R, Ferrannini E, Buse J, Stern M. The metabolic syndrome: time for a critical appraisal. Diabetes Care 2005; 28:2289–2304.
11. Yusuf S, Hawken S, Ounpuu S, et al. On behalf of the INTERHEART Investigators. Effect of potentially modifiable risk factors associated with myocardial infarction in 52 countries (the INTERHEART study): case-control study. Lancet 2004; 364:937–952.
12. Grundy SM, Brewer HB Jr, Cleeman JI, et al. American Heart Association, and National Heart, Lung and Blood Institute. Definition of metabolic syndrome: Report of the National Heart, Lung, and Blood Institute/American Heart Association conference on scientific issues related to definition. Circulation 2004; 109(3):433–438.
13. Laaksonen DE, Lakka HM, Niskanen LK, et al. Metabolic syndrome and development of diabetes mellitus: application and validation of recently suggested definitions of the metabolic syndrome in a prospective cohort study. Am J Epidemiol 2002; 156 (11):1070–1077.
14. Malik S, Wong ND, Franklin SS, et al. Impact of the metabolic syndrome on mortality from coronary heart disease, cardiovascular disease, and all causes in United States adults. Circulation 2004; 110:1245–1250.
15. Eckel RH, Grundy SM, Zimmet PZ. The metabolic syndrome. Lancet 2005; 365(9468):1415–1428.
16. Payne D. Medical students learn to cater for healthy appetites. Lancet 2002; 359(9313):1220.
17. Chobanian AV, Bakris GL, Black HR, et al. Joint National Committee on Prevention, Detection Evaluation and Treatment of High Blood Pressure. Seventh report of the Joint National Committee on Prevention, Detection, Evaluation, And Treatment Of High Blood Pressure. Hypertension 2003; 42(6):1206-1252.
18. Todaro JF, Con A, Niaura R, et al. Combined effect of the metabolic syndrome and hostility on the incidence of myocardial infarction (the Normative Aging Study). Am J Cardiol 2005; 96(2):221–226.
19. Grundy SM, Cleeman JI, Merz CN, et al.; Coordinating Committee of the National Cholesterol Education Program. Implications of recent clinical trials for the National Cholesterol Education Program Adult Treatment Panel III Guidelines. J Am Coll Cardiol 2004; 44(3):720–732.
20. American Diabetes Association, Inc. Position Statement Standards of Medical Care for Patients With Diabetes Mellitus American Diabetes Association. Diabetes Care 2002; 25:S33–S49.
21. Van Gaal LF, Rissanen AM, Scheen AJ, et al.; For the RIO-Europe Study Group. Effects of the cannabinoid-1 receptor blocker rimonabant on weight reduction and

cardiovascular risk factors in overweight patients: 1-year experience from the RIO-Europe study. Lancet 2005; 365:1389–1397.

22. www.hearthighway.org/cvd/obesity/ObesityTrends2003.pdf (Accessed 11.07.2005).

23. http://www.iuns.org/features/obesity/obesity.htm (Accessed 11.07.2005.)

24. Grundy SM, Cleeman JI, Daniels SR, et al. Diagnosis and Management of the Metabolic Syndrome. An American Heart Association/National Heart, Lung, and Blood Institute Scientific Statement. Circulation 2005; 112:2735–2752.

25. Abood DA, Black DR, Feral D. Nutrition education worksite intervention for university staff: application of the health belief model. J Nutr Educ Behav 2003; 35(5):260–267.

26. Sorensen M. Maintenance of exercise behavior for individuals at risk for cardiovascular disease. Percept Mot Skills 1997; 85:867–880.

27. Fu D, Fu H, McGowan P, et al. Implementation and quantitative evaluation of chronic disease self-management programme in Shanghai, China: randomized controlled trial. Bull World Health Organ 2003;174–183.

28. Wdowik MJ, Kendall PA, Harris MA, et al. Development and evaluation of an intervention program: control on campus. Diabetes Educ 2000; 26(1):94–104.

29. Glanz K, Rimer BK, Lewis FM. Health Behavior and Health Education. Theory, Research and Practice. San Fransisco: Wiley & Sons, 1992.

30. Prochaska JO, DiClemente CC. Stages of change in the modification of problem behaviors. Prog Behav Modif 1992; 28:183–218.

31. Smith DE, Heckemeyer CM, Kratt PP, et al. Motivational interviewing to improve adherence to a behavioral weight-control program for older obese women with NIDDM. A pilot study. 1. Diabetes Care 1997; 20:52–54.

32. Logue EE, Jarjoura DG, Sutton KS, Smucker WD, Baughman KR, Capers CF. Longitudinal relationship between elapsed time in the action stages of change and weight loss. Obes Res 2004; 12(9):1499–1508.

33. Steptoe A, Kerry S, Rink E, et al. The impact of behavioral counseling on stage of change in fat intake, physical activity, and cigarette smoking in adults at increased risk of coronary heart disease. Am J Public Health 2001; 91(2):265–269.

34. Jeffery RW, French SA, Rothman AJ. Stage of change as a predictor of success in weight control in adult women. Health Psychol 1999; 18(5):543–546.

35. Rollnick S, Miller WR. What is motivational interviewing? Behav Cogn Psychother 2005; 23:325–334.

36. Woollard J, Beilin L, Lord T, et al. A controlled trial of nurse ounseling on lifestyle change for hypertensives treated in general practice: preliminary results. Clin Exp Pharmacol Physiol 1995; 22(6–7):466–468.

37. Goldberg JH, Kiernan M. Innovative techniques to address retention in a behavioral weight-loss trial. Health Educ Res 2005; 20(4):439–447.

38. Colby SM, Monti PM, O'Leary Tevyaw T, et al. Brief motivational intervention for adolescent smokers in medical settings. Addict Behav 2005; 30(5):865–874.

39. Knowler WC, Barrett-Connor E, Fowler SE, et al.; Diabetes Prevention Program Research Group. Reduction in the incidence of Type 2 diabetes with lifestyle intervention or metformin. N Engl J Med 2002; 346:393–403.

40. Kappagoda CT, Amsterdam EA. Multiple Intervention. Studies in Secondary Prevention. In: Gaziano JM, Braunwald EA, eds. Atlas of Cardiovasular Risk Factors. Philadelphia, Pennsylvania: Gauvent Medicine LLC, 2006;303–318.

41. Kappagoda CT, Ma A, Cort DA, et al. Cardiac event rate in a lifestyle modification program for patients with chronic coronary artery disease. Clin Cardiol. 2006; 29(9):319–321.
42. ACE Fitness Matters. Vol. 1. Number 4, 1995.
43. Frank LL, Sorensen BE, Yasui Y, et al. Effects of exercise on metabolic risk variables in overweight postmenopausal women: a randomized clinical trial. Obes Res 2005; 13(3):615–625.
44. Orchard TJ, Temprosa M, Goldberg R, et al.; Diabetes Prevention Program Research Group. The effect of metformin and intensive lifestyle intervention on the metabolic syndrome: the Diabetes Prevention Program randomized trial. Ann Intern Med 2005; 142(8):611–619.
45. Food and Nutrition Board (FNB), Institute of Medicine IOM. Dietary Reference Intakes for Energy, Carbohydrate, Fiber, Fat, Fatty Acids, Cholesterol, Protein, and Amino Acids (Macronutrients). Washington: National Academy Press, 2002.
46. Scott R, Kritz-Silverstein D, Barrett-Connor, E et al. The association of non-insulin-dependent diabetes mellitus and cognitive function in an older cohort. J Am Geriatr Soc 1998; 46(10):1217–1222.
47. Wu JH, Haan MN, Liang J, et al. Impact of diabetes on cognitive function among older Latinos: a population-based cohort study. J Clin Epidemiol 2003; 56(7):686–693.
48. Elias MF, Elias PK, Sullivan, et al. Lower cognitive function in the presence of obesity and hypertension: The Framingham heart study. Int J Obes Relat Metab Disord 2003; 27(2):260–268.
49. Trento M, Passera P, Borgo E, et al. A 5-year randomized controlled study of learning, problem solving ability, and quality of life modifications in people with Type 2 diabetes managed by group care. Diabetes Care 2004; 27(3):670–675.
50. Messier C, Tsiakas M, Gagnon M, et al. Effect of age and glucoregulation on cognitive performance. Neurobiol Aging 2003; 24(7):985–1003.
51. Stewart R, Liolitsa D. Type 2 diabetes mellitus, cognitive impairment and dementia. Diabet Med 1999; 16(2):93–112.
52. Lacroix A, Assal J-P. Therapeutic Education of Patients. 2nd ed. Editions Maloines, 2003.
53. Tuomilehto J, Lindstrom J, Eriksson JG. Finnish Diabetes Prevention Study Group. Prevention of Type 2 diabetes mellitus by changes in lifestyle among subjects with impaired glucose tolerance. N Engl J Med 2003; 344:1343–1350.
54. Eddy DM, Schlessinger L, Kahn R. Clinical outcomes and cost-effectiveness of strategies for managing people at high risk for diabetes. Ann Intern Med 2005; 143(4):251–264.
55. Herman WH, Hoerger TJ, Brandle M, et al.; Diabetes Prevention Program Research Group. The cost-effectiveness of lifestyle modification or metformin in preventing Type 2 diabetes in adults with impaired glucose tolerance. Ann Intern Med 2005; 142(5):323–332.
56. Engelgau MM. Trying to predict the future for people with diabetes: a tough but important task. Ann Intern Med 2005; 143(4):301–302.
57. Schlessinger L, Eddy DM. Archimedes: a new model for simulating healthcare systems—the mathematical formulation. J Biomed Inform 2002; 35(1):37–50.
58. Eddy DM, Schlessinger L. Validation of the rchimedes diabetes model. Diabetes Care 2003; 26(1):3102–3110.

Index

Milton Keynes UK
Ingram Content Group UK Ltd.
UKHW031135141024
449569UK00006B/159